# ATLAS OF CLINICAL
# ENDOCRINOLOGY

# ATLAS OF CLINICAL ENDOCRINOLOGY

## Series Editor
## Stanley G. Korenman, MD

Professor and Associate Dean
Department of Medicine
UCLA School of Medicine
UCLA Medical Center
Los Angeles, California

## Volume III
# OSTEOPOROSIS

## Volume Editor
## Robert Marcus, MD

Professor
Department of Medicine
Stanford University School of Medicine
Stanford, California;
Director, Aging Study Unit
Geriatrics Research, Education, and Clinical Center
Veterans Affairs Medical Center
Palo Alto, California

*With 18 contributors*

**Blackwell Science**

Developed by Current Medicine, Inc., Philadelphia

# Current Medicine

400 Market Street
Suite 700
Philadelphia, PA 19106

| | |
|---|---|
| Developmental Editor: | *Marian A. Bellus* |
| Editorial Assistant: | *Forrest Rian Perry* |
| Design and Layout: | *Christopher Allan* |
| Illustrators: | *Nicole Mock, Paul Schiffmacher, Larry Ward, Debra Wertz* |
| Director of Product Development: | *Mary Kinsella* |
| Associate Art Director: | *Jerilyn Kauffman* |
| Art Department Manager: | *Debra Wertz* |
| Production: | *Lori Holland, Amy Giuffi* |
| Indexing: | *Dorothy Hoffman* |

Osteoporosis / volume editor, Robert Marcus
      p. cm.—(Atlas of clinical endocrinology; v. 3)
      Includes bibliographical references and index.

    ISBN 0-632-04403-9
    1. Osteoporosis Atlases.       I. Marcus, Robert, 1940-  II. Series

    Atlas of Clinical Endocrinology; 3.
    RC931.O73 O75 1999
    616.7'16—dc21
    for Library of Congress              99—34891
                                      CIP

Printed in Hong Kong by Paramount Printing Group Limited

10  9  8  7  6  5  4  3  2  1

DISTRIBUTED WORLDWIDE BY BLACKWELL, SCIENCE, INC.

# Series Preface

The human body depends on information even more than energy. The means of information transfer are chemical, whether at synapses or through the mediation of hormones at a distance (endocrine), between adjacent cells (paracrine), or within a single cell (autocrine). The body seems to be able to utilize any available molecule for signaling, including gases like nitric oxide and nutrients such as calcium and glucose. In endocrinology, the physician deals with signaling and its disorders, and in nutrition and metabolism, both signaling and energetics.

Endocrinology has been at the forefront of scientific medicine because the molecules involved are so potent that they produce measurable responses at low concentration, and the syndromes produced by an absence or an excess of hormones can be characterized. Furthermore, researchers purified hormones and elucidated their properties very early in the development of scientific medicine, which led to their introduction as pharmaceuticals for both diagnostic and therapeutic purposes. As new hormones and signaling and molecular response processes are elucidated, endocrinology continues to expand and become more sophisticated. Because the available knowledge is so extensive, it is relatively simple to place new information in context. Providing information to clinicians in an atlas format is particularly suitable for the field of endocrinology because the syndromes are often dramatic, molecular and metabolic pathways are well described, and algorithms for diagnosis and therapy can be developed. In fact, the reader will be struck by the remarkable thoroughness achievable in depicting this field in an atlas, namely, the *Atlas of Clinical Endocrinology*.

The *Atlas of Clinical Endocrinology* series includes five volumes: Thyroid Diseases, Diabetes, Osteoporosis, Neuroendocrinology and Pituitary Diseases, and Human Nutrition and Obesity. In each field, outstanding experts have contributed not only "state of the art" information but also their expert perspectives on the problems they cover. Throughout the field of endocrinology, major advances have strengthened the scientific base, the diagnostic armamentarium, and the therapeutic options.

In the Thyroid Diseases volume, the recent advances in our understanding of the thyroid hormone economy shed light on the alterations that occur with chronic illness, drugs, and aging. The contributors thoroughly illustrate the dilemmas associated with the management of thyroid nodules and thyroid cancer as well as thyroid disease in pregnancy and the complications of Graves' disease.

Advances in diabetes research and treatment have been dramatic. The volume on Diabetes illustrates the great advances in our understanding of the regulation of insulin secretion and the multiple mechanisms of its action. These advances, as well as the epidemiologic and genetic research that is covered, provide a strong foundation for understanding and managing the consequences of long-term hyperglycemia on the eye, kidney, nerves, and lipids, and on the cardiovascular system. Algorithms are provided for clinical treatment of deficient insulin action with newer agents as well as insulin in both types of diabetes.

Therapy to prevent osteoporotic fractures has become a mainstay in the health care of older women and now older men as well. The Osteoporosis volume describes the bone economy and illustrates the various syndromes leading to loss of bone mineral and the consequences of osteoporotic fracture. The authors describe and justify approaches to preventive and postfracture therapy, using both medications and nonpharmaceutical means.

In the Neuroendocrinology and Pituitary Diseases volume, major advances in understanding of the interrelationships between the central nervous system and control of pituitary and hypothalamic function are illustrated. Individuals with disorders of growth are characterized. The role of medical treatment in the management of acromegaly and prolactinomas and the approach toward the diagnosis of Cushing's syndrome are elucidated.

Disorders of nutrition, particularly obesity, are the most common disorders in advanced societies. In the Human Nutrition and Obesity volume, the regulation of appetite and eating is addressed; the nutritional requirements for growth and development are characterized; and the impact of diet on clinical conditions such as diabetes, hypertension, cardiovascular disease, cancer, aging and digestive diseases is discussed. The growing use of nutritional supplements is addressed and an integrated program for the management of obesity given.

We are grateful to Current Medicine and especially to Abe Krieger who saw the *Atlas of Clinical Endocrinology* as a dramatic and efficient medium for providing information about endocrinology and metabolism.

**Stanley G. Korenman, MD**

# Preface

The recent explosion of interest in osteoporosis reflects a realization by both physicians and the public of the societal and personal cost of fragility-related fractures. Once restricted to endocrinologists and rheumatologists, osteoporosis now occupies the interest of scientists representing such diverse fields as mechanical engineering, cell biology, pediatrics, and epidemiology.

These changes were enabled by several technical advances in noninvasive bone-mass measurement, in histomorphometry, in fundamental bone biology, and in therapeutics. The interested reader can now consult at least four nonorthopedic journals primarily devoted to bone health, as well as a number of books dedicated to this topic. This volume attempts to provide exposure to a variety of topics of great importance to an understanding of osteoporosis but which are not generally considered in most discussions of this condition. The latest information is provided about the role of peak bone mass, mechanical loading of the skeleton, bone biomechanics, and falls, which complements other more traditional areas, such as the role of nutrition, reproductive hormones, and pharmacologic therapies.

Since first promulgated by Albright in 1948, the entrenched view of osteoporosis has held it to be a specific entity due either to exaggerated loss of bone following the menopause or to "involutional" or "senile" changes associated with progressive aging. This concept has been restated as "Type I and Type II osteoporosis," reflecting the specific consequence of menopausal estrogen deprivation (Type I) versus a composite effect of age-related changes in intestinal, renal, and hormonal function on bone (Type II). An alternative model may be proposed, in which osteoporosis is considered to be a condition of global skeletal fragility of sufficient magnitude to increase the risk for fracture. By this model, a person's skeletal condition reflects all the factors that influenced his or her acquisition, maintenance, and loss of bone throughout life. These factors would include genetic constitution as well as lifelong exposure to environmental influences, such as hormonal milieu, diet and exercise, tobacco and ethanol, and illness and medication. In other words, osteoporosis can be viewed as a nonspecific end-result that can be achieved by myriad routes. The implication of such a definition is that, like fingerprints, the underlying basis of osteoporosis differs for each individual. By this construction it is easier to understand why osteoporotic patients frequently show substantial overlap with age-matched "normal" populations for bone mass, rates of bone turnover, or bone histomorphometry. The final word on this topic has not been written, but information in this volume describing the skeletal effects of numerous genetic and environmental factors should give readers a solid basis to reach their own decisions, or even to formulate their own models.

**Robert Marcus, MD**

# Contributors

**LAURA BACHRACH, MD**
Associate Professor
Department of Pediatrics
Stanford Medical School
Stanford, California

**GABRIELLE BERGMAN, MD**
Assistant Professor
Department of Radiology
Stanford Medical School
Stanford, California

**MARY BOUXSEIN, PHD**
Instructor
Department of Orthopedics
Harvard Medical School;
Senior Research Associate
Beth Israel Deaconess Medical Center
Boston, Massachusetts

**ALAN L. BURSHELL, MD**
Chairman of Endocrinology Fellowship
Department of Endocrinology
Alton Ochsner Medical Foundation
New Orleans, Louisiana

**JANE A. CAULEY, DrPH**
Associate Professor
Department of Epidemiology
Graduate School of Public Health
Pittsburgh, Pennsylvania

**LORRAINE A. FITZPATRICK, MD**
Professor
Department of Internal Medicine and Endocrinology
Mayo Medical School;
Consultant in Endocrinology and Metabolism
Mayo Clinic
Rochester, Minnesota

**DOUGLAS P. KIEL, MD, MPH**
Assistant Professor
Department of Medicine
Harvard Medical School;
Associate Director of Medical Research
Hebrew Rehabilitation Center for Aged
  Research and Training Institute
Boston, Massachusetts

**B. JENNY KIRATLI, PhD**
Research Health Scientist
Spinal Cord Injury Center
VA Palo Alto Health Care System
Palo Alto, California

**ROBERT F. KLEIN, MD**
Assistant Professor
Department of Medicine
Oregon Health Sciences University;
Staff Physician
Portland VA Medical Center
Portland, Oregon

**PHILIPP LANG, MD**
Assistant Professor
Department of Radiology
Stanford Medical School
Stanford, California

**ROBERT MARCUS, MD**
Professor
Department of Medicine
Stanford University School of Medicine
Stanford, California;
Director, Aging Study Unit
Geriatrics Research, Education, and Clinical Center
Veterans Affairs Medical Center
Palo Alto, California

# Contributors, *continued*

**PAUL D. MILLER, MD**

Clinical Professor
Department of Medicine
University of Colorado Health Science Center
Denver, Colorado

**RICHARD L. PRINCE, MD, FRACP**

Associate Professor
Department of Medicine
University of Western Australia School of Medicine
Perth, Western Australia;
Associate Professor
Sir Charles Gairdner Hospital
Nedlands, Western Australia

**CLIFFORD J. ROSEN, MD**

Professor of Nutrition
University of Maine
Orono, Maine;
Director
Maine Center for Osteoporosis Research
    and Education at St. Joseph's Hospital
Bangor, Maine

**LORAN M. SALAMONE, PhD**

Assistant Professor
Department of Epidemiology
Graduate School of Public Health
Pittsburgh, Pennsylvania

**JAN VANDEVENNE, MD**

Fellow
Musculoskeletal Section
Department of Radiology
Stanford University Medical Center
Stanford, California

**SONIA M. VICTORES, MD**

Universidad Central del Este
San Pedro de Macoris
Dominican Republic;
Endocrinology Fellow
Ochsner Clinic
New Orleans, Louisiana

**NELSON B. WATTS, MD**

Professor
Department of Medicine
Emory University;
Director, Osteoporosis and Bone Health Program
The Emory Clinic
Atlanta, Georgia

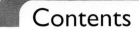

# Contents

# Contents, *continued*

## Contents, *continued*

# THE NATURE OF OSTEOPOROSIS

## Robert Marcus

The recent emergence of osteoporosis as a major focus of investigation in fields as diverse as mechanical engineering, pediatrics, and epidemiology has led to many important advances in understanding and therapeutics. Whereas the topic of osteoporosis formerly occupied just a few paragraphs in standard texts, it is now the primary focus of several journals and textbooks. This volume provides current information regarding skeletal health and its disruption. Attention is given to bone acquisition during growth years, mechanisms of adult bone loss, and new developments in osteoporosis diagnostics and therapeutics.

In the final analysis, osteoporosis is a condition of bone, a complex tissue that undergoes physiologic repair throughout life. The study of bone transcends a simple measurement of its amount or mineral density to encompass aspects of its physical properties and geometry. This chapter introduces the reader to the "nature" of osteoporosis, ie, the physical characteristics of healthy and porotic bone. In addition, some of the important geometric features of bone that substantially influence bone strength are discussed. Finally, the gross and cellular features of normal and disordered bone remodeling are described. Bone modeling is a continuous renewal process that underlies the basis for changes in bone mass during adult life.

## Osteoporotic Bone

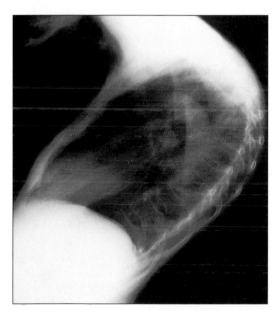

**FIGURE 1-1.** Lateral chest radiograph showing a classic spine deformity called kyphosis. Kyphosis is the end result of multiple vertebral compression fractures. Osteoporosis is defined as a skeletal condition of decreased bone quantity accompanied by abnormalities in the microscopic architecture of bone that renders a person more likely to sustain a fracture with little or no trauma. Osteoporosis frequently is considered in the context of specific fracture syndromes, including vertebral compression, Colles' (distal radial) fracture, and hip fracture. However, osteoporosis truly is a disease of global skeletal fragility, with increased risk for low-trauma fractures in all portions of the skeleton. (Copyright © R. Marcus.)

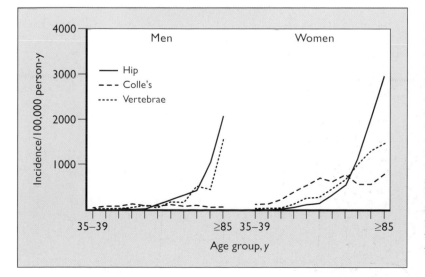

**FIGURE 1-2.** Incidence of osteoporotic fractures. The clinical consequence of bone fragility is fracture. Shown here are curves representing the age-related incidences of vertebral, forearm, and hip fractures in North American men and women. The incidence of fractures is about twice as great in women as it is in men. However, osteoporosis is not a disorder exclusive to women. The incidence of hip fracture is increasing most rapidly in men over 70 years of age. One third of vertebral fractures result in pain sufficient to cause the patient to seek medical attention; however, many occur without obvious symptoms, becoming apparent only as a loss of height or development of curvature. Wrist fractures typically occur at an earlier age than do hip fractures. This fact is explained by differences in the types of falls that occur. Wrist fractures occur when a person standing upright falls forward and attempts to break the fall by arm extension. Hip fractures are more likely to occur when a person attempts to rise from a seated position but fails to generate adequate momentum to elevate the center of gravity to a stable position. A backward fall results, with direct impact on the femoral trochanter. Thus, the occurrence of fracture in patients with osteoporosis is a function not only of intrinsic bone strength but also of factors conducive to falls. (*From* Cooper and Melton [1]; with permission.)

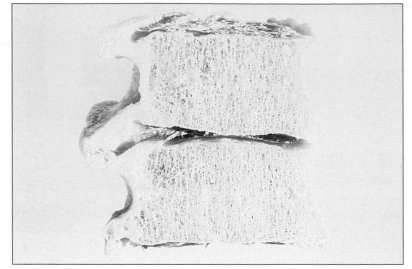

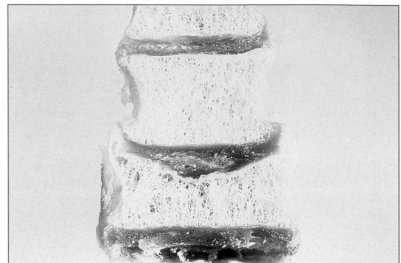

**FIGURE 1-3.** (*see* Color Plate) Normal vertebral bodies. Contained within a thin cortical shell, about 35% of vertebral bodies by weight and 80% by surface are comprised of a honeycomb of vertical and horizontal bars, or trabeculae. In adults, trabecular interstices of the axial (central) skeleton constitute the primary repository for red bone marrow. Events leading to loss of bone occur on bone surfaces. The surfaces of trabecular bone are great in extent and lie in close proximity to the marrow-derived cells that participate in bone turnover. Therefore, changes in bone mass occur earlier and to a greater extent than they do in regions of the skeleton that are primarily cortical. (Copyright © R. Marcus.)

**FIGURE 1-4.** (*see* Color Plate) Osteoporotic vertebral bodies. The term *porosis* means spongelike. Weakness of the trabecular structure has resulted in mechanical failure, with collapse of the intervertebral disk into the underlying bony substance. This weakness reflects a decrease in the total amount of bone within the vertebral body and also a disruption of the normal trabecular micro-architecture, as evidenced by the appearance of several large holes. A formal definition of the term *osteoporosis* is a skeletal condition characterized by low bone mass and abnormal micro-architecture, leading to increased risk for fracture with minimal trauma. (Copyright © R. Marcus.)

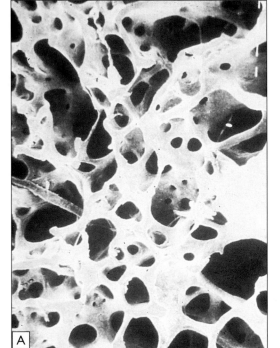

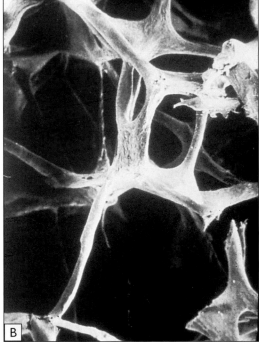

**FIGURE 1-5.** (*see* Color Plate) Scanning electron micrograph of normal (**A**) and osteoporotic (**B**) trabecular structures. In osteoporosis, the platelike normal trabeculae have been replaced by thin rods, and trabecular perforation has disrupted trabecular continuity. (*Courtesy of* J. Kosek.)

# Bone Mass Measurement

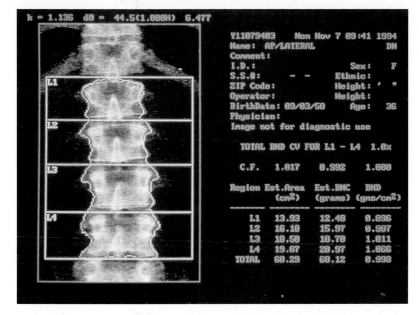

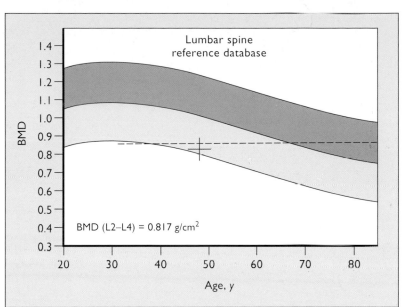

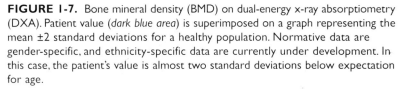

**FIGURE 1-6.** Printout from a lumbar spine bone density examination. Although both low bone mass and architectural disruption are essential components of the diagnosis of osteoporosis, current widely applicable diagnostic tools provide measurements of bone mass (the amount of bone) only, and do not address micro-architectural disruption or other "qualitative" aspects of bone fragility. Dual-energy x-ray absorptiometry (DXA) is a technique that exploits the ability of bone mineral to attenuate the passage of photons through the body to provide estimates of the mineral density of bone. Machine software estimates the area and mineral content of bones in the region scanned. A calculated areal bone mineral density (measured in $g/cm^2$) is generated for the scanned region. For clinical purposes, the scanned regions generally include the lumbar spine, proximal femur, forearm, and whole body. For research purposes, any skeletal region can be assessed.

**FIGURE 1-7.** Bone mineral density (BMD) on dual-energy x-ray absorptiometry (DXA). Patient value (*dark blue area*) is superimposed on a graph representing the mean ±2 standard deviations for a healthy population. Normative data are gender-specific, and ethnicity-specific data are currently under development. In this case, the patient's value is almost two standard deviations below expectation for age.

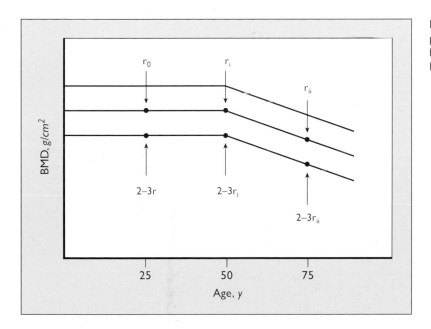

**FIGURE 1-8.** Implications of low bone mineral density (BMD). Based on prospective observational studies, it is estimated that each standard deviation below the age-predicted mean value imposes a two- to threefold increase in long-term fracture risk.

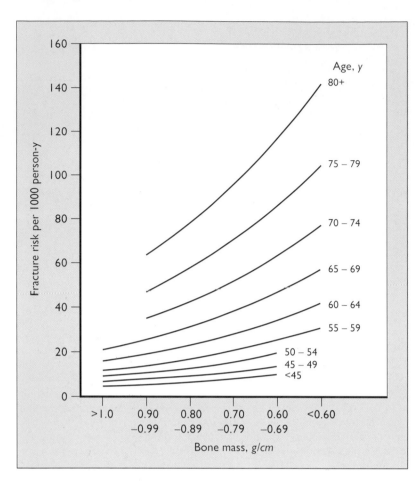

**FIGURE 1-9.** Interaction of age and bone mineral density (BMD) on fracture incidence. A large cohort of women were followed over time. Fracture incidence is shown on the vertical axis, and the women are stratified by bone density along the horizontal axis. In addition, women are stratified by age, represented by a family of curves. At any given BMD, fracture incidence is higher with progressive age. In fact, the slope of this relationship to fracture is steeper for age than it is for BMD, which would not be expected if BMD itself were the sole determinant of fracture risk. For the oldest women, the incidence of falls is greater and contributes to the added fracture experience. However, falls do not account for the age effect at younger ages. Thus, attention has been paid to so-called qualitative factors affecting bone fragility that are not accounted for in the BMD measurement. (*From* Hui *et al.* [2]; with permission.)

# Qualitative Abnormalities in Osteoporotic Bone

**BONE QUALITY
IN OSTEOPOROSIS**

Altered mineral composition
Cement lines
Cortical porosity
Fatigue accumulation
Trabecular disruption

**FIGURE 1-10.**
Qualitative abnormalities in osteoporotic bone are provided.

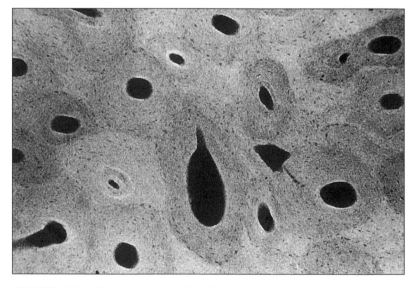

**FIGURE 1-11.** Microradiograph of qualitative abnormalities in osteoporotic cortical bone. Note the substantial heterogeneity of haversian canal dimensions. The gray levels indicate patchy differences in mineralization, with white representing the highest level [3].

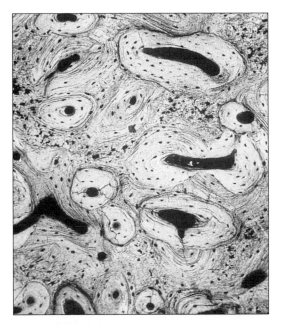

**FIGURE 1-12.** Micrograph of a biopsy specimen of the iliac crest showing qualitative abnormalities in bone. Cortical porosity is seen in this specimen from an 80-year-old man. Note the occurrence of large haversian canals in several osteons. Also note the very high prevalence of haversian systems, indicating an extensive lifelong history of remodeling events [4].

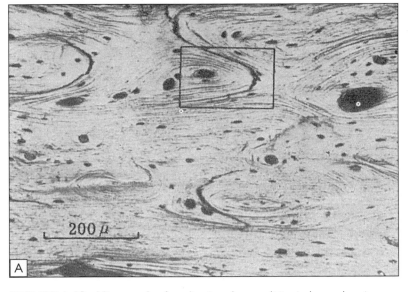

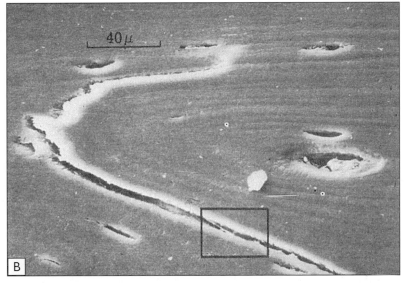

**FIGURE 1-13.** Micrograph of qualitative abnormalities in bone showing cement lines. Cement lines are the residue of a previous bone resorption event. Composed of a filigree of woven rather than dense lamellar collagen, cement lines create an area of weakened resistance to structural failure.

**A,** Cement lines forming the base of osteonal units. **B,** Dehiscence of a cement line after application of a bending force to the whole bone. When bone fractures, fracture lines propagate from one cement line to the next [5].

# Bone Geometry

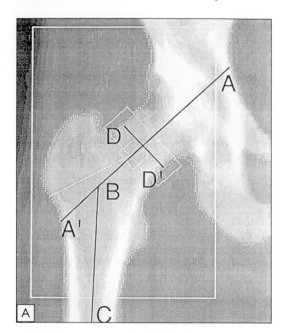

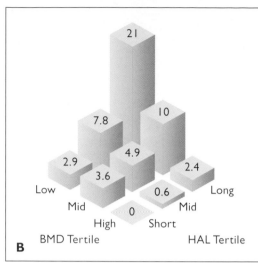

**FIGURE 1-14.** Geometric contributions to bone strength and fracture risk. Despite an undisputed relationship between bone mineral density (BMD) and fracture incidence, factors independent of BMD make important contributions to fracture. Of particular importance are bone geometry and the occurrence of falls (*see* Chapter 12). To illustrate the role of macroscopic bone geometry, these two figures show the importance a measurement called the hip axial length (HAL) has on hip fracture risk. **A,** HAL is the length of a straight line connecting the inferior surface of the greater trochanter to the inner surface of the hip acetabulum. **B,** Results of a large prospective observational study of elderly women showing that the incidence of hip fracture is heavily dependent on HAL. At any level of BMD, women with longer HAL had significantly greater risk of hip fracture. Indeed, women with BMD in the lowest tertile who also had HAL in the longest tertile experienced a 21-fold increased relative risk for hip fracture. (*Part B from* Faulkner *et al.* [6]; with permission.)

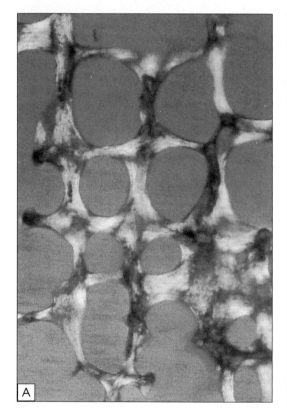

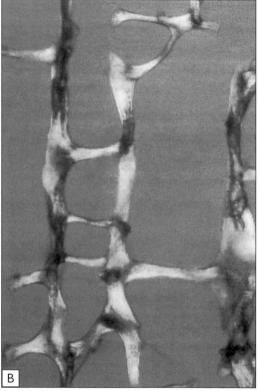

**FIGURE 1-15.** (*see* Color Plate) Geometric contributions to bone strength and fracture risk. Illustrated is the pattern of trabecular loss with age in which progressive loss of horizontal trabeculae is more exaggerated than is that of vertical trabeculae. The microscopic architecture is shown in a 50-year old man **A**, 58-year old man **B**,

(*Continued on next page*)

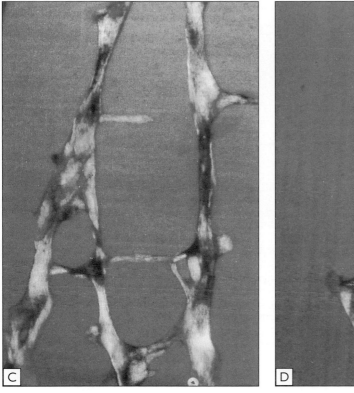

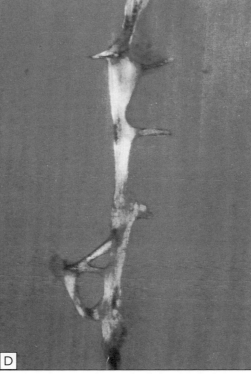

**FIGURE 1-15.** (*Continued*) 76-year-old man **C**, and an 80-year old woman **D** [7].

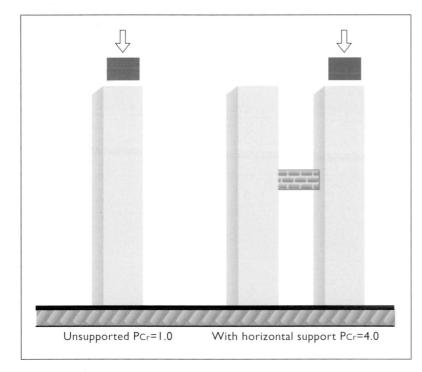

Unsupported Pcr=1.0    With horizontal support Pcr=4.0

**FIGURE 1-16.** Diagram of geometric contributions to bone strength and fracture risk showing the consequences of horizontal trabecular loss. A single horizontal connecting strut increases by fourfold the maximum load (Pcr) that can be carried by a vertical bar without buckling. Thus, loss of horizontal trabeculae with age has a profound independent effect on vertebral trabecular strength. (*From* Snow-Harter and Marcus [8]; with permission.)

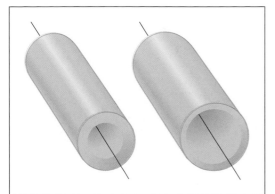

**FIGURE 1-17.** Diagram of geometric contributions to bone strength and fracture risk showing the effect of mass distribution on bone strength. Assume that two cylinders have equal mass. The one on the right shows the distribution of mass further away from the bending axis, *ie*, increased cross-sectional moment of inertia (CSMI), resulting in substantially increased resistance to bending along this axis. The long bones of men are generally larger than are those of women. Therefore, the increased CSMI of the bones of men confers on them relative protection against fracture at any given value of bone mineral density. One adaptive response that occurs with aging is a compensation for bone loss by increasing the CSMI of the long bones, a process that appears to be more efficient in men than it is in women. (*From* Snow-Harter and Marcus [8]; with permission.)

# Role of Remodeling in Lifelong Acquisition and Loss of Bone

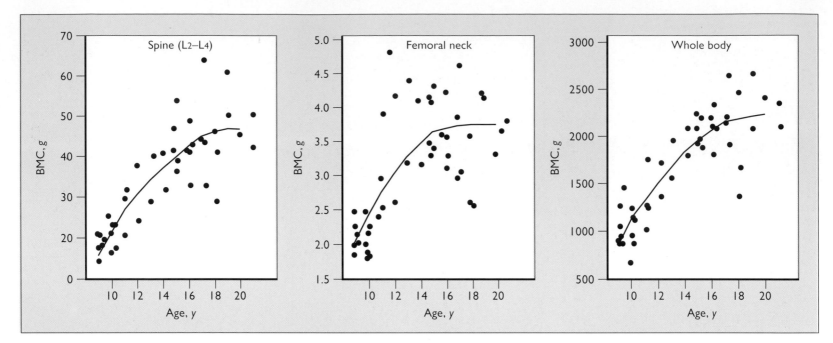

**FIGURE 1-18.** Acquisition of bone during adolescence. At any time during adult life bone mass reflects bone that has been gained during years of growth minus bone that subsequently has been lost. Previous theories about osteoporosis have not adequately considered the role of bone acquisition in determining lifelong fracture risk. This study of healthy white girls aged 9 to 21 years shows that about 60% of final adult "peak" bone mass is acquired during the adolescent growth spurt. Only about 5% of peak bone mass is acquired after aged 18 years. Thus, adolescence constitutes a window of opportunity when genetic, dietary, hormonal, and other factors determine the magnitude of bone gain. About 80% of peak bone mass is genetically determined. Important environmental factors include dietary calcium intake, reproductive endocrine status, and habitual physical activity. In contrast, adolescence is a window of vulnerability when inadequate attention to these same factors can lead to low bone mass at skeletal maturity. Persons who have not gained adequate bone mass would not need to lose very much bone in adulthood to have a substantially increased risk for osteoporosis and fracture. Of particular concern are dietary calcium intake, which is generally low in American teenaged girls; a relatively sedentary lifestyle; and the high prevalence of anorexia nervosa and other eating disorders. (*From* Katzman *et al.* [9]; with permission.)

**FIGURE 1-19.** Acquisitional osteopenia. This is a partial list of childhood conditions known to occur in adults with low bone mass. Low bone mass puts adults at increased risk of fracture.

## ACQUISITIONAL OSTEOPENIA

Delayed puberty
Immobilization or therapeutic rest
Specific disorders:
   Anorexia nervosa
   Cystic fibrosis
   Intestinal or renal disease
   Marfan syndrome
   Osteogenesis imperfecta

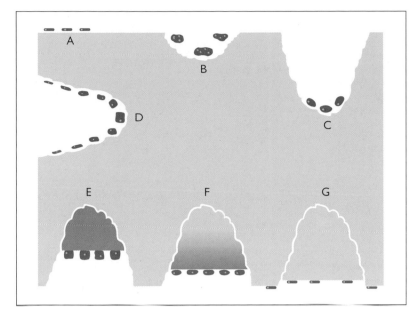

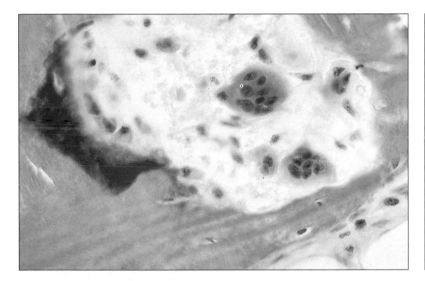

**FIGURE 1-20.** Bone remodeling. Once new bone is laid down, it is subject to a continuous process of breakdown and renewal called *remodeling* that continues throughout life. After linear growth stops and peak bone mass has

been reached, remodeling constitutes the final common pathway by which bone mass is adjusted throughout adult life. Remodeling is carried out by thousands of individual and independent "bone remodeling units" on the surfaces of bone throughout the skeleton.

**A,** About 90% of bone surface is normally inactive, covered by a thin layer of lining cells. **B,** In response to physical or biochemical signals, recruitment of marrow precursor cells to a site at the bone surface results in their fusion into the characteristic multinucleated osteoclasts that resorb, or dig a cavity into the bone. In cortical bone, resorption creates tunnels within haversian canals, whereas trabecular resorption creates scalloped areas of the bone surface called Howship lacunas. **C,** On termination of the resorption phase, a 60μ cavity remains and is bordered at its deepest extent by a cement line, a region of loosely organized collagen fibrils. **D,** Completion of resorption is followed by ingress of preosteoblasts derived from marrow stromal stem cells into the base of the resorption cavity. **E,** These cells develop the characteristic osteoblastic phenotype and begin to replace the resorbed bone by elaborating new bone matrix constituents, such as collagen, osteocalcin, and other proteins. **F,** Once the newly formed osteoid reaches a thickness of about 20μ, mineralization begins.

The remodeling cycle normally is completed in about 6 months. No net change in bone mass occurs as a result of remodeling when the amount of resorbed bone replaced equals the amount removed. Persistence of small bone deficits on completion of each cycle, however, reflects an inefficiency in remodeling dynamics. Lifelong accumulation of remodeling deficits underlies the phenomenon of age-related bone loss. (*From* Marcus [10]; with permission.)

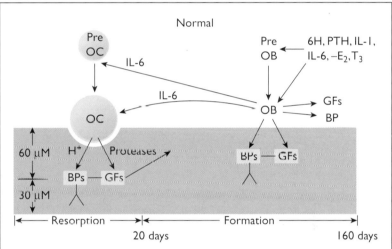

**FIGURE 1-21.** (see Color Plate) Bone biopsy specimen from the iliac crest showing the cellular participants in bone remodeling. Large multinucleated cells seen in the middle of the field are osteoclasts. Derived from a mononuclear macrophage precursor, these cells migrate to a locus on the bone surface, become adherent to the surface with participation of a number of adherence molecules, and resorb bone (both organic matrix and mineral) from the bone. The layer of cuboidal mononuclear cells at the bone surface are osteoblasts, and the thick red band beneath them represents organic matrix that has not yet been mineralized (osteoid). Mineralized bone is olive in color (Goldner stain). (*Courtesy of* J. Kosek.)

**FIGURE 1-22.** Close-up view of bone remodeling. The proximate target cells for hormones and cytokines that regulate bone remodeling are osteoblasts (OB). Osteoblasts possess specific high-affinity receptors for estradiol, thyroid hormone, parathyroid hormone (PTH), and calcitriol. After interactions of these agents with their receptors, osteoblasts secrete other molecules, such as interleukins 6 and 11 (IL-6, IL-11), which initiate proliferation and maturation of osteoclast (OC) precursors. Also shown are some of the matrix-embedded growth factors (GFs) released during the process of resorption thought to promote ingress of new osteoblastic precursors that arise within the bone marrow stroma. BPs—binding proteins; $E_2$—estradiol; H—hydrogen; $T_3$—triiodothyronine. (*Courtesy of* C. Rosen.)

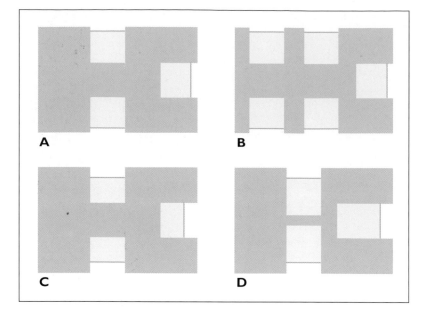

**FIGURE 1-23.** Perturbations in remodeling. Alterations in remodeling activity represent the final pathway through which diverse stimuli such as dietary insufficiency, hormones, and drugs affect bone balance. A change in the whole-body remodeling rate can be brought about through distinct perturbations in remodeling dynamics.

A representation of normal remodeling is shown. **A,** Three areas of remodeling activity, each with identical resorption lacunas that have filled in with new bone (*blue*). Identical small bone deficits are shown with each remodeling area, reflecting remodeling inefficiency (described previously). **A,** Increased remodeling owing to an increase in the activation, or birthrate, of remodeling units. Examples include hyperthyroidism, hyperparathyroidism, and hypervitaminosis D. **B,** Exaggerated inefficiency of osteoblastic response. The number of remodeling units in play is unchanged; however, the magnitude of bone deficit is increased. Such changes are typical of osteoblastic toxins, such as ethanol, and glucocorticosteroids. Progressive age also may be associated with increasing deficits in osteoblast recruitment and function. **C,** Exaggerated osteoclastic activity. Estrogen deficiency may augment osteoclastic resorptive capacity. If the resorption cavities perforate the trabeculae, no scaffold remains for new bone formation to take place. Such resorption becomes a permanent loss of bone.

At any given time a transient deficit in bone exists called the *remodeling space*, which represents sites of bone resorption that have not yet been filled. In response to any stimulus that alters the birthrate of new remodeling units, the remodeling space will either increase or decrease accordingly until a new steady state is established. This adjustment is seen as an increase or decrease in bone mass. (*From* Marcus [10]; with permission.)

**FIGURE 1-24.** Age-related bone loss. This graph represents a large cross-sectional study of cortical bone mineral density (BMD) in men and women across the adult lifespan. At any time in adult life, BMD in men is higher than is that of women. However, this fact represents an artefact of bone size, which is larger in men. If 1-cm cubes of bone from average young men and women were compared, mineral content would be equal. It is not trivial that bone diameters in men are larger than those in women because bone strength is a function of BMD squared times the bone cross-sectional area. Thus, with bones of equal true BMD, larger cross-sectional areas confer relative protection against fracture on men (*see* Fig. 1-17).

Bone mineral density (BMD) remains stable until about aged 50 years, when both men and women show progressive loss. BMD loss is more rapid in women aged 50 to 60 years, reflecting the impact of menopausal loss of estrogen production. Subsequently, age-related loss of BMD is similar for men and women. Although bone loss detectable by densitometric methods is generally detected only after 50 years of age, more sensitive methods (albeit invasive, such as iliac crest biopsy) show the beginning of age-related bone loss as early as the third decade [7].

Maintenance of bone mass through adult life requires meeting a number of challenges imposed by both physiologic and environmental factors. From the principles of bone remodeling, discussed previously, it can be seen that any factors tending to increase overall bone remodeling will promote bone loss, whereas factors that reduce remodeling activity may lower the rate of bone loss. Listed are only a few of the important factors that may promote bone remodeling and bone loss in elderly persons: loss of reproductive function in all women and in a sizable number of elderly men; age-related increases in circulating parathyroid hormone, which may reflect a decreased calcium nutritional state either from limited nutrient intake or age-imposed deficits in vitamin D status and intestinal calcium absorption efficiency; and age-related decrease in habitual physical activity and recreational exercise. (*From* Meema and Meema [11]; with permission.)

---

**REQUIREMENTS FOR MAINTENANCE OF SKELETAL INTEGRITY**

Nutrient adequacy
Physical activity
Reproductive hormone status

**FIGURE 1-25.** Requirements for maintenance of skeletal integrity. Skeletal integrity requires adequacy of habitual mechanical environment (physical activity), reproductive hormone status, and nutrients. Overzealous attention to any two of these factors does not suffice when the third factor is neglected. Thus, an immobilized patient loses bone even when both reproductive hormone and nutritional status are more than adequate. Similarly, a woman athlete who exercises to the point of development of amenorrhea (and low estrogen status) loses bone, despite a high mechanical environment and calcium supplementation.

# References

1. Cooper C, Melton LJ III: Epidemiology of osteoporosis. *Trends Endocrinol Metab* 1992, 3:224–229.

2. Hui SL, Slemenda CW, Johnston CC Jr: Age and bone mass as predictors of fracture in a prospective study. *J Clin Invest* 1988, 81:1804–1809.

3. Grynpas M: Age and disease-related changes in the mineral of bone. *Calcif Tiss Int* 1993, 53(suppl 1):S57–S64.

4. Marcus R: The nature of osteoporosis. In *Osteoporosis*. Edited by Marcus R, Feldman D, Kelsey J. San Diego: Academic Press; 1996:647–659.

5. Carter DR, Hayes WC: Compact bone fatigue damage. A microscopic examination. *Clin Orthop Rel Res* 1977, 127:265–274.

6. Faulkner K, Cummings S, Black D: Simple measurement of femoral geometry predicts hip fracture: the study of osteoporotic fractures. *J Bone Miner Res* 1993, 8:1211–1217.

7. Mosekilde Li: Age related changes in vertebral trabecular bone architecture-assessed by a new method. *Bone* 1988, 9:247–250.

8. Snow-Harter C, Marcus R: Exercise, bone density, and osteoporosis. *Exerc Sports Sci Rev* 1991, 19:351–388.

9. Katzman DK, Bachrach LK, Carter DR, Marcus R: Clinical and anthropometric correlates of bone mineral acquisition in healthy adolescent girls. *J Clin Endocrinol Metab* 1991, 73:1332–1339.

10. Marcus R: Normal and abnormal bone remodeling in man. *Annu Rev Med* 1987, 38:129–141.

11. Meema H, Meema S: Compact bone mineral density of the normal human radius. *Acta Radiol Oncol* 1978, 17:342–350.

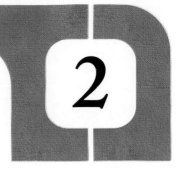

# BONE ACQUISITION AND PEAK BONE MASS

## Laura Bachrach

The foundation of bone health is established in the first three decades of life [1]. Peak bone mass acquired by early adulthood serves as the bone bank for the remainder of life. The more robust the skeletal mass at its peak, the greater the bone loss (from aging, menopause, and other factors) that can be tolerated without clinical signs of osteoporosis. The pace of bone mineral acquisition is similar to that of linear bone growth, with rapid gains in infancy, slower increases during childhood, and major gains at puberty [2]. At least half of adult bone mineral density is gained during the teenage years, making this a critical period to optimize conditions for skeletal health. Unlike growth patterns, however, peak bone mineral acquisition lags a year behind peak height velocity [3]. Furthermore, gains in bone mineral density continue into the third decade after bone growth has ceased [4].

Bone mineral density acquired by early adulthood is a key determinant of the lifetime risk of osteoporosis. Peak bone mass accounts for at least half of the variability in skeletal mass in the elderly, with the remainder attributable to subsequent bone loss [1]. To a large extent, peak bone mass is predetermined by heritable factors. Family and twin studies suggest that 60% to 80% of the differences in peak bone mass between individuals can be attributed to genetics [5,6]. Ethnic and racial differences in bone mass also have been observed [7]. Although some of these differences appear to be artifacts of densitometry techniques, healthy blacks have been shown to achieve greater true bone density during adolescence than do nonblacks [8,9]. The gene or genes linked to osteoporosis have not yet been identified, although several have been considered, including the vitamin D and estrogen receptors [10].

Lifestyle factors also have a substantial influence on bone acquisition, explaining 20% to 40% of the variability in the skeletal mass of young adults. Maximal gains in bone mineral density occur only when nutrition, physical activity, and hormone production are adequate. Body mass is a consistent correlate of bone mineral density in healthy youths, perhaps because weight is an indicator of overall nutritional status [11]. Other researchers have suggested that body mass fosters bone accrual through mechanical loading on the skeleton [12]. Calcium influences rates of bone accrual, as has been shown in several calcium supplementation trials; children given calcium supplementation gained more bone mineral than did those in the control group [13,14]. The recommended daily calcium intakes for children and adolescents were increased in 1997, reflecting these recent findings [15]. Weight-bearing physical activity also appears to stimulate rates of bone mineral accrual and may even modify bone size [3,16,17]. Several studies have shown that active children and adults may gain 5% to 10% more bone mineral density than do their sedentary peers [18]. Other studies have failed to find a correlation between exercise patterns and bone mass. For this reason, the amount and type of activity needed to foster bone accrual remain controversial. Furthermore, activity may boost bone acquisition only when calcium intake is sufficient [19]. Normal endocrine function also is important for optimal bone mineral acquisition. Bone mass in adolescents is more highly correlated with pubertal stage than with chronologic age, reflecting the pivotal role of sex steroids in bone accrual [20]. Peak bone mass is reduced in patients with deficiency or resistance in sex steroids [21]. Growth hormone deficiency, hyperthyroidism, and glucocorticoid excess also have been associated with low bone mass in children and adults [22–25].

The annual cost of treating osteoporotic fractures already has reached $13.8 billion, an amount that is projected to double over the next 25 years [26]. Stemming the rise of these costs will require effective intervention directed at increasing peak bone mass and reducing subsequent bone loss. A bone health program for all youths includes maintaining adequate body weight, appropriate calcium intake, and regular physical activity. Unfortunately, in the United States, the gap continues to widen between the recommended and actual intake of calcium; over 90% of girls and 50% of boys consume less than the optimal amount of calcium during their teenage years [27]. In addition, American youth have become less active over time; only half of teenagers (aged 12 to 21 years) exercise vigorously on a regular basis, and 25% report no vigorous physical activity [28]. Girls are less active than are boys, and black girls are less active than are white girls. Skeletal health is a more immediate concern for a youth with a variety of chronic disorders associated with early deficits in bone mass [22]. Anorexia nervosa, exercise-associated amenorrhea, cystic fibrosis, and steroid-dependent disorders may reduce gains or accelerate loss of bone mineral, resulting in osteopenia (low bone mass for age) or osteoporosis (more profound deficits that may lead to fracture). Whether these deficits can be reversed with early recognition and treatment remains uncertain. Continued efforts are needed to define ways to optimize peak bone mass and then deliver the message that osteoporosis prevention begins in childhood.

# Bone Mineral Acquisition

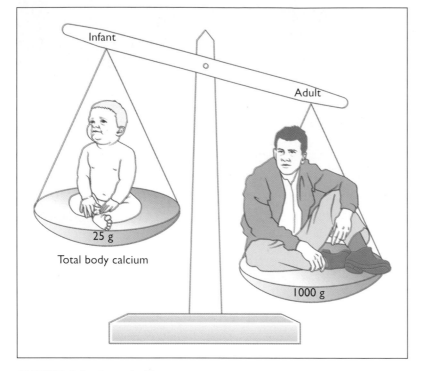

**FIGURE 2-1.** Accrual of bone mass during childhood and adolescence. Total skeletal calcium increases dramatically from infancy until adulthood. Half of these gains occur during adolescence, making this period critical in establishing bone health [2,3]. Peak bone mass is reached during the third decade and serves as the bone bank for the remainder of adult life [4,29].

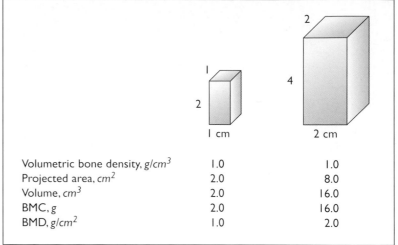

| | 1 cm | 2 cm |
|---|---|---|
| Volumetric bone density, $g/cm^3$ | 1.0 | 1.0 |
| Projected area, $cm^2$ | 2.0 | 8.0 |
| Volume, $cm^3$ | 2.0 | 16.0 |
| BMC, $g$ | 2.0 | 16.0 |
| BMD, $g/cm^2$ | 1.0 | 2.0 |

**FIGURE 2-2.** Noninvasive measurement of bone mineral. Dual-energy x-ray absorptiometry (DXA) is the most commonly used means of determining bone mineral content(BMC, measured in g) and bone mineral density (BMD, measured in $g/cm^2$). DXA corrects for the area but not the thickness of bone in the region studied. Both BMC and BMD are influenced by bone size. The two blocks have the same material properties (or volumetric density); however, the reported BMC and BMD are greater in the larger block. Models of volumetric bone density (termed *bone mineral apparent density*, or BMAD, measured in $g/cm^3$) have been developed to reduce the influence of bone size on bone mineral measurements [30,31]. BMAD is useful in examining bone mineral accrual during childhood and adolescent growth. (*From* Carter *et al.* [30].)

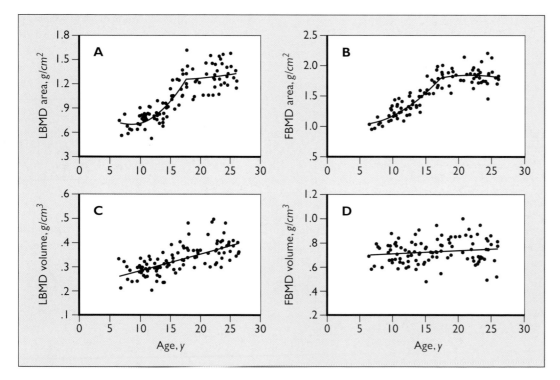

**FIGURE 2-3.** Bone mineral acquisition reflects bone growth. Gains in bone mineral during childhood and adolescence vary by skeletal site and the measurement term used [31–33]. **A** and **B,** Areal bone density (BMD area) increases with age at all sites, including the lumbar spine (L) and femoral neck (F). **C** and **D,** In contrast, volumetric bone density (BMD volume) increases at the spine but not at the femoral neck. These findings suggest that gains in bone mass during adolescence are due largely to bone expansion, although trabecular bone mass within the vertebrae increases as well [34]. Data from healthy males are shown; similar differences in areal and volumetric BMD are observed in females [31]. (*From* Lu *et al.* [31]; with permission.)

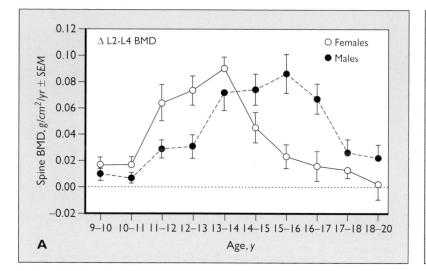

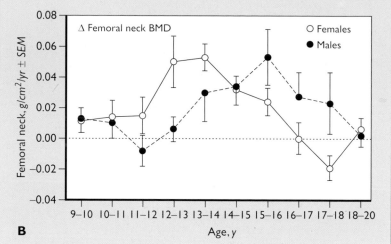

**FIGURE 2-4.** Bone mineral acquisition during puberty. The tempo of bone mineral acquisition during adolescence is more closely linked to pubertal development than to chronologic age [2,3]. Spine (L2–4) (**A**) and femoral neck (**B**) bone mineral density (BMD) increase most rapidly between the ages of 11 and 14 years in girls and 14 and 17 years in boys, reflecting the later onset of puberty in boys [29]. Gains in BMD are greater at the spine and hip than they are in the forearm or shaft of the femur. Girls reach 95% of their adult bone mineral content by the age of 18 years and have only modest gains during the third decade of life [4,35]. SEM—standard error of the mean. (*From* Theintz *et al.* [29]; with permission.)

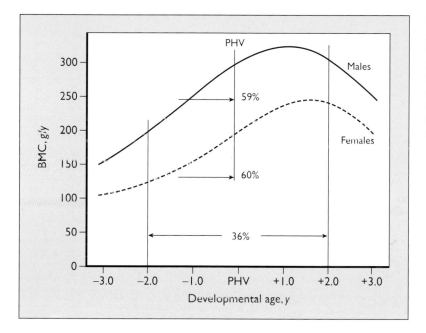

**FIGURE 2-5.** Bone mineral acquisition lags behind linear growth. The most rapid gains in total-body bone mineral content occur approximately 1 year after peak height velocity (PHV) is reached [3]. At the age of PHV (11.6 years of age for girls and 13.5 for boys), adolescents have reached 90% of adult height but only 60% of adult total-body bone mineral content (BMC), 60% of adult BMC for the spine, and 70% of adult BMC at the femoral neck. The discrepancy between bone size and mineral content during the adolescent growth spurt results transiently in relative bone weakness, possibly contributing to the higher incidence of fracture at this age [36]. (*From* Bailey [37]; with permission.)

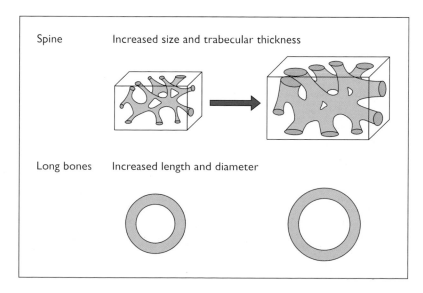

**FIGURE 2-6.** Adolescent changes in bone geometry. Changes in bone geometry accompany gains in bone size and mineral throughout childhood as medullary cavity expands. Spinal vertebrae increase not only in size but also in the thickness of trabeculae within the bone [34]. Long bones increase in length and in cross-sectional area. The increases in cortical thickness are largely proportional to the increase in bone diameter so that volumetric bone density of long bones changes little throughout childhood and adolescence [34]. Hip axial length (HAL) increases during puberty; however, the ratio of HAL to height does not change [38]. These skeletal changes are important clinically because bone size and shape influence bone strength, independent of bone mineral [39,40]. (*Modified from* Seeman [34]; with permission.)

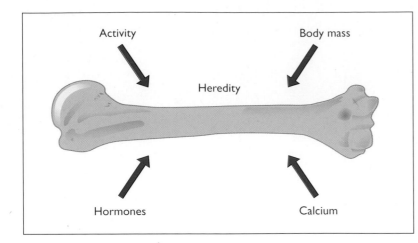

**FIGURE 2-7.** Determinants of peak bone mass. Peak bone mass is largely determined by genetic factors, which account for 60% to 80% of the observed variance in adult bone mineral [5,6]. Several lifestyle factors influence the remaining 20% to 40%. Weight-bearing physical activity stimulates bone accrual, whereas immobility leads to accelerated bone loss [3,17]. Body mass is highly correlated with bone mass, perhaps because weight reflects bone size and nutritional status [11,12]. Additionally, body weight may act as a mechanical load to the skeleton. Calcium intake modifies rates of bone gain and resorption [13,14]. Finally, sex steroids and growth hormone contribute to bone mineral accrual, whereas glucocorticoids, thyroid hormone, and parathyroid hormone in excess may result in bone loss [21–25].

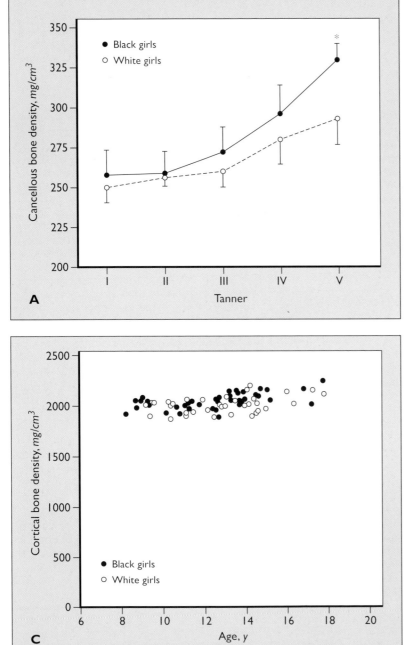

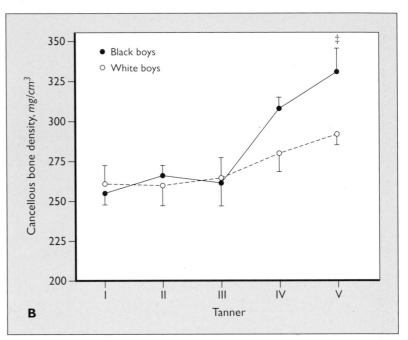

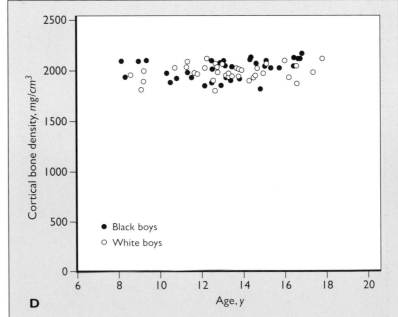

**FIGURE 2-8.** Racial differences in bone mass. There are few racial differences in bone mass between Asians, Hispanic, and white youths once adjustments are made for bone size [38]. By late adolescence, however, black youths have significantly greater bone mass than do white youths [8]. Using quantitative computed tomography (QCT), Gilsanz and colleagues [8] found racial differences in bone density but not bone size at the spine (**A** and **B**). In contrast, bone density at the femoral shaft (**C** and **D**) did not differ by race; however, blacks had greater cross-sectional area at that site than did whites. The observed differences in bone density and size likely contribute to the lower incidence of osteoporosis in blacks [7]. (*From* Gilsanz *et al.* [8]; with permission.)

## CANDIDATE GENES FOR OSTEOPOROSIS

| Gene | Role in Bone Metabolism | Polymorphisms |
|---|---|---|
| Vitamin D receptor | Vitamin D acts through its receptor to influence calcium absorption, bone differentiation, and mineralization. | *Bsml/Apal/Taq* I. Intronic polymorphisms, function unknown. *Fok* I alters VDR translational start site and receptor protein size. |
| Estrogen receptor | Estrogen acts through its receptor to influence skeletal growth, maturation, and bone loss after menopause. | *Pvu* II/*Xba* I intronic polymorphism, function unknown. |
| Collagen I α I | Major protein in bone. Mutations occur in type I collagen genes in osteogenesis imperfecta. | COLIAI polymorphism, function unknown. |
| Transforming growth factor (TGF) | Present in bone matrix. May regulate osteoblast-osteoclast coupling. | Polymorphism, function unknown. |
| Interleukin 6 | Regulates osteoclast growth and differentiation. May mediate effects of sex steroids on bone. | Polymorphism, function unknown. |

*Adapted from Hobson and Ralston [10]; with permission.*

**FIGURE 2-9.** Candidate genes for osteoporosis. Heritable factors are major determinants of peak bone mass, explaining an estimated 60% to 80% of the variability in peak bone mass between individuals [5,6]. Racial, ethnic, and familial similarities in bone mineral density have been observed, supporting the contribution of genetics in bone acquisition. The osteoporosis gene or genes have not yet been identified [10]. The genes listed have been considered as candidates because gene polymorphisms have been associated with bone mass, the gene product plays a role in bone metabolism, or for both reasons. VDR—vitamin D receptor.

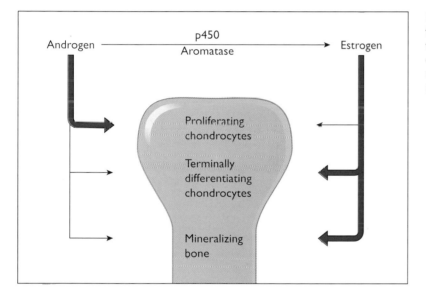

**FIGURE 2-10.** Estrogen and bone acquisition. Estrogen appears to be essential for normal bone maturation and mineral acquisition in girls and boys. Patients with rare disorders of estrogen resistance or impaired synthesis (aromatase deficiency) have osteopenia and delayed epiphyseal closure [21]. Estrogen therapy results in skeletal maturation and increases bone mineral acquisition [41]. (*From* Bachrach and Smith [21]; with permission.)

# Calcium Economics and Bone Health

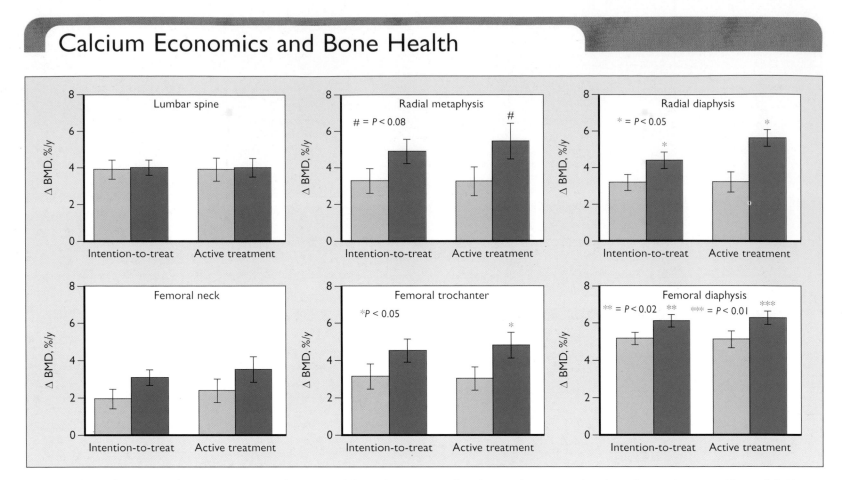

**FIGURE 2-11.** Calcium supplementation increases bone accrual. Several controlled trials have shown that increasing calcium intake in childhood and adolescence results in gains in bone mineral density [13,14]. In the study results shown, girls who consumed foods supplemented with milk protein gained significantly more bone mineral at the radius, trochanter, and femoral diaphysis than did those in the unsupplemented control group [14]. The greatest gains occurred in girls whose habitual diet contained less than 880 mg/d without supplementation. (*From* Bonjour *et al.* [14]; with permission.)

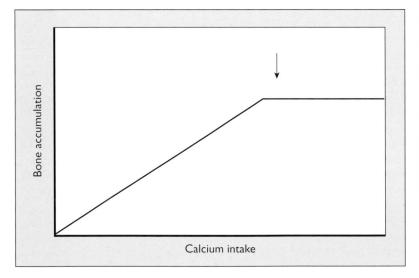

**FIGURE 2-12.** Optimal calcium intake for skeletal health. Calcium retention and bone accrual increase with greater calcium intake until a threshold is reached. Calcium balance studies indicate that calcium retention plateaus at a daily intake of 1200 to 1500 mg/d [42]. Bone mineral acquisition also reaches a maximum at an intake of 1100 to 1200 mg/d based on calcium supplementation studies (*see* Fig. 2-11) [13,14].

## DIETARY REFERENCE INTAKE FOR CALCIUM

| Age, y | Calcium Intake, *mg/d* |
|--------|------------------------|
| 1–3 | 500 |
| 4–8 | 800 |
| 9–18 | 1300 |
| 19–50 | 1000 |
| 51+ | 1200 |

**FIGURE 2-13.** Dietary reference intake for calcium. In 1997, the National Academy of Science issued new dietary guidelines for substances related to bone health, including calcium, phosphorus, magnesium, vitamin D, and fluoride. The recommended intake of calcium for each age group is shown. The calcium recommendations for children and adolescents were raised, based on data linking increased calcium with greater bone accrual [15]. Calcium intake of 1300 mg/d is the equivalent of 4.3 glasses of milk.

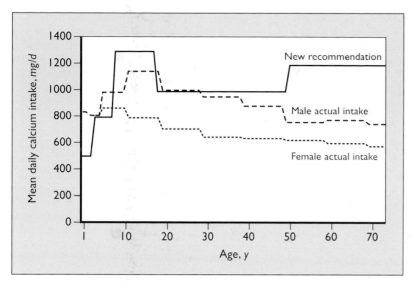

**FIGURE 2-14.** The gap in calcium intake. The mean daily calcium intake falls well below the recommended level, especially during adolescence. Data shown here from the 1994–95 Continuing Survey of Food Intakes by Individuals (CSI) indicate that 86% of girls and 65% of boys aged 12 to 18 years failed to meet the previous recommended daily calcium allowance of 1200 mg/d [27]. Because the optimal intake for calcium has now been set at 1300 mg/d, the gap between the recommended and actual intake of dietary calcium has widened in American youth.

## CALCIUM CONTENT OF COMMON FOODS

| Foods | Serving Size | Calcium Content, *mg* |
|---|---|---|
| Dairy products | | |
| Milk | 1 cup | 300 |
| Yogurt | 1 cup | 345 |
| Cheese | 1-1/2 oz | 300 |
| Ice cream | 1/2 cup | 100 |
| Frozen yogurt* | 1/2 cup | 60–100 |
| Macaroni and cheese | 1/2 cup | 180 |
| Cheese pizza | 1 slice | 100 |
| Nondairy foods: | | |
| Calcium-fortified orange juice | 1 cup | 300 |
| Calcium-fortified cereal* | 1 oz | 160–250 |
| Almonds | 1 oz | 80 |
| Broccoli | 1/2 cup | 35 |
| Soybeans (dry-roasted) | 1/2 cup | 230 |
| Kale | 1 cup | 180 |
| Salmon (canned with bones) | 2 oz | 130 |
| Sardines (canned with bones) | 3-3/4 oz | 380 |
| Tofu (with calcium)* | 1/2 cup | 50–250 |

*Calcium content varies by brand.*

**FIGURE 2-15.** Calcium content of common foods. Meeting the recommended daily intake of calcium is challenging without consuming dairy products. Calcium-fortified products offer a means to boost calcium consumption through nondairy foods.

## BARRIERS TO CALCIUM INTAKE

| Avoidance of Dairy Products | Limited Intake from Nondairy Sources |
|---|---|
| Substitution of soft drinks for milk | Ethnic dietary preferences |
| Fear of fat | Low calcium content or bioavailability of many foods |
| Lactose intolerance | Paucity of calcium fortified foods |
| Ethnic dietary preferences | |
| Concerns regarding environmental toxins | |

**FIGURE 2-16.** Barriers to calcium intake. Dairy products provide 75% of the dietary calcium consumed in the American diet. Several factors that contribute to the declining intake of dairy products can be addressed. Low-fat or fat-free milk, yogurt, and cheeses can be substituted for whole-milk products without reducing the calcium content. Furthermore, most lactose-intolerant persons can consume dairy products in small amounts without symptoms. Nondairy sources of calcium such as breads, cereals, vegetables, and fish generally have a lower content or less bioavailable form of calcium. Some calcium-rich foods such as tofu, turnip greens, and sardines are not part of the standard American diet.

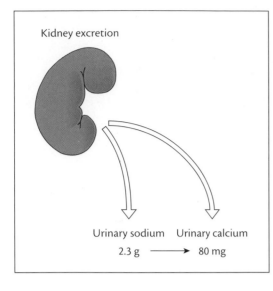

Kidney excretion

Urinary sodium    Urinary calcium
2.3 g  ⟶  80 mg

**FIGURE 2-17.** Calcium economics and sodium intake. The net amount of calcium available for bone metabolism reflects the balance of calcium intake, absorption, and excretion. Calcium consumption has declined in recent years, and only 30% to 40% of what is consumed is absorbed [43]. To compound these problems, urinary calcium losses are likely to be on the rise because of increased sodium intake. Calcium and sodium excretion are linked, with 80 mg of calcium lost for every 2.3 g of urinary sodium [44]. Americans are consuming more sodium contained within prepackaged and fast foods. Decreased calcium intake coupled with increased urinary losses may translate to inadequate calcium for optimal bone acquisition.

# Physical Activity and Bone Mass

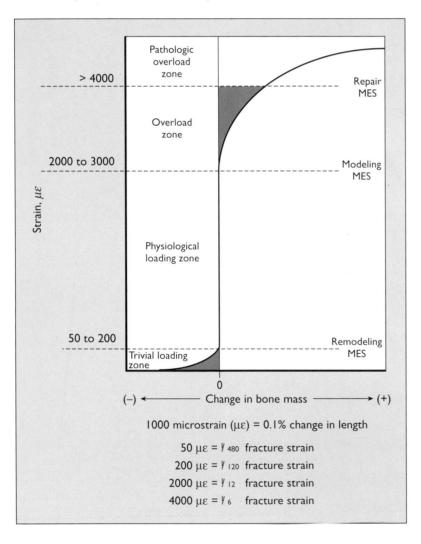

1000 microstrain (με) = 0.1% change in length

50 με = ¹⁄₄₈₀ fracture strain

200 με = ¹⁄₁₂₀ fracture strain

2000 με = ¹⁄₁₂ fracture strain

4000 με = ¹⁄₆ fracture strain

**FIGURE 2-18.** The effects of mechanical loading on bone acquisition. The effect of physical strain on the growing skeleton varies across a range of intensity. According to biomechanical models, when skeletal loading is trivial (as in immobilization), the stimulus for acquisition is insufficient and bone loss occurs. With more moderate (physiologic) loading, neither loss nor gain of bone occurs. In the overload zone, increased strain stimulates bone gain; still greater loading results in formation of poorly constructed bone mineral. MES—minimum effective strain. (*Adapted from* Bailey *et al.* [3]; with permission.)

## PHYSICAL ACTIVITY AND BONE MINERAL ACQUISITION

| Bone Mineral Density | Multiple Regression Coefficients | | | |
| --- | --- | --- | --- | --- |
| | Physical Activity | Gender | Change in Height | Change in Weight |
| Radius | 0.012 ± 0.005* | 0.040 ± 0.018* | 0.011 ± 0.003† | -0.003 ± 0.002 |
| Spine | 0.028 ± 0.007† | 0.018 ± 0.019 | 0.004 ± 0.003 | 0.009 ± 0.003‡ |
| Femoral neck | 0.025 ± 0.004† | 0.030 ± 0.010* | 0.010 ± 0.002† | 0.002 ± 0.002 |
| Trochanter | 0.023 ± 0.008‡ | 0.010 ± 0.022 | 0.006 ± 0.002‡ | 0.006 ± 0.002‡ |

*P < 0.05
†P < 0.001
‡P < 0.01.

**FIGURE 2-19.** Physical activity and bone mineral acquisition. Physical activity has been linked with bone accrual, although the effects of exercise is less well established that is that of calcium [3,18]. In a 3-year longitudinal study, Slemenda and colleagues [18] found activity to be a significant predictor of bone mineral density (BMD) at all skeletal sites in prepubertal children. Bone mass is more consistently correlated with activity than it is with gender or body size. At puberty, weight and height are strong predictors of change in BMD. Intensive exercise before puberty may increase bone size and mineral acquisition. Kannus and colleagues [16] found that young elite tennis players had larger forearm bones in their dominant arm. (*Adapted from* Slemenda [18]; with permission.)

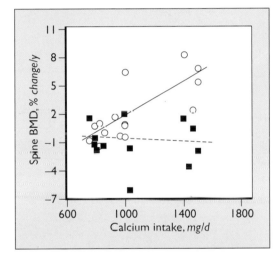

**FIGURE 2-20.** The interaction between calcium and activity. Calcium intake modulates the bone response to physical activity. In a meta-analysis of exercise intervention studies in adults, Specker [19] found that persons in the control group who maintained their usual activity patterns experienced no change in bone mass across a range of calcium intakes. Women assigned to the exercise intervention groups had gains in spinal bone mineral density (BMD) but only if their calcium intake exceeded 1000 mg/d. These studies underscore the important interaction of diet and physical activity in bone health. (*From* Specker [19]; with permission.)

## EFFECTS OF ACTIVITY OR DIETARY CALCIUM INTAKE ON GAINS IN SPINAL BONE DENSITY IN YOUNG WOMEN

Activity level varied (3–7 counts/h), calcium intake was constant (800 mg/d):
The change in BMD/decade = +0.3% to + 8.4%.

Activity level was constant (5 counts/h), calcium intake varied (200–2100 mg/d):
The change in BMD/decade = -1.0% to +16.4%.

**FIGURE 2-21.** Effects of activity or dietary calcium intake on gains in spinal bone density in young women. Varying calcium intake or activity patterns may alter bone mineral gains by approximately 5% to 10% in both children and young adults. In a longitudinal study of young women aged 19 to 29 years, Recker and colleagues [4] examined the contribution of these lifestyle factors on rates of bone mineral acquisition. When calcium intake was held constant in the statistical model, increasing activity (measured by accelerometer) accounted for up to 8% of the differences in the amount of bone gained in the third decade. With activity held constant, gains in bone mass ranged from -1% to +16% with increasing calcium intake. Studies in children suggest that greater activity and calcium intake may increase gains in bone mineral density by 3% to 8% [13,14,18]. BMD—bone mineral density. (*Adapted from* Recker [4]; with permission.)

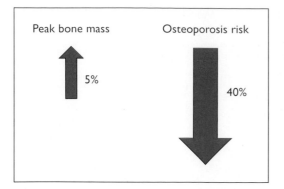

Peak bone mass    Osteoporosis risk

5%

40%

**FIGURE 2-22.** Small differences in peak bone mass mean major differences in skeletal health. The gains in bone mass associated with increasing calcium intake or activity are modest but sufficient to influence skeletal health. A 5% increase in peak bone mass reduces the lifetime risk of osteoporosis by 40%. Conversely, the risk of osteoporotic fracture doubles for each standard deviation (10%) that bone mass falls below the mean value for healthy adults [45].

## FOSTERING SKELETAL HEALTH

Nutrition:

  Avoid high sodium intake

  Maintain daily calcium intake at recommended level

  Maintain healthy body weight

Physical activity

  Avoid excessive exercise (exercise-associated amenorrhea)

  Exercise 30 min or more daily

  Perform a variety of weight-bearing activities

Avoid smoking cigarettes and alcohol use

**FIGURE 2-23.** Fostering skeletal health. Even the modest gains in bone mass seen in persons with a healthy lifestyle may produce a measurable benefit. Although it may be difficult to convince youths of the relevance of bone health, health care professionals, educators, and the media need to spread the word that osteoporosis prevention begins in childhood.

# Acquisitional Osteopenia

## EXAMPLES OF ACQUISITIONAL OSTEOPENIA

Anorexia nervosa

Endocrinopathies

  Cushing syndrome and iatrogenic glucocorticoid excess

  Diabetes

  Growth hormone deficiency

  Hyperprolactinemia

  Hyperthyroidism

  Hypogonadism

Exercise-associated amenorrhea

Idiopathic juvenile osteoporosis

Systemic diseases

  Asthma

  Celiac disease

  Cystic fibrosis

  Leukemia

  Post–organ transplantation

  Rheumatologic disorders

**FIGURE 2-24.** Examples of acquisitional osteopenia. A variety of chronic conditions have been associated with low bone mass in the first two decades of life [22]. In some cases, such as in patients with diabetes and growth hormone deficiency, the deficits may be mild. Osteoporosis and atraumatic fractures have been reported in patients with anorexia nervosa, cystic fibrosis, and glucocorticoid excess, and after organ transplantation. Idiopathic juvenile osteoporosis is a poorly understood syndrome of bone pain and low bone mass that improves spontaneously at puberty.

## COMMON RISK FACTORS FOR OSTEOPENIA

Endocrine:
  Glucocorticoid excess
  Sex steroid deficiency
Immobility
Nutritional:
  Calcium deficiency
  Calorie deficiency
  Malabsorption
  Protein deficiency
  Vitamin D deficiency

**FIGURE 2-25.** Common risk factors for osteopenia. The varied disorders associated with acquisitional osteopenia share common risk factors. These nutritional, mechanical, and hormonal factors reduce the amount of bone mineral acquired, contribute to increased bone loss, or both. Early deficits range in severity from osteopenia (low bone mass for age) to osteoporosis, a more profound deficit in bone mineral with disruption of bone architecture that results in pathologic fractures.

## DEFINING OSTEOPENIA IN CHILDHOOD

Normative data are limited
Adjust for
  Bone size
  Ethnicity and race
  Pubertal stage
  Skeletal maturation

**FIGURE 2-26.** Pitfalls to defining osteopenia in childhood. The interpretation of densitometry data in children and adolescents is considerably more challenging than it is in adults. The software provided by most manufacturers of dual-energy x-ray absorptiometry (DXA) equipment either lacks or includes only limited pediatric data; to interpret the bone mineral density (BMD) results, clinicians must refer to published norms collected using similar DXA equipment (see Fig. 2-23). Furthermore, bone growth and pubertal stage should be considered when interpreting BMD results. Patients with chronic disease often have growth retardation as well as delayed sexual and skeletal maturation, which result in lower BMD values. It may be more appropriate to compare the BMD results from these patients on the basis of bone age or pubertal stage rather than chronological age. To correct for smaller bone size, volumetric bone density can be estimated and compared with published values [31,38].

## PEDIATRIC DATA FOR DUAL-ENERGY X-RAY ABSORPTIOMETRY

| Study | Equipment | Number | Age, y | Sex | Ethnicity | Sites |
|---|---|---|---|---|---|---|
| 46 | Hologic 1000 | 218 | 1—19 | Male, female | Black, white | Whole body |
| 47 | Hologic 1000 | 207 | 9—18 | Male, female | White (Switzerland) | Femoral neck, spine (L2–4) |
| 48 | Hologic 2000 Array Mode | >650 | 8—17 | Male, female | Mostly white (Canada) | Femoral neck, whole body, spine (L1–4) |
| 38 | Hologic 1000W Pencil Beam | 423 | 9—25 | Male, female | Asian, black, Hispanic, white | Femoral neck, whole body, spine (L2–4) |
| 49 | ODX-240 | 574 | 10—24 | Female | White (France) | Spine (L2–4) |
| 50 | Lunar DPXL/PED | 500 | 4—20 | Male, female | White (Netherlands) | Whole body, spine (L2–4) |

**FIGURE 2-27.** Pediatric reference data for dual energy x-ray absorptiometry (DXA). Normative pediatric data are now available using a variety of dual-energy x-ray absorptiometry (DXA) equipment and software [31,38,46–50]. When using these data to interpret bone mineral density (BMD) results, it is important to select reference data collected with the same software and equipment used to study patients, because there are systematic differences in results [51]. Standard deviation scores will vary, depending on the normative data employed [52]. In particular, the percentage of persons defined as osteopenic (over two standard deviations below normal) is greater when gender-specific data are not employed.

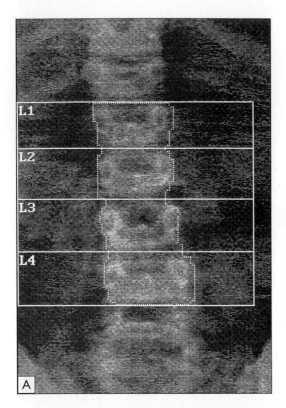

A

### B. BONE MINERAL DENSITY

| Region | Estimated area, $cm^2$ | Estimated BMC, g | BMD, $g/cm^2$ |
|--------|------------------------|------------------|---------------|
| L2 | 8.40 | 3.57 | 0.425 |
| L3 | 9.13 | 4.14 | 0.454 |
| L4 | 9.80 | 5.27 | 0.537 |
| Total | 27.33 | 12.98 | 0.475 |

*Total BMD CV for L2–L4, 1.0%.*

### C. BONE MINERAL DENSITY

| Region | BMD | T (%) |
|--------|-----|-------|
| N/A | | |
| L2 | 0.425 | -5.48 (41) |
| L3 | 0.454 | -5.73 (42) |
| L4 | 0.537 | -5.26 (48) |
| L2–L4 | 0.475 | -5.49 (44) |

*T—peak bone mass, 30.0.*
*BMD L2–L4, 0.475 g/cm².*

**FIGURE 2-28.** Osteopenia in a 15-year-old girl with cystic fibrosis (CF) The patient suffered an atraumatic fracture of the left forearm at age 90. This patient had been treated with pancreatic enzymes and vitamin D (for malabsorption), calcium supplements, and alternate-day prednisone (for pulmonary disease). Her spinal bone mineral density (BMD) testing using dual-energy x-ray absorptiometry was more than two standard deviations below that expected for her age. She was treated with pancreatic enzymes and vitamin D (for malabsorption), calcium supplements, and alternate-day prednisone (for pulmonary disease). Despite increased calcium and caloric supplementation and efforts to wean her steroid dose, she had continued to lose bone density. At aged 15 years, her spinal BMD was more than four standard deviations below normal [53]. BMC—bone mineral content; CV—coefficient of variation.

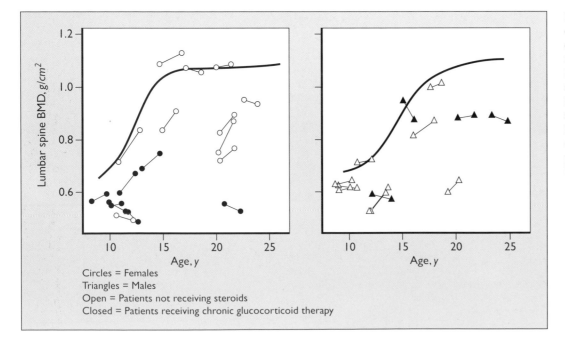

Circles = Females
Triangles = Males
Open = Patients not receiving steroids
Closed = Patients receiving chronic glucocorticoid therapy

**FIGURE 2-29.** The spectrum of bone mineral density (BMD) in cystic fibrosis. Osteopenia is common in several chronic disorders because of reduced bone acquisition or increased bone loss. Bhudhikanok and colleagues [53] found that lumbar spine (LS) BMD was below the mean for age (dark line) in many young patients with cystic fibrosis at study entry. At follow-up 1.5 years later, most patients had gained bone mineral density but failed to reach expected values. Bone loss was more common in patients on glucocorticoid therapy. (*From* Bhudhikanok *et al.* [53]; with permission.)

## DETERMINANTS OF SKELETAL STATUS IN ATHLETES

Age at onset of training

Body mass

Menstrual status

Skeletal site

  Trabecular vs cortical bone

  Weight-bearing vs non–weight-bearing

Sport

  Ballet

  Gymnastics

  Running

  Swimming

**FIGURE 2-30.** Determinants of skeletal status in the athlete. Exercise-associated amenorrhea is another frequent cause of early osteopenia. The risk of low bone mass in young women who train intensively is dependent on a number of variables. The most profound deficits have been observed as part of the "athletic triad" of disordered eating, amenorrhea, and osteoporosis [54]. Earlier onset of training, low body mass, and delayed or absent menses have been identified as risk factors for low bone mass. Deficits in bone mineral density have been observed at the spine, hip, femoral shaft, and tibia, indicating that weight-bearing activity may not be sufficient to protect against the deleterious effects of hypogonadism [55]. Finally, the risk of osteopenia is not equal for all activities. Female gymnasts have greater spinal and hip bone mass (after correcting for bone size) than do runners and nonathletes, despite a high incidence of menstrual dysfunction [56]. In contrast, elite swimmers have no greater bone mass at these sites than do persons in the nonathletic control group [57]. These observations underscore the importance of high-impact activity as a stimulus for bone formation (see Fig. 2-18).

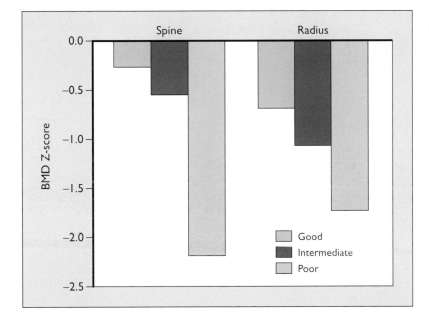

**FIGURE 2-31.** Recovery from osteopenia in anorexia nervosa. Skeletal status after anorexia nervosa in adolescents and young adults is related to the adequacy of recovery from this disorder. Herzog and colleagues [58] examined the bone mineral density (BMD) of 51 women an average of 11.7 years after their first hospitalization for anorexia nervosa [58]. BMD standard deviations (z scores) were significantly related to recovery of weight and menstrual function. However, even those women with a good clinical outcome had persistently low BMD, particularly at the forearm. Low BMD also has been observed in younger persons after recovery from anorexia nervosa, indicating that early deficits in bone mass may not be fully reversible [59,60].

## EVALUATION OF OSTEOPENIA IN CHILDHOOD

History

  Activity patterns

  Calorie, protein, and calcium intake

  Medications

Laboratory tests

  1,25-dihydroxyvitamin D (to test conversion to active form)

  25-hydroxyvitamin D (to assess stores)

  Calcium, phosphorus, creatinine, and alkaline phosphatase

  Estradiol and testosterone

  Genetic studies

  Intact parathyroid hormone

  Thyroid function

Bone densitometry (DXA)

**FIGURE 2-32.** Evaluation of osteopenia in childhood. The cause of osteopenia may be apparent from the clinical history, such as chronic glucocorticoid use, anorexia nervosa, and cystic fibrosis. When the cause of osteopenia is unknown, laboratory studies may be indicated to rule out endocrine and renal disorders. The diagnosis of inherited disorders of bone metabolism (such as osteogenesis imperfecta) is established from DNA analysis of skin biopsy specimens. Bone densitometry is indicated to determine the severity of osteopenia and establish a baseline before initiation of therapy. Currently, dual-energy x-ray absorptiometry is the preferred method to assess bone mass in children.

## THERAPY FOR ACQUISITIONAL OSTEOPENIA

Risk-free Therapies
  Address nutritional deficits
    Increase calorie and protein intake
    Supplement calcium intake
    Supplement vitamin D intake
  Treat endocrinopathies
    Cushing syndrome
    Diabetes
    Growth hormone deficiency
    Hyperthyroidism
  Avoid immobility
Possible Beneficial Therapy
  Sex steroids
Experimental Therapies
  Antiresorptive agents
  Bisphosphonates
  Calcitonin
  Anabolic agents
  Fluoride
  Parathyroid hormone

**FIGURE 2-33.** Therapy for acquisitional osteopenia. Treatment of acquisitional osteopenia begins by addressing recognized multiple nutritional and hormonal risk factors. Weight-bearing physical activity should be encouraged, when possible, balancing the risks of slower weight gain or pathologic fracture against the benefits of mechanical loading. Sex steroid replacement therapy should be considered for patients with hypogonadism; however, this therapy has not proved sufficient to correct the osteopenia associated with anorexia nervosa [61]. Furthermore, in a controlled trial, estrogen replacement therapy has not been shown to increase bone mass or prevent fractures in athletes with amenorrhea. The antiresorptive agents have not been proved safe or effective in children and remain experimental. In theory, anabolic agents may prove to be of greater benefit because osteopenia acquired early in life is likely to reflect a failure to gain bone with or without increased bone loss.

# References

1. Hui SL, Slemenda CW, Johnston CC: The contribution of bone loss to post menopausal osteoporosis. *Osteoporosis Int* 1990, 1:30–34.

2. Bonjour JP: Bone mineral acquisition in adolescence. In *Osteoporosis*. Edited by Marcus R, Feldman D, Kelsey J. San Diego: Academic Press; 1996:465–476.

3. Bailey DA, Faulkner RA, McKay HA: Growth, physical activity, and bone mineral acquisition. *Exerc Sports Sci Rev* 1996, 24:233–266.

4. Recker RR, Davies M, Hinders SM, *et al.*: Bone gain in young adult women. *JAMA* 1992, 268:2403–2408.

5. Kelly PJ, Eisman JA, Sambrook PN: Interaction of genetic and environmental influences on peak bone density. *Osteoporosis Int* 1990, 1:56–60.

6. Krall EA, Dawson-Hughes B: Heritable and lifestyle determinants of bone mineral density. *J Bone Miner Res* 1993, 8:1–9.

7. Villa ML, Nelson L: Race, ethnicity, and osteoporosis. In *Osteoporosis*. Edited by Marcus R, Feldman D, Kelsey J. San Diego: Academic Press; 1996:435–447.

8. Gilsanz V, Skaggs DL, Kovanlikaya A, *et al.*: Differential effect of race on the axial and appendicular skeletons of children. *J Clin Endocrinol Metab* 1998, 83:1420–1427.

9. Seeman E: Growth in bone mass and size: Are racial and gender differences in bone mineral density more apparent than real? [editorial]. *J Clin Endocrinol Metab* 1998, 83:1414–1419.

10. Hobson EE, Ralston SH: The genetics of osteoporosis. *The Endocrinologist* 1997, 7:429–435.

10. Miller JZ, Slemenda CW, Meaney FJ, *et al.*: The relationship of bone mineral density and anthropometric variables in healthy male and female children. *Bone Miner* 1991, 14:137–152.

12. Moro M, van der Meulen MCH, Kiratli BJ, *et al.*: Body mass is the primary determinant of midfemoral bone acquisition during adolescent growth. *Bone* 1996, 19:519–526.

13. Johnston CC Jr, Miller JZ, Slemenda CW, *et al.*: Calcium supplementation and increases in bone mineral density in children. *N Engl J Med* 1992, 327:82–87.

14. Bonjour J-Ph, Carrie A-L, Ferrari S, *et al.*: Calcium-enriched foods and bone mass growth in prepubertal girls: a randomized, double-blind, placebo-controlled trial. *J Clin Invest* 1997, 99:1287–1294.

15. National Institutes of Health: Optimal calcium intake. NIH Consensus Statement. 1994, 12:1–31.

16. Kannus P, Haaspasalo H, Sankelo M, *et al.*: Effect of starting age on bone mass in the dominant arm of tennis and squash players. *Ann Intern Med* 1995, 12:27–31.

17. Ferretti JL, Schiessl H, Frost HM: On new opportunities for absorptiometry. *J Clin Densitometry* 1998, 1:41–53.

18. Slemenda CW, Reister TK, Sui SL, *et al.*: Influences on skeletal mineralization in children and adolescents: evidence of varying effects of sexual maturation and physical activity. *J Pediatr* 1994, 125:201–207.

19. Specker BL: Evidence for an interaction between calcium intake and physical activity on changes in bone mineral density. *J Bone Miner Res* 1996, 11:1539–1544.

20. Rubin K, Schirduan V, Gendreau P, *et al.*: Predictors of axial and peripheral bone mineral density in healthy children and adolescents, with special attention to the role of puberty. *J Pediatr* 1993, 123:863–870.

21. Bachrach BE, Smith EP: The role of sex steroids in bone growth and development: evolving new concepts. *The Endocrinologist* 1996, 6:362–368.

22. Bachrach LK: Osteopenia in childhood and adolescence. In *Osteoporosis*. Edited by Marcus R, Feldman D, Kelsey J. San Diego: Academic Press; 1996:785–800.

23. Saggese G, Baroncelli BI, Bertelloni S, *et al.*: Effects of long-term treatment with growth hormone on bone and mineral metabolism in children with growth hormone deficiency. *J Pediatr* 1993, 122:37–45.

24. Kotaniemi A, Savolainen A, Kautiainen H, Kroger H: Estimation of central osteopenia in children with chronic polyarthritis treated with glucocorticoids. *Pediatr* 1993, 91:1127–1129.

25. Radetti G, Castellan C, Tato L, *et al.*: Bone mineral density in children and adolescent females treated with high doses of L-thyroxine. *Horm Res* 1993, 3:127–131.

26. Ray NF, Chan JK, Thamer M, Melton LJ III: Medical expenditures for the treatment of osteoporotic fractures in the United States in 1995: Report from the National Osteoporosis Foundation. *J Bone Miner Res* 1997, 12:24–35.

27. USDA Continuing Survey of Food Intakes by Individuals, 1994–95: Agricultural Research Service, US Department of Agriculture, Washington, DC.

28. US Department of Health and Human Services: Physical activity and health. A report of the Surgeon General, Washington, DC. 1996.

29. Theintz G, Buchs B, Rizzoli R, et al.: Longitudinal monitoring of bone mass accumulation in healthy adolescents: evidence for a marked reduction after 16 years of age at the levels of lumbar spine and femoral neck in female subjects. *J Clin Endocrinol Metab* 1992, 75:1060–1065.

30. Carter DR, Bouxsein ML, Marcus R: New approaches for interpreting projected bone densitometry data. *J Bone Miner Res* 1992, 7:137–145.

31. Lu PW, Cowell CT, Lloyd-Jones SA, et al.: Volumetric bone mineral density in normal subjects, aged 5–27 years. *J Clin Endocrinol Metab* 1996, 81:1586–1590.

32. Katzman DK, Bachrach LK, Carter DR, Marcus R: Clinical and anthropometric correlates of bone mineral acquisition in healthy adolescent girls. *J Clin Endocrinol Metab* 1991, 73:1332–1339.

33. Kroger H, Kotaniemi A, Vainio P, Alhava E: Bone densitometry of the spine and femur in children by dual-energy x-ray absorptiometry. *Bone Miner Res* 1992, 17:75–85.

34. Seeman E: From density to structure: growing up and growing old on the surfaces of bone. *J Bone Miner Res* 1997, 12:509–521.

35. Teegarden D, Proulx WR, Martin BR, et al.: Peak bone mass in young women. *J Bone Miner Res* 1995, 10:711–715.

36. Blimkie CJR, Levevre J, Beunen GP, et al.: Fractures, physical activity, and growth velocity in adolescent Belgian boys. *Med Sci Sports Exerc* 1993, 25:801–808.

37. Bailey DA: The Saskatchewan pediatric bone mineral accrual study: bone mineral acquisition during the growing years. *Int J Sports Med* 1997, 18:S191–S194.

38. Wang M-C, Aguirre M, Bhudhikanok GS, et al.: Bone mass and hip axis length in healthy Asian, Black, Hispanic and White American youths. *J Bone Miner Res* 1997, 12:1922–1935.

39. Gilsanz V, Loro ML, Roe TF, et al.: Vertebral size in elderly women with osteoporosis: mechanical implications and relationship to fractures. *J Clin Invest* 1995, 95:2332–2337.

40. Faulkner KG, Cummings SR, Black D, et al.: Simple measurement of femoral geometry predicts hip fracture: the study of osteoporotic fractures. *J Bone Miner Res* 1993, 8:1211–1217.

41. Bilezikian JP, Morishima A, Bell J, Grumbach MM: Increased bone mass a result of estrogen therapy in a man with aromatase deficiency. *N Engl J Med* 1998, 339:599–603.

42. Matkovic V, Heaney RP: Calcium balance during human growth: evidence for threshold behavior. *Am J Clin Nutr* 1992, 55:992–996.

43. Abram SA, O'Brien KO, Liang LK, Stuff JE: Differences in calcium absorption and kinetics between black and white girls aged 5–16 years. *J Bone Miner Res* 1995, 10:829–833.

44. Matkovic V, Ilich JZ, Andon MB, et al.: Urinary calcium, sodium, and bone mass of young females. *Am J Clin Nutr* 1995, 62:417–425.

45. Hui SL, Slemenda CS, Johnson CC Jr: Age and bone mass as predictors of fracture in a prospective study. *J Clin Invest* 1988, 81:1804–1809.

46. Southard RN, Morris JD, Maha JD, et al.: Bone mass in healthy children: measurement with quantitative DXA. *Radiology* 1991, 179:735–738.

47. Bonjour JP, Theintz G, Buchs B, et al.: Critical years and stages of puberty for spinal and femoral bone mass accumulation during adolescence. *J Clin Endocrinol Metab* 1991, 73:555–563.

48. Faulkner RA, Bailey DA, Drinkwater DT, et al.: Bone densitometry in Canadian children 8–17 years of age. *Calcif Tissue Int* 1996, 59:344–351.

49. Sabatier J-P, Guaydier-Souquieres G, Laroche D, et al.: Bone mineral acquisition during adolescence and early adulthood: a study in 574 healthy females 10–24 years of age. *Osteoporosis Int* 1996, 6:141–148.

50. Boot AM, De Ridder MAJ, Pols HAP, et al.: Bone mineral density in children and adolescents: relation to puberty, calcium intake, and physical activity. *J Clin Endocrinol Metab* 1997, 82:57–62.

51. Genant HK: Universal standardization for dual x-ray absorptiometry: patient and phantom cross-calibration results. *J Bone Miner Res* 1995, 10:997 998.

52. Leonard MB, Propert KJ, Zemel BS, et al.: Comparability of pediatric bone mineral density (BMD) normative data in the assessment of children at risk. *J Bone Miner Res* 1997, 12(suppl):S250.

53. Bhudhikanok GS, Wang M-C, Marcus R, et al.: Bone acquisition and loss in children and adults with cystic fibrosis: a longitudinal study. *J Pediatr* 1998, 133:18–27.

54. Snow-Harter CM: Bone health and prevention of osteoporosis in active and athletic women. *Clin Sports Med* 1994, 13:389–404.

55. Young N, Formica C, Szmukler G, Seeman E: Bone density at weight-bearing and nonweight-bearing sites in ballet dancers: the effects of exercise, hypogonadism, and body weight. *J Clin Endocrinol Metab* 1994, 78:449–454.

56. Robinson TL, Snow-Harter C, Taaffe DR, et al.: Gymnasts exhibit higher bone mass than runners despite similar prevalence of amenorrhea and oligomenorrhea. *J Bone Miner Res* 1995, 10:26–35.

57. Taaffe DR, Snow-Harter C, Connolly DA, et al.: Differential effects of swimming versus weight-bearing activity on bone mineral status of eumenorrheic athletes. *J Bone Miner Res* 1995, 10:586–593.

58. Herzog W, Minne H, Deter C, et al.: Outcome of Bone mineral density in anorexia nervosa 11.7 years after first admission. *J Bone Miner Res* 1993, 8:597–605.

59. Bachrach LK, Katzman DK, Litt IF, et al.: Recovery from osteopenia in adolescent girls with anorexia nervosa. *J Clin Endocrinol Metab* 1991, 72:602–606.

60. Kooh SW, Noriega E, Leslie K, et al.: Bone mass and soft tissue composition in adolescents with anorexia nervosa. *Bone* 1996, 19:181–188.

61. Klibanski A, Biller BMK, Schoenfeld DA, et al.: The effects of estrogen administration on trabecular bone loss in young women with anorexia nervosa. *J Clin Endocrinol Metab* 1995, 80:898–904.

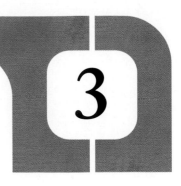

# ADULT BONE MAINTENANCE

## Douglas P. Kiel

From the time of peak bone mass, which occurs between the ages of 20 and 30 years, women lose approximately 42% of their spinal and 58% of their femoral bone mass. Surprisingly, the rates of bone loss in the eighth and ninth decades of life may exceed those found in the immediate perimenopausal period in part because uncoupling occurs in the remodeling cycle. Several contributing factors to adult bone loss are the focus of this chapter, including those related to diet, hormones, and physical activity.

One of the most significant dietary factors that contributes to bone health is calcium. Dietary calcium deficiency is very common and results in secondary hyperparathyroidism, which leads to an increase in bone resorption. Bone resorption often is compounded by vitamin D deficiency, especially in northern latitudes. Numerous clinical trials have demonstrated the benefit of calcium and vitamin D repletion on skeletal health. Based on the results of these clinical trials the National Academy of Sciences recommended an increase in the minimal daily requirement for calcium intake in persons over aged 65 years to 1500 mg/d, and in the vitamin D requirement to 600 IU/d.

In addition to calcium and vitamin D, other nutritional factors may play a role in age-related osteoporosis. Malnutrition or even low dietary protein intake may lead to increases in bone loss. Considerable controversy surrounds the notion that too much dietary protein leads to bone loss through an increase in acid load from protein metabolism. Vitamin K deficiency may contribute to an increased risk of osteoporotic fractures and bone loss, although the findings in studies have been inconsistent. Another interesting dietary component that may influence bone remodeling and bone loss are the phytoestrogens, specifically the isoflavones, which are the most common form of phytoestrogen. In fact, ipriflavone, which is a derivative of naturally occurring isoflavones, has been shown to retard bone loss when compared with placebo. Other dietary components that may influence bone health include magnesium, potassium, and vitamin C, all of which contribute to bone metabolism.

Estrogen deficiency has long been recognized as a major cause of bone loss in the first decade after menopause. More recently, a link has been established between endogenous estrogen levels and bone mass in both women and men. Although the link between estrogen and bone health in women has long been recognized, a series of studies have demonstrated a strong association between estradiol levels and bone mineral density in men. In some of these studies, testosterone in men also has been associated with bone mass; however, the findings are less consistent than are those for estradiol. In addition to the role of sex hormones in skeletal health, changes in the growth hormone–insulin-like growth factor-I (IGF-I) axis may contribute to age-related bone loss. Growth hormone secretion declines with age, leading to lower serum levels of IGF-I and alterations in the IGF-I binding proteins with age. Finally, the adrenal androgens dehydroepiandrosterone (DHEA) and DHEA-S also have been implicated in adult bone loss, although the data are limited.

Physical activity has been shown to have clear beneficial effects on the skeleton. A recent meta-analysis of studies examining the relationship between physical activity and bone mass concluded that a positive association clearly exits. What is not precisely defined is the intensity and frequency of the activity necessary to maintain bone mass at various ages over the lifespan. The role of nutritional factors, hormonal influences, smoking cigarettes, alcohol consumption, and physical activity in the maintenance of the adult skeleton are reviewed.

## Nutritional Influences on Bone

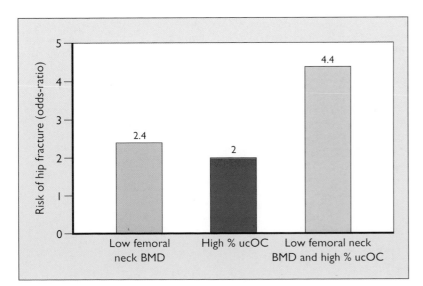

**FIGURE 3-1.** Bone mineral density and undercarboxylated osteocalcin levels to predict hip fracture. The undercarboxylation of osteocalcin owing to vitamin K deficiency has been hypothesized to affect bone mass because vitamin K plays an important role in the $\gamma$-carboxylation of glutamic acid residues in pro-osteocalcin, which is essential for the mineralization of osteoid. Vergnaud and colleagues [1] studied 104 elderly women with hip fracture, using 255 women (average age, 82 years) with hip fracture as the control group. Both femoral neck bone mineral density (BMD) and levels of undercarboxylated osteocalcin (ucOC) are equal predictors of fracture, when using BMD as the lowest quartile and high ucOC as the highest quartile. Those women with both low BMD and high ucOC were at the highest risk of hip fracture. (*From* Vergnaud *et al.* [1].)

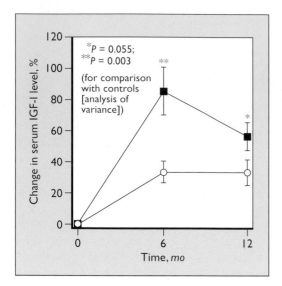

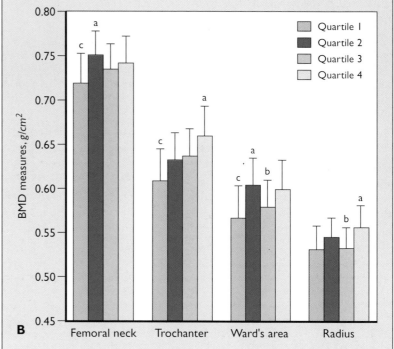

**FIGURE 3-2.** Protein supplementation in patients with hip fracture improves bone mass. Protein restriction has been shown to reduce plasma levels of insulin-like growth factor-I (IGF-I) by inducing resistance to the action of growth hormone in the liver and increasing the metabolic clearance rate of the growth factor. Furthermore, evidence shows that protein depletion may blunt the effect of IGF-I on organs such as bone. Thus, low protein intake in elderly persons, such as those recovering from hip fracture, may be detrimental to skeletal health. In a recent randomized controlled trial of a protein supplement given to patients recuperating from hip fracture (n = 41 treated; 41 in the control group), supplements increased IGF-I levels significantly and slowed the loss of BMD compared with placebo. The *solid line* represents patients who received protein supplements; the *dashed line* represents patients in the control group. (*From* Schurch et al. [2]; with permission.)

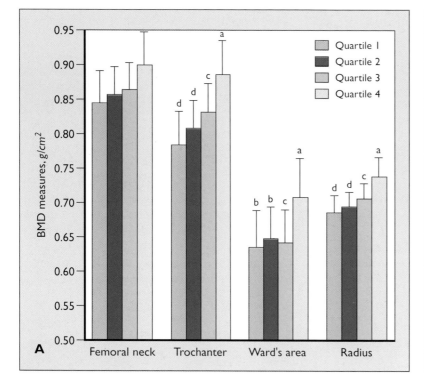

**FIGURE 3-3.** Dietary magnesium, potassium, and bone mass. Bone mineral serves as a buffer for the acid loads from the metabolism of certain nutrients such as animal protein. Some researchers have suggested that a diet favoring "alkaline ash" would lessen the acid load and lead to better maintenance of adult bone mass. Such a diet would emphasize the ingestion of fruits, vegetables, vegetable protein, and moderate amounts of milk. Two specific nutrients that may have buffering effects are potassium and magnesium, which are found in a variety of whole unrefined foods, including fruits and vegetables. As part of the Framingham Osteoporosis Study, dietary and supplement intakes were assessed by a food frequency questionnaire and bone mineral density (BMD) as measured at three hip sites and one forearm site. Because potassium and magnesium intakes are highly correlated, the nutrient intakes were summed using standardized z scores to adjust for the different scales of the two variables. Quartiles of the combined intake of magnesium and potassium were then created. As can be seen in the graphs for men (**A**) and for women (**B**), at every skeletal site except the femoral neck, greater intakes of magnesium and potassium were associated with greater BMD after adjusting for multiple covariates such as age, body mass index, physical activity, alcohol consumption, cigarette smoking, total energy intake, dietary calcium intake, dietary vitamin D intake, use of a calcium supplement, use of a vitamin D supplement, season of bone measurement, and current estrogen replacement therapy in women. (a > b, $P < 0.1$; a > c, $P < 0.05$; a > d, $P < 0.01$). (*From* Tucker et al. [3]; with permission.)

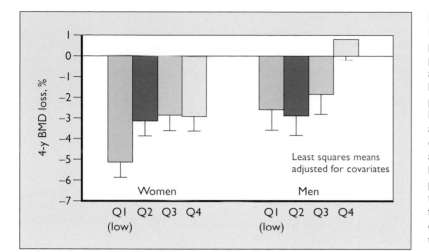

**FIGURE 3-4.** Protein intake and bone loss in elderly men and women. Evidence suggests that protein undernutrition may be associated with osteoporotic fractures. In contrast, evidence also exists that diets rich in animal protein may actually result in negative calcium balance, which would result in acceleration of bone loss. These considerations notwithstanding, there have been no longitudinal studies of protein intake and bone loss among older persons, who may be consuming less protein than the amounts previously linked to negative calcium balance. Such a study recently has been completed as part of the Framingham Osteoporosis Study. Four-year longitudinal data on dietary intake and bone mineral density (BMD) were collected on 391 women and 274 men who were members of the original Framingham Heart Study between the 1988 and 1992. Both men and women in the lowest quartile of protein intake had greater losses of bone mass at the femoral neck than did those in the highest quartile of protein intake. This was true after adjustment for multiple covariates including age, weight, cigarette smoking, caffeine intake, calcium intake, physical activity, alcohol consumption, and estrogen replacement therapy in women. (*From* Hannan *et al.* [4]; with permission.)

## Hormonal Effects on Bone

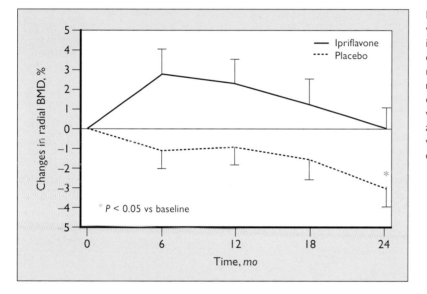

**FIGURE 3-5.** Clinical trial of ipriflavone to prevent bone loss in postmenopausal women. Ipriflavone, 7-isopropoxy-isoflavone, is a derivative of naturally occurring isoflavones, which are considered phytoestrogens. The precise effects of phytoestrogens on the skeleton are not well established. These results are from a 2-year randomized double-blind placebo-controlled trial. This trial enrolled 255 postmenopausal women between the ages of 50 and 65 years, with bone mineral density (BMD) at the distal radius one standard deviation below the mean value of age-matched healthy women. After 2 years of administration of this agent, BMD was maintained and was statistically significantly higher compared with the placebo group, which lost bone over the 2 years. All women received calcium supplementation. (*From* Adami *et al.* [5]; with permission.)

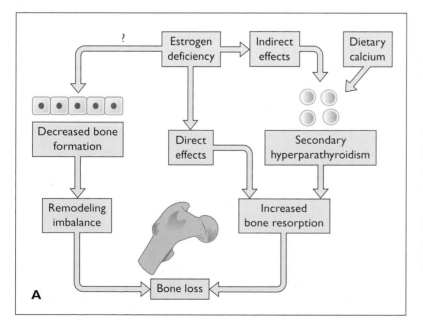

**FIGURE 3-6. A,** Unitary model for bone loss in postmenopausal women. Based on recent studies of the relation between sex hormones and bone metabolism, an essential role for estrogen has emerged in involutional bone loss in both men and women. In this new unitary model proposed by Riggs and colleagues [6], estrogen deficiency plays a central role in the pathophysiology of both phases of involutional bone loss in women and plays a major contributory role in the continuous phase of bone loss in men. At menopause, the acute loss of the restraining effects of estrogen on bone cell activity leads to an accelerated phase of loss of predominantly cancellous bone lasting up to 20 years. The slow phase of bone loss, which also begins at menopause, then becomes dominant, involves loss of both cancellous and cortical bone, and continues throughout the remainder of life. The effects of loss of estrogen on extraskeletal calcium homeostasis lead to decreased intestinal calcium absorption, increased calcium wasting, effects on vitamin D metabolism, and loss of a direct effect on the parathyroid gland that ordinarily decreases parathyroid hormone secretion. The resulting increase in parathyroid hormone causes increased bone resorption and bone loss. Estrogen deficiency also may cause an impairment in bone formation by the loss of estrogen-stimulated synthesis of bone matrix proteins by osteoblasts, although the evidence for this is lacking.

(Continued on next page)

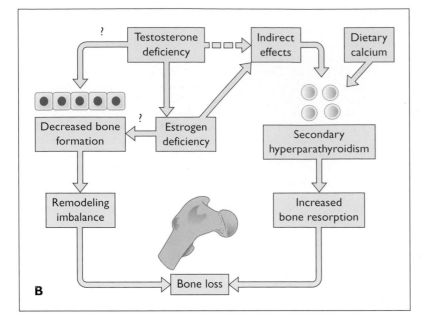

**FIGURE 3-6.** (*Continued*) **B,** Unitary model for bone loss in aging men. Recent data in men suggest that estrogen regulates bone metabolism as much or more than does testosterone. Elderly men have low levels of serum bioavailable estrogen, and thus estrogen may contribute to bone loss in men. This gradual induction of estrogen deficiency in aging men leads to bone loss by mechanisms similar to those in women (*Panel A*). In men, testosterone itself may exert effects on the skeleton directly or indirectly through conversion to estrogen. (*From* Riggs *et al.* [6]; with permission.)

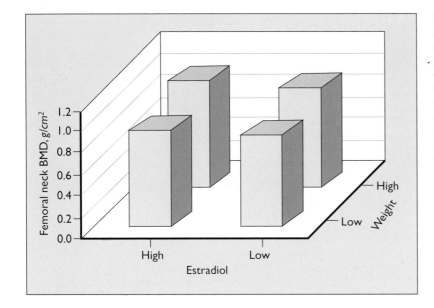

**FIGURE 3-7.** Serum estradiol, weight, and bone mineral density (BMD) in older men. Because the focus of research in osteoporosis has been on women, much less is known regarding those factors that may influence bone mass or loss in older men. Studies of sex steroids and gonadal function in men have focused primarily on androgens and are much less common than are studies in women. These studies of androgens in men have found either weak correlations or no correlation with bone mass. Estrogens in men have not been well characterized with regard to bone mass. In this study, 93 healthy men, an average of 67 years of age, had an average testosterone level of 4.2 ng/mL and an average estradiol (E2) level of 35 pg/mL. The greatest femoral neck BMD was observed in men above the median E2 level and weight group. The lowest BMD was observed in men below the median E2 level and weight group. Intermediate values were seen in men in the low-E2-level high-weight group or high-E2-level low-weight group. These findings underscore the role of E2 in the aging skeletons of men. (*From* Slemenda *et al.* [7].)

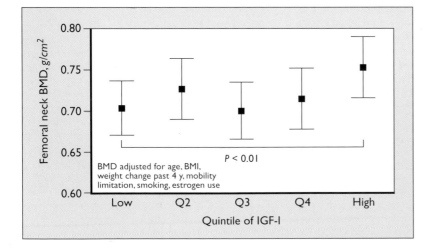

**FIGURE 3-8.** Insulin-like growth factor-I (IGF-I) and bone mineral density (BMD) in women. IGF-I is one of the most abundant growth factors in bone and has been shown to stimulate bone formation. Declines in skeletal and serum IGF-I levels with age parallel decreases in bone mass with age; however, few studies have been done in elderly persons. In this study, 425 women members of the Framingham Osteoporosis Study had determinations made of BMD of the hip and serum IGF-I levels. High IGF-I levels were associated with greater BMD after adjustment for age, body mass index (BMI), weight change in the past 4 years, mobility limitation, smoking cigarettes, and estrogen replacement therapy. Women in the highest quintile of IGF-I levels had significantly higher BMD than did women in the lowest quintile ($P$ 0.01). The figure shows mean/67 of 95% confidence intervals (*From* Langlois *et al.* [8]; with permission.)

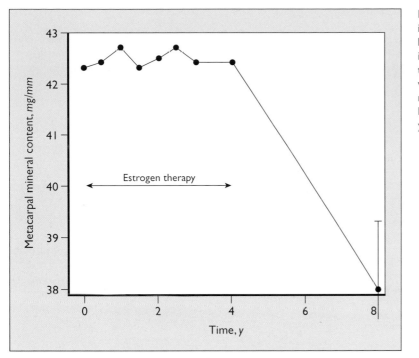

**FIGURE 3-9.** Withdrawal of estrogen replacement therapy (ERT) and bone loss in postmenopausal women. It is well recognized that ERT after menopause prevents bone loss for as long as it is taken. When ERT is discontinued, bone turnover increases and bone loss quickly returns to the levels of those of nonusers. In this classic study by Lindsay and colleagues [9], 14 women with oophorectomy who had been taking mestranol for 4 years discontinued ERT and had bone mass measured approximately 8 years from the time of cessation. The rate of bone loss per year was 2.5%, equivalent to that of women in the first 1 or 2 years after bilateral oophorectomy. (*From* Lindsay *et al.* [9]; with permission.)

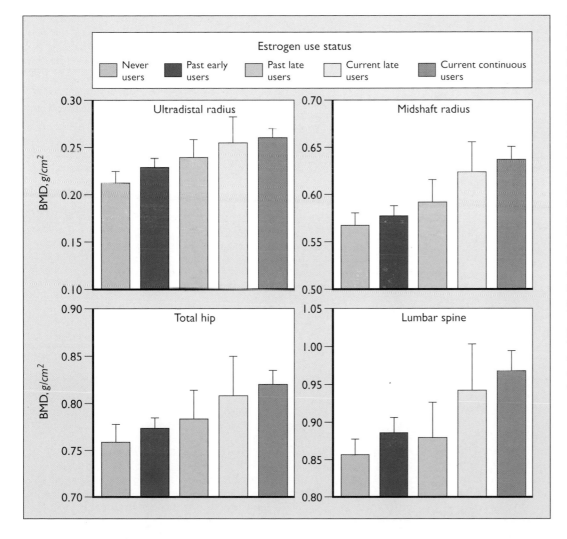

**FIGURE 3-10.** Timing of estrogen replacement therapy (ERT) and bone mass in postmenopausal women. Observations have been made that discontinuing ERT leads to resumption of bone loss and even prolonged ERT in the early postmenopausal years may not protect the skeleton in advanced age. Because of these two observations, attempts have been made to ascertain the timing of ERT to maximize bone mineral density (BMD) at the ages when fractures are more common. In this study of 740 women aged 60 to 98 years, current users of ERT who began therapy at menopause had the highest BMD levels. In these women, BMD levels were significantly higher than those in women who had never had ERT and those in women who previously had ERT beginning at menopause (with 10 years' duration of use). However, among current users, no significant difference in BMD levels at any site was observed between those who started ERT at menopause (with 20 years' use) and those who started after aged 60 years (with 9 years' use). These data suggest that ERT initiated after menopause and continued into late life is associated with the highest BMD. However, ERT begun after aged 60 years and continued confers substantial benefits on the aging skeletons in women. (*From* Schneider *et al.* [10].)

# Physical Activity and Bone

## EFFECT SIZES FOR INDIVIDUAL STUDIES AND COMBINED EFFECTS FOR ALL POSSIBLE PARAMETER-SPECIFIC AND ANATOMIC SITE–SPECIFIC GROUPS FOR THE PREVENTION OF BONE LOSS

| Site | Parameter, site | Study | Hedges and Olkin's effect size (95% CI) |
|---|---|---|---|
| Lumbar spine | BMC, L2–4 | Dalsky et al. [11] | 0.0147 (–1.3251–1.3545) |
| | BMD, L2–4 | Sinaki et al. [12] | –0.0988 (–0.5858–0.3883) |
| | | Nelson et al. [13] | 0.4799 (–0.4573–1.4171) |
| | | Prince et al. [14] | –0.9904 (–1.4655– –0.5154) |
| | | Grove and Londeree [15] | |
| | | High-impact group | 0.7794 (–0.5064–2.0652) |
| | | Low-impact group | 0.6867 (–0.5889–1.9623) |
| | | Lau et al. [16] | 0.0647 (–0.7537–0.8830) |
| | | Pruitt et al. [17] | 1.1373 (0.2233–2.0512)* |
| | | Hatori et al. [18] | |
| | | High-intensity group | 0.9484 (0.1045–1.7924)* |
| | | Moderate intensity group | 0.2294 (–0.6377–1.0964) |
| | | Nelson et al. [19] | 0.1828 (–0.4464–0.8120) |
| | | Kohrt et al. [20] | 1.3248 (0.2426–2.4070)* |
| | BMD, L1–2 | Cavanaugh and Cann [21] | –0.4026 (–1.3645–0.5594) |
| | BMD, L1–3 | Nelson et al. [13] | 1.0177 (0.0057–2.0296)* |
| | BMD, L1–4 | Bloomfield et al. [22] | 1.9619 (0.6361–3.2878)* |
| | | Tsukhara et al. [23] | |
| | | Newcomers group | 0.2142 (–0.4072–0.8356) |
| | | Veterans group | 0.5241 (–0.0510–1.0992) |
| Hip | BMD, femoral neck | Nelson et al. [13] | 0.2560 (–0.6717–1.1837) |
| | | Lau et al. [16] | –0.4028 (–1.2291–0.4236) |
| | | Pruitt et al. [17] | –0.3828 (–1.2063–0.4408) |
| | | Nelson et al. [19] | 0.1611 (–0.4678–0.7901) |
| | | Kohrt et al. [20] | 2.8364 (1.4485–4.2242)* |
| | BMD, femur | Bloomfield et al. [22] | 0.7323 (–0.3499–1.8145) |
| | BMD, intertrochanteric area | Lau et al. [16] | –0.0136 (–0.8317–0.8046) |
| | | Kohrt et al. [20] | 1.1451 (0.0879–2.2024)* |
| | BMD, Ward's triangle | Lau et al. [16] | –0.2024 (–1.0227–0.6178) |
| | | Kohrt et al. [20] | 1.1125 (0.0594–2.1656)* |
| Heel | BMC, heel | Rundgren et al. [27] | 0.7434 (0.0589–1.4279)* |

*$P < 0.05$

**FIGURE 3-11.** Meta-analysis of the relationship between physical activity and bone mineral density (BMD). Although basic bone biology recognizes the importance of skeletal loading to bone formation, a review of the literature on physical activity and osteoporosis demonstrates inconsistent conclusions regarding the effects of such activities. Useful conclusions about the role of physical activity on bone health can be derived from a synthesis, or meta-analysis, of results from multiple prospective intervention trials. The *effect size* is defined as the ratio of the average difference in post-treatment means observed in the exercise and control groups to the weighted standard deviation. The effect sizes are given for 13 individual studies and the combined effects for all possible parameter-specific and anatomic site–specific groups for bone loss prevention. Taking into account the frequency, duration, compliance rate, and average age of those enrolled in the study, the programs were judged of moderate intensity and focused on walking, running, physical conditioning, and aerobics. In studies published after 1991, a significant effect of physical activity on the BMD at the L2–4 level of the lumbar spine was detected. However, no effect could be seen on femoral bone mass. BMC—bone mineral content. (*From* Berard et al. [24]; with permission.)

# Aging and Gender Effects on Bone

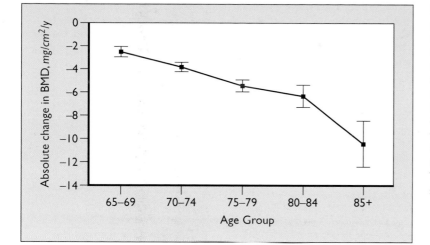

**FIGURE 3-12.** Bone loss increases with advancing age in women. Large cross-sectional studies have found a strong inverse relationship between age and bone mass. Potential biases in cross-sectional data, however, could substantially underestimate or overestimate the actual rate of loss. These data are from the Study of Osteoporotic Fractures, a longitudinal study of 8116 women 65 years of age and older, 5698 of whom returned in 3 years for a second measurement of bone mineral density (BMD) of the hip. These data demonstrate that the rate of decline in total hip BMD steadily increased from 2.5 mg/cm$^2$/y in women 67 to 69 years old to 10.4 mg/cm$^2$/y in those aged 85 and older. The average loss of bone from the total hip is sufficient to increase the risk of hip fracture by 21% per 5 years in women aged 80 years and older. This fact underscores the concept that bone loss continues unabated into very old age and may in fact increase with aging. The same pattern of bone loss with aging has been reported in a longitudinal study of men from Australia [25]. (*From* Ensrud *et al.* [26]; with permission.)

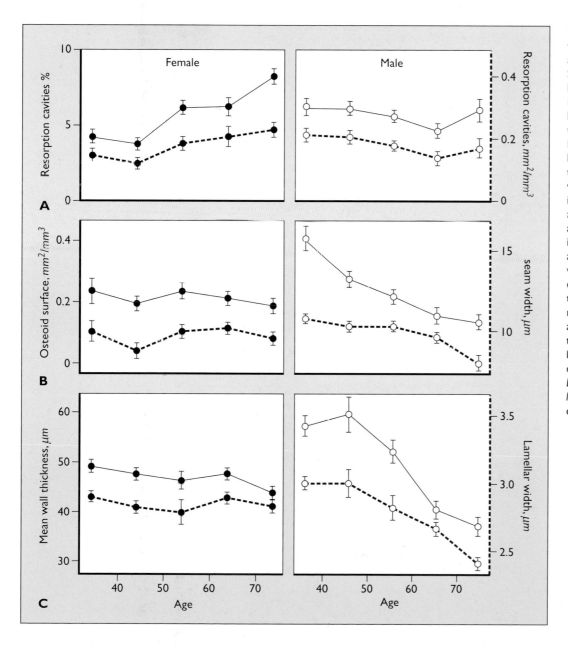

**FIGURE 3-13.** Sex differences in trabecular bone with aging (**A** to **C**). A loss of trabecular bone with age is common to both sexes and similar in extent. Significant differences in static indices of remodeling, however, can be demonstrated between the sexes. In men, the extent of resorption cavities changes little with age when expressed either in absolute terms or as a percentage of total trabecular surface. In contrast, in women, an increase from initially low levels is apparent in the sixth decade. In women, the extent of osteoid borders shows little change with age in absolute or relative terms. Conversely, in men, progressive decline occurs in both absolute and relative terms. The decrease in osteoid tissue in aging men also is associated with a decline not only in mean wall thickness but in both lamellar number and width. These changes were not seen in the women, in whom the variables remained almost constant. From these findings it can be concluded that in the aging woman increased resorption occurs, resulting in a loss of trabeculae rather than progressive attenuation. In the aging man, however, it appears that the ramifications of the trabecular network are largely maintained and the width of trabeculae diminishes as a result of decreased bone formation. *Dashed lines*—read the values on the right; *solid lines*—read the values on the left. SE—standard error. (*From* Aaron *et al.* [27]; with permission.)

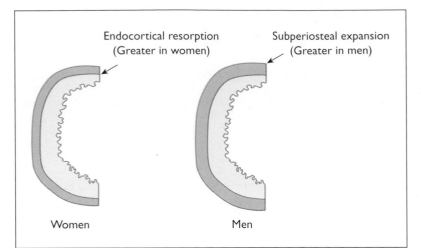

FIGURE 3-14. Sex differences in cortical bone remodeling with age. The diminution in cortical bone density is less in men because endocortical bone resorption is less and periosteal appositional growth is greater. The greater periosteal bone formation may be a more important means of preserving bone strength than is the lesser endosteal bone resorption because placing bone distant from the neutral or long axis of bone is biomechanically advantageous. This greater age-related increase in periosteal bone formation in men than in women has been shown for the vertebral body, proximal femur, and midtibia. (From Ruff and Hayes [28].)

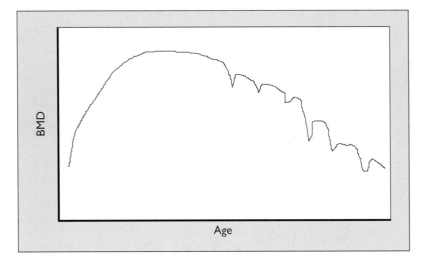

FIGURE 3-15. A proposed model for age-related bone loss: the contribution of catabolic illness. Age-related bone loss occurs because of the cumulative effects of resorption exceeding formation after peak bone mass is achieved. Obviously, many genetic and environmental factors influence the balance between resorption and formation. One potentially important contributor, however, is the periodic occurrence of a catabolic event such as surgery, medical illness, or injury. This contributor results in diminished caloric intake, diminished physical activity, and muscle atrophy. These events contribute to an increase in the imbalance between bone resorption and bone formation. It is likely that recovery of the lost bone mass never fully occurs. If this model of bone loss is shown to be clinically important, treatment strategies should be targeted toward these periods of time. BMD—bone mineral density.

# Smoking, Alcohol, and Bone

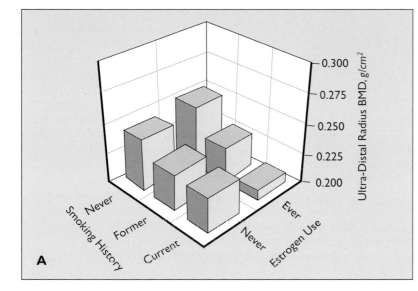

**A**

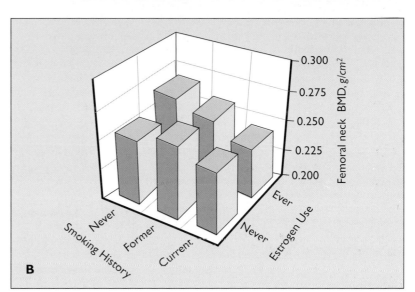

**B**

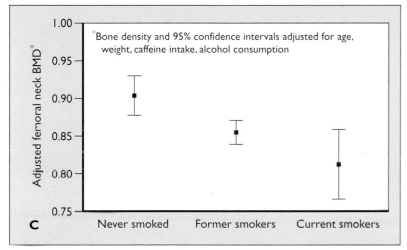

*Bone density and 95% confidence intervals adjusted for age, weight, caffeine intake, alcohol consumption

**C**

**FIGURE 3-16. A** and **B,** Deleterious effects of cigarette smoking on the skeleton in women. The negative effects of smoking cigarettes on skeletal health have long been recognized; however, the results of studies have not all been in agreement. One possible factor that may interact with cigarette smoking in women is estrogen status. Because cigarette smoking accelerates the 2-hydroxylation of estone to an inactive metabolite, 2-hydroxy estrone, a biologic mechanism exists that may explain why women who take estrogen replacement therapy (ERT) and smoke have a lower bone mineral density (BMD) than do women who take ERT and do not smoke. Women who had used ERT had higher BMD than did nonusers only if they had never smoked. Use of ERT did not confer any advantage in BMD among current smokers. **C,** The deleterious effects of smoking cigarettes on the skeleton in men. In men, cigarette smoking clearly results in lower BMD. In this study of 348 elderly men, current smokers had lower BMD at the femoral neck than did those who did not smoke [29].(*From Kiel* et al. *[29]; with permission.*)

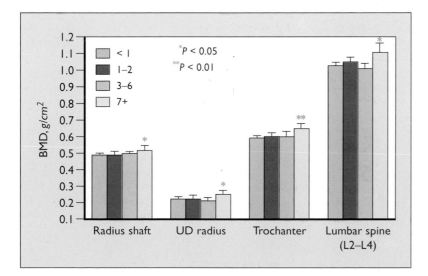

**FIGURE 3-17.** Moderate alcohol intake is associated with increased bone mineral density (BMD). Although persons who are alcoholics suffer from osteoporosis and increased risk of fracture, the consumption of lesser amounts of alcohol may favorably impact the skeletal status of women. One mechanism for this may be the recognized effects of alcohol on increasing endogenous estrogen levels or even adrenal androgen levels. In this study of 384 women, BMD was higher in those who drank at least 7 oz/wk of alcohol than it was in those who drank less than 1 oz/wk. This difference was not explained by differences in age, weight, height, age at menopause, smoking cigarettes, and years of estrogen replacement therapy, which were adjusted for in this analysis [30]. UD—ultra distal. (*From Felson* et al. *[30]; with permission.*)

# References

1. Vergnaud P, Garnero P, Meunier PJ, et al.: Undercarboxylated osteocalcin measured with a specific immunoassay predicts hip fracture in elderly women: The EPIDOS study. *J Clin Endocrinol Metab* 1997, 82:719–724.

2. Schurch MA, Rissoli R, Slosman D, et al.: Protein supplements increase serum insulin-like growth factor-I levels and attenuate proximal femur bone loss in patients with recent hip fracture a randomized, double-blind, placebo-controlled trial. *Ann Intern Med* 1998, 128:801–809.

3. Tucker KT, Hannan MT, Chen H, et al.: Potassium, magnesium, and fruit and vegetable intakes are associated with greater bone mineral density in older men and women. *Am J Clin Nutr* 1999, 69:727–736.

4. Hannan M, Dawson-Hughes B, Felson D, Kiel D: Effect of dietary protein on bone loss in elderly men and women: the Framingham Osteoporosis Study. *J Bone Miner Res* 1997, 12:S151.

5. Adami S, Bufalino L, Cervetti R, et al.: Ipriflavone prevents radial bone loss in postmenopausal women with low bone mass over 2 years. *Osteoporosis Int* 1997, 7:119–125.

6. Riggs BL, Khosla S, Melton LJ: A unitary model for involutional osteoporosis: estrogen deficiency causes both type I and type II osteoporosis in postmenopausal women and contributes to bone loss in aging men. *J Bone Miner Res* 1998, 13:763–773.

7. Slemenda CW, Longcope C, Zhou L, et al.: Sex steroids and bone mass in older men positive associations with serum estrogens and negative associations with androgens. *J Clin Invest* 1997, 100:1755–1759.

8. Langlois JA, Visser M, Rosen CJ, et al.: Insulin-like growth factor-I and bone mineral density in older women and men. *J Clin Endocrinol Metab* 1998, 83:4257–4262.

9. Lindsay R, MacLean A, Kraszewski A, et al.: Bone response to termination of oestrogen treatment. *Lancet* 1978, i:1325–1327.

10. Schneider DL, Barrett-Connor EL, Morton DJ: Timing of postmenopausal estrogen for optimal bone mineral density the Rancho Bernardo study. *JAMA* 1997, 277:543–547.

11. Dalsky G, Stocke K, Ehsani A: Weight-bearing exercise training and lumbar bone mineral content in postmenopausal women. *Ann Intern Med* 1988, 108:824–828.

12. Sinaki M, Wahner H, Offord K, Hodgson S: Efficacy of nonloading exercises in prevention of vertebral bone loss in postmenopausal women: a controlled trial. *Mayo Clin Proc* 1989, 64:762–769.

13. Nelson M, Fisher E, Dilmanian F, et al.: A walking program and increased dietary calcium in postmenopausal women: effects on bone. *Am J Nutr* 1991, 53:1304–1311.

14. Prince R, Smith M, Dick I, et al.: A comparative study of exercise, calcium supplementation, and hormone-replacement therapy. *N Engl J Med* 1991, 325:1189–1195.

15. Grove K, Londeree B: Bone density in postmenopausal women: high impact vs low impact exercise. *Med Sci Sports Exerc* 1992, 24:1190–1194.

16. Lau E, Woo J, Leung P, et al.: The effects of calcium supplementation and exercise on bone density in elderly Chinese women. *Osteoporosis Int* 1992, 2:168–173.

17. Pruitt L, Jackson R, Bartels R, Lehnhard H: Weight-training effects on bone mineral density in early postmenopausal women. *J Bone Miner Res* 1992, 7:179–185.

18. Hatori M, Hasegawa A, Adachi H, et al.: The effects of walking at the anaerobic threshold level on vertebral bone loss in postmenopausal women. *Calcif Tissue Int* 1993, 52:411–414.

19. Nelson M, Fiatarone M, Morganti C, et al.: Effects of high-intensity strength training on multiple risk factors for osteoporotic fractures: a randomized controlled trial. *JAMA* 1994, 272:1909–1914.

20. Kohrt W, Snead D, Slatopolsky E, Birge SJ: Additive effects of weight-bearing exercise and estrogen on bone mineral density in older women. *J Bone Miner Res* 1995, 10:1303–1311.

21. Cavanaugh D, Cann C: Brisk walking does not stop bone loss in post-menopausal women. *Bone* 1988, 9:201–204.

22. Bloomfield S, Williams N, Lamb D, Jackson R: Non-weightbearing exercise may increase lumbar spine bone mineral density in healthy post-menopausal women. *Am J Phys Med Rehabil* 1993, 72:204–209.

23. Tsukahara N, Toda A, Goto J, Ezawa I: Cross-sectional and longitudinal studies on the effect of water exercise in controlling bone loss in Japanese postmenopausal women. *J Nutr Sci Vitaminol* 1994, 40:37–47.

24. Berard A, Bravo G, Gauthier P: Meta-analysis of the effectiveness of physical activity for the prevention of bone loss in postmenopausal women. *Osteoporosis Int* 1997, 7:331–337.

25. Ensrud KE, Palermo L, Black DM, et al.: Hip and calcaneal bone loss increase with advancing age: longitudinal results from the study of osteoporotic fractures. *J Bone Miner Res* 1995, 10:1778–1787.

26. Jones G, Nguyen T, Sambrook P, et al.: Progressive loss of bone in the femoral neck in elderly people: longitudinal findings from the Dubbo osteoporosis epidemiology study. *BMJ* 1994, 309:691–695.

27. Aaron JE, Makins NB, Sagreya K: The microanatomy of trabecular bone loss in normal aging men and women. *Clin Orthop Rel Res* 1987, 215:260–271.

28. Ruff CB, Hayes WC: Sex differences in age-related remodeling of the femur and tibia. *J Orthop Res* 1988, 6:886–896.

29. Kiel DP, Zhang Y, Hannan MT et al.: The effect of smoking at different life stages on bone mineral density in elderly men and women. *Osteoporosis Int* 1996, 6:240–248.

30. Felson DT, Zhang Y, Hannan MT et al.: Alcohol intake and bone mineral density in elderly men and women. The Framingham Study. *Am J Epidemiol* 1995, 142:485–492.

# EPIDEMIOLOGY OF OSTEOPOROSIS AND ASSOCIATED FRACTURES

## Loran M. Salamone and Jane A. Cauley

Osteoporosis is a metabolic bone disease characterized by low bone mass and microarchitectural deterioration of bone tissue, leading to enhanced bone fragility and a consequent increase in fracture risk [1]. Osteoporosis is the most prevalent metabolic bone disease in the United States and in other developed countries. In the United States, up to 54% (16.8 million) of postmenopausal white women have low bone mass or osteopenia and another 30% (9.4 million) have osteoporosis. Among 50-year-old white women and men, the estimated lifetime fracture risk is 40% in women and 13% in men [2].

Osteoporotic fractures are directly related to age with a rising incidence of fractures in women starting at about the age of 50. In women, the incidence of most fractures increase with age after menopause; there is a similar age-related increase in men, although the total number of fractures is approximately half that seen in women [4]. Hip fractures result in the highest morbidity and mortality with a mortality rate of 10% to 20% during the first year following a fracture, with most of the deaths occurring within 6 months of the fracture [5].

The risk for osteoporosis can be defined in terms of bone mineral density (BMD) or by the occurrence of fractures. Bone mineral density is a useful risk factor by which to categorize people according to the degree of fracture risk. Bone density measurements are safe and noninvasive and not only can assess differences in risk between individuals, but also can monitor changes in risk within individuals over time. BMD is essential in predicting the risk of fracture and monitoring progress of intervention strategies. It has been estimated that a decline of 1 standard deviation (SD) decline in BMD is equivalent to a 1.5-fold to 2.5-fold increase in fracture risk for women and men [6,7].

Alternatively, one can describe the impact of osteoporosis by assessing the prevalence and incidence of fractures. *Prevalence* refers to the number of people in the population who at a given time have already had fractures related to osteoporosis, whereas *incidence* refers to the number of new fractures occurring in a population within a specified period of time. Osteoporosis fractures are characterized by higher incidence rates among women than among men, rates that increase sharply with age, and a greater propensity for fractures in skeletal sites containing large amounts of cancellous bone [8]. The hip, spine and distal forearm, which share these characteristics, are recognized as the most common sites affected in osteoporosis. Most fractures in older women are in fact due to low bone mass [9]. Since bone loss is an asymptomatic process, diagnosis often is made only after fracture has occurred. It is critical to gain a broader recognition of the extent of this public health problem to allow earlier detection, prevention, and better management of this increasingly important disease among the growing elderly population.

This chapter summarizes epidemiologic data related to the frequency of osteoporosis and its related fractures, and discusses the societal impact of this disease. More specifically, it focuses on the magnitude of the health problem, encompassing prevalence and incidence patterns of both low bone mass and fractures across cultural groups; the evaluation of fracture risk including an over-view of identifiable risk factors, the role of bone density and the risk of falling; and the economic consequences of osteoporotic fractures.

# Epidemiology of Osteoporosis

**DIAGNOSTIC CRITERIA FOR OSTEOPOROSIS ESTABLISHED BY THE WORLD HEALTH ORGANIZATION BASED ON COMPARISON TO YOUNG ADULT MEAN BONE DENSITY***

Normal

  Bone density is within 1 SD (standard deviation) of the young adult mean.

Osteopenia

  Bone density is within 1 to 2.5 SD below the young adult mean.

Osteoporosis

  Bone density is 2.5 SD or more below the young adult mean.

Severe (established) osteoporosis

  Bone density is more than 2.5 SD below the young adult mean and there has been one or more osteoporotic fractures.

*One standard deviation represents about a 10–12% decline in bone density.*

**FIGURE 4-1.** Diagnostic criteria established by the World Health Organization based on comparison to young adult mean bone density. (*reprinted from* Kanis *et al.* [10]; with permission.)

**RISK FACTORS FOR OSTEOPOROSIS**

Age or age-related

  Each decade associated with 1.4–1.8-fold increased risk

Genetic

  Ethnicity: whites and Asians > African-Americans

  Gender female > male

  Family history

Environmental

  Nutrition: calcium deficiency, vitamin D deficiency, excess dietary protein

  physical activity and mechanical loading

  Medications, *eg*, corticosteroids

  Smoking

  Alcohol

  Falls (trauma)

Endogenous hormones and chronic diseases

  Estrogen deficiency

  Androgen deficiency

  Chronic conditions, *eg*, hyperthyroidism, gastrectomy, cirrhosis, hypercortisolism

Physical characteristics of bone

  Density (mass)

  Size and geometry

  Microarchitecture

  Composition

**FIGURE 4-2.** Risk factors for osteoporosis. (*Reprinted from* Wasnish [11]; with permission.)

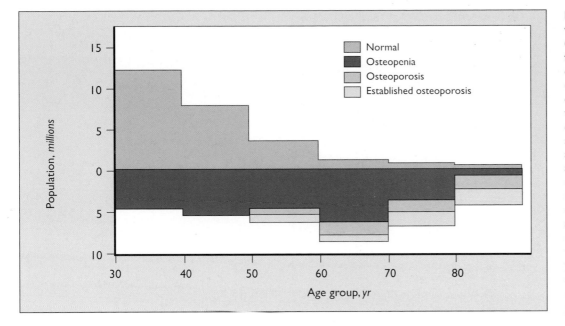

**FIGURE 4-3.** Estimated skeletal status of white women in the United States in 1990 by age group. *Osteopenia* is bone density of the hip, spine or distal forearm more than 1.0 but less than 2.5 standard deviations (SD) below the mean in young adults (ages 30–40 years). *Osteoporosis* is bone density at one or more of these sites more than 2.5 SD below the young adult mean (ages 30–40 years). *Established osteoporosis* is bone density at one or more of these sites more than 2.5 SD below the young adult mean and at least one osteoporotic fracture. Numbers above the middle line 0 represent women with normal bone density, numbers below the middle line represent the women in the three categories of osteopenia and osteoporosis. Most women under age 50 have normal bone density at all four skeletal sites, although with advancing age, a greater proportion have osteopenia or osteoporosis. At age 80 years and over, only 3% have normal bone density at all four sites, 27% have osteopenia at one skeletal site or another, and 70% have osteoporosis. (*Reprinted from* Cooper and Melton [8]; with permission.)

## PROPORTION (%) OF ROCHESTER, MINNESOTA, WOMEN WITH BONE MINERAL MEASUREMENTS MORE THAN 2.5 STANDARD DEVIATIONS BELOW THE MEAN FOR YOUNG NORMAL WOMEN

| Age Group, y | Lumbar Spine, % | Either Hip Site, % | Midradius, % | Spine, Hip, or Midradius, % |
|---|---|---|---|---|
| 50–59 | 7.6 | 3.9 | 3.7 | 14.8 |
| 60–69 | 11.8 | 8.0 | 11.8 | 21.6 |
| 70–79 | 25.0 | 24.5 | 23.1 | 38.5 |
| ≥80 | 32.0 | 47.5 | 50.0 | 70.0 |
| Total | 16.5 | 16.2 | 17.4 | 30.1 |

**FIGURE 4-4.** Proportion of women in Rochester, Minnesota with bone mineral measurements more than 2.5 standard deviations below the mean for young normal women. The mean is derived from 48 subjects under age 40 who were randomly sampled from the Rochester, Minnesota, population. None of them was known to have any disorder that might influence bone metabolism. The total is age-adjusted to the population structure of 1990 United States white women 50 years of age and older. (*Reprinted from* Melton [3]; with permission.)

**FIGURE 4-5.** Prevalence of low femoral bone density in noninstitutionalized United States women ages 50 and older, according to NHANES III 1988–1994. (*Reprinted from* Looker [12]; with permission.)

## PREVALENCE OF LOW FEMORAL BONE DENSITY IN NONINSTITUTIONALIZED UNITED STATES WOMEN AGES 50 AND OLDER (NHANES III 1988–1994)

| Region of Interest | Osteoporosis Prevalence† | Osteoporosis 95% CI† | Osteoporosis Millions‡ |
|---|---|---|---|
| Non–Hispanic Whites | | | |
| Femur neck | 20(17) | 17,22 | 6 |
| Trochanter | 13(12) | 11,15 | 4 |
| Intertrochanter | 15(13) | 13,17 | 4 |
| Total femur | 17(15) | 15,19 | 5 |
| Non–Hispanic Blacks | | | |
| Femur neck | 5(6) | 4,7 | 0.2 |
| Trochanter | 7(7) | 5,8 | 0.2 |
| Intertrochanter | 7(7) | 5,10 | 0.2 |
| Total femur | 8(8) | 6,10 | 0.3 |
| Mexican Americans | | | |
| Femur neck | 10(14) | 7,13 | 0.1 |
| Trochanter | 12(15) | 7,16 | 0.1 |
| Intertrochanter | 11(14) | 7,14 | 0.1 |
| Total femur | 12(16) | 8,16 | 0.1 |

*Prevalences shown in parenthesis are age-adjusted to the 1980 U.S. census population.

†Pertain to unadjusted prevalences.

‡Based on the average of undercount-adjusted population estimates from the March 1990 and March 1993 Current Population Surveys.

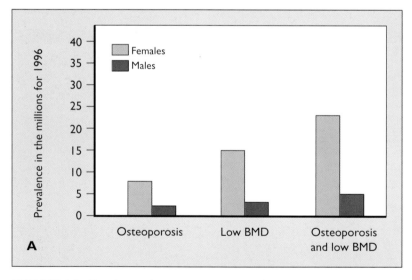

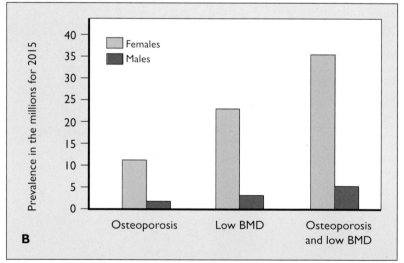

**FIGURE 4-6.** For this study, osteoporosis was defined as bone density values more than 2.5 standard deviations (SD) below those of a non-Hispanic white female reference group mean age 20–29 years. Low bone mass was defined as bone density values between 1 and 2.5 SD below a non-Hispanic white female reference group (mean aged 20–29 years). Research summaries from NHANES III were used as the basis for extrapolations of prevalence data. **A**, Osteoporosis prevalence figures for 1996 in the United States population of women and men age 50 and over [13]. Osteoporosis: women = 8,021,036; men = 2,081,950. Low bone mass or osteopenia: women = 15,434,059; men = 3,122,926. Total women and men with osteoporosis and low bone mass: women = 23,455,096; men = 5,204,875. **B**, Estimated prevalence of osteoporosis for 2015 in the United States population of women and men age 50 and over. Osteoporosis: women = 11,914,236; men = 2,461,927. Low bone mass, or osteopenia: women = 23,115,835; men = 2,461,927. Total with osteoporosis and low bone mass: Women = 35,030,069; men = 6,154,825. BMD—bone mineral density. (*Data from* National Osteoporosis Foundation [14]; with permission.).

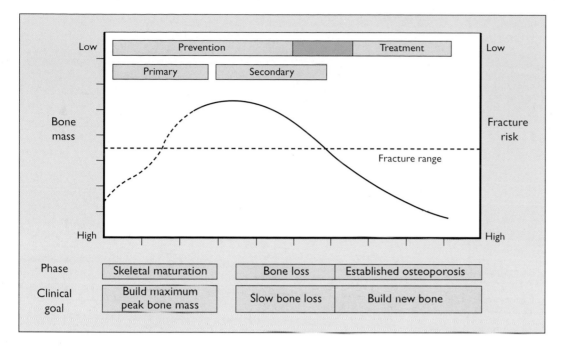

**FIGURE 4-7.** Bone mass and risk of fracture over the lifespan. (*Reprinted from* Wasnish [11]; with permission.)

# Fracture Epidemiology

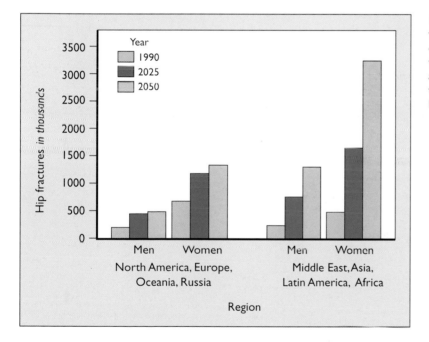

**FIGURE 4-8.** The estimated number of fractures (in thousands) for men and women in different regions of the world in 1990, 2025, and 2050. The number of hip fractures worldwide is projected to increase from 1.66 million in 1990 to 6.26 million by 2050. Currently, about half of all hip fractures occur in Europe and North America; by 2050 these regions will account for only one fourth of the total, and the majority of hip fractures are expected to occur in Asia and Latin America. (*Reprinted from* Cooper et al. [15]; with permission.)

## INCIDENCE OF HIP FRACTURE (RATES PER 100,000) IN 1990 BY AGE, SEX AND REGION

| Region | Men: Age, y | | | | | | |
|---|---|---|---|---|---|---|---|
| Europe | 50–54 | 55–59 | 60–64 | 65–69 | 70–74 | 75–79 | 80+ |
| Western Europe | 28 | 33 | 67 | 103 | 203 | 331 | 880 |
| Southern Europe | 10 | 16 | 34 | 55 | 81 | 190 | 534 |
| Eastern Europe | 38 | 38 | 88 | 88 | 194 | 194 | 475 |
| Northern Europe | 58 | 66 | 97 | 198 | 382 | 682 | 1864 |
| North America | 33 | 33 | 81 | 123 | 119 | 338 | 1230 |
| Oceania | 20 | 34 | 63 | 92 | 180 | 445 | 1157 |
| Asia | 19.5 | 19.5 | 36.5 | 46.5 | 102 | 150 | 364 |
| Africa | 6.0 | 10.0 | 14.0 | 27.0 | 8.0 | 0 | 116 |
| Latin America | 25 | 40 | 40 | 106 | 106 | 327 | 327 |
| World | 22.5 | 24.5 | 47.3 | 68.7 | 119.1 | 219.4 | 630.2 |
| | Women: Age, y | | | | | | |
| Europe | 50–54 | 55–59 | 60–64 | 65–69 | 70–74 | 75–79 | 80+ |
| Western Europe | 33 | 54 | 115 | 184 | 362 | 657 | 1808 |
| Southern Europe | 11 | 21 | 47 | 100 | 170 | 380 | 1075 |
| Eastern Europe | 58 | 58 | 155 | 155 | 426 | 426 | 1251 |
| Northern Europe | 74 | 78 | 190 | 327 | 612 | 1294 | 2997 |
| North America | 60 | 60 | 117 | 252 | 437 | 850 | 2296 |
| Oceania | 31 | 63 | 112 | 204 | 358 | 899 | 2476 |
| Asia | 14 | 14 | 38 | 74.5 | 155.5 | 252 | 562.5 |
| Africa | 4.0 | 12 | 17 | 12 | 16 | 50 | 80 |
| Latin America | 19.5 | 50 | 50 | 162.5 | 162.5 | 622 | 622 |
| World | 23.9 | 28.4 | 69.1 | 121.6 | 239.8 | 457.7 | 1289.3 |

**FIGURE 4-9.** Incidence of hip fracture (per 100,000) in 1990 by age, sex, and region. (*Reprinted from* Gullberg et al. [16]; with permission.)

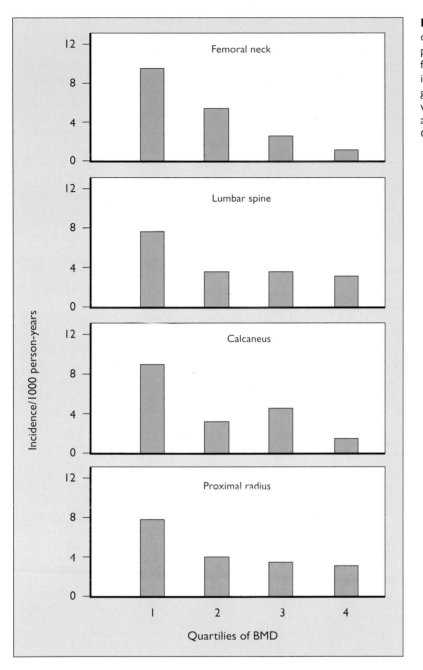

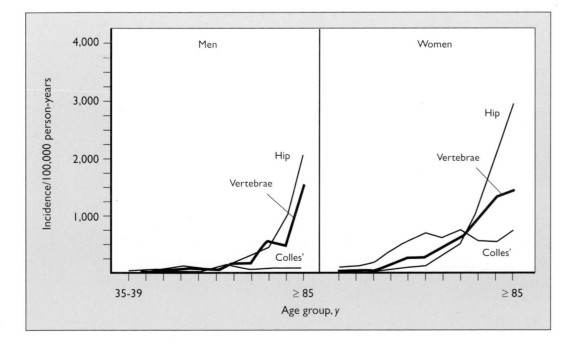

**FIGURE 4-10.** Incidence of hip fracture by age-adjusted quartile of bone mineral density (BMD). Bone mineral density measured in any of the regions of the proximal femur is more strongly associated with the subsequent risk of hip fracture than BMD measured in the radius, calcaneus or spine. An older woman in the lowest quartile of femoral neck BMD had a risk of hip fracture 8.5 times greater than that of those in the highest quartile of BMD. Data based on 65 women who had hip fractures during 1.8 years of follow-up after the second annual clinic examination in the Study of Osteoporotic Fractures. (*Reprinted from Cummings et al.* [17]; with permission.)

**FIGURE 4-11.** Age-specific incidence rates for hip, vertebral, and distal forearm (Colles') fractures in men and women in Rochester, Minnesota. As the population ages, there will be a dramatic increase in the number of fractures that occur due to the exponential relationship of fracture rate to age. (*Reprinted from Cooper and Melton* [18]; with permission.)

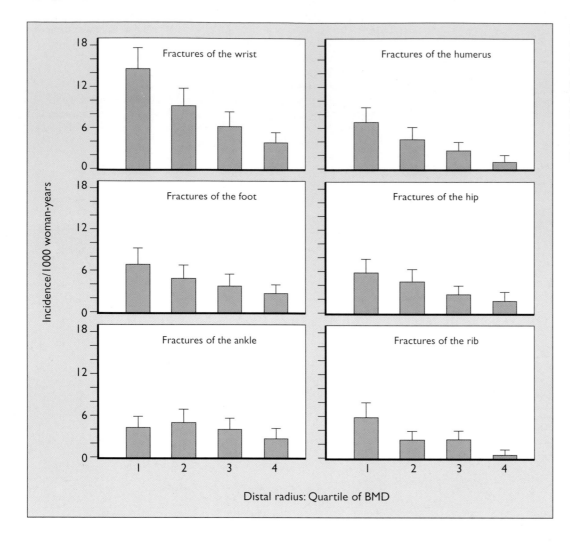

**FIGURE 4-12.** Rates of nonspinal fractures for each age-adjusted quartile of distal radius bone mass. Decreased bone mass was associated with increased risk in a graded manner for fractures of the wrist, foot, humerus, hip and rib. Each quartile represents approximately 4900 woman-years of follow-up from ambulatory, nonblack women 65 years of age and older enrolled in the Study of Osteoporotic Fractures. BMD—bone mineral density. (*Reprinted from Seeley et al.* [9]; with permission.)

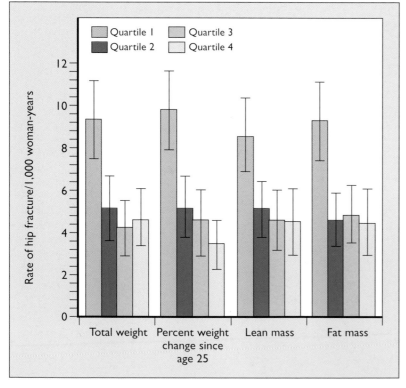

**FIGURE 4-13.** Rate of hip fracture by quartile of body size measures. Fracture rates are adjusted for age. Vertical bars denote 95% confidence intervals. Quartile cutpoints: total weight (kg): 57.8, 64.9, 73.3; percent weight since age 25 (%): 5.0, 16.4, 29.6; lean mass (kg): 36.6, 39.3, 42.4; fat mass (kg): 20.6, 25.5, 31.6. Women with smaller body size (women in the first quartile of each measurement) had a higher risk of hip fracture than women with average and larger body sizes (women in the second, third and fourth quartile of each measurement) who had similarly lower risks of hip fracture. Data based on 8011 ambulatory, nonblack women 65 years of age and older enrolled in the Study of Osteoporotic Fractures. (*Reprinted from* Ensrud et al. [19]; with permission.)

**OBSERVED PREVALENCE, SMOOTHED PREVALENCE, AND ESTIMATED INCIDENCE OF VERTEBRAL DEFORMITIES AMONG AN AGE-STRATIFIED RANDOM SAMPLE OF ROCHESTER, MINNESOTA WOMEN, AGED 50 YEARS AND OVER, COUNTING ALL DEFORMITIES**

| Age, y | No. Sampled | No. with Deformities | Observed Prevalence (per 100) | Smoothed Prevalence (per 100)* | Estimated Incidence (per 100)† |
|---|---|---|---|---|---|
| 50–54 | 106 | 11 | 10.4 | 7.6 | 5.8 |
| 55–59 | 137 | 16 | 11.7 | 10.8 | 8.2 |
| 60–64 | 112 | 14 | 12.5 | 15.1 | 11.4 |
| 65–69 | 107 | 18 | 16.8 | 20.8 | 15.4 |
| 70–74 | 80 | 24 | 30.0 | 27.8 | 20.4 |
| 75–79 | 100 | 33 | 33.0 | 36.2 | 26.1 |
| 80–84 | 59 | 33 | 55.9 | 45.5 | 32.1 |
| 85–89 | 49 | 24 | 49.0 | 55.1 | 37.7 |
| >90 | 12 | 9 | 75.0 | 64.3 | — |
| Total | 762 | 182 | 23.9 | 25.3‡ | 17.8§ |

*Smoothed age-specific prevalence (%) of one or more vertebral deformities, as determined by the method of Leske et al. [20].

†Estimated age-specific incidence per 1000 person-years, as determined form smoothed prevalence rates by the method of Leske et al. [20].

‡Overall prevalence directly age-adjusted to the population structure of 1990 Rochester women 50 years of age and over.

§Overall incidence directly age-adjusted to the population structure of 1990 Rochester women 50 years of age and over, assuming the 85–89 year rate applies to the whole population aged 85 years and over.

**FIGURE 4-14.** Observed prevalence, smoothed prevalence and estimated incidence of vertebral deformities among an age-stratified random sample of Rochester, Minnesota women, aged 50 years and over, counting all deformities. An age-stratified sample of 762 Rochester, Minnesota women aged 50 and over underwent columbar radiography. Height ratios were used to characterize three types of vertebral deformity: anterior wedge deformity; concavity (or end plate) deformity, and compression (or crush) deformity. (*Data from* Leske, *et al.* [20] and Melton, *et al.* [21].)

# Risk Factors for Osteoporotic Fractures

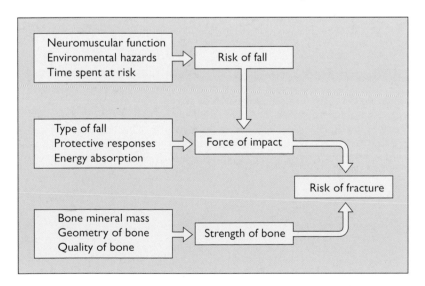

**FIGURE 4-15.** Determinants of fracture risk. (*Reprinted from* Kanis and McCloskey [22]; with permission.)

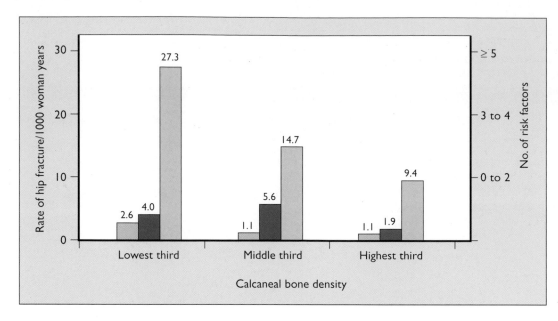

**FIGURE 4-16.** Annual risk of hip fracture according to number of risk factors and age-specific calcaneal bone density. Risk factors were assessed in 9516 white women 65 years of age or older who had no previous hip fracture and who were enrolled in the Study of Osteoporotic Fractures. Women were followed at 4-month intervals for an average of 4.1 years to determine frequency of hip fracture. Risk factors included: age ≥ 80 years; maternal history of hip fracture; any fracture (except hip fracture) since the age of 50; fair, poor, or very poor health; previous hyperthyroidism; anticonvulsant therapy; current long-acting benzodiazepine therapy; current weight less than at age 25; height at the age of 25 ≥ 168 cm; present caffeine intake more than the equivalent of two cups of coffee per day; on feet ≤ 4 hours per day; no walking for exercise; inability to rise from a chair without using arms; lowest quartile of depth perception (SD > 2.44); lowest quartile of contrast sensitivity (SD > 0.70 unit); and pulse rate > 80 per minute. (*Reprinted from* Cummings et al. [23]; with permission.)

## RISK FACTORS FOR OSTEOPOROTIC FRACTURE IN ELDERLY MEN

| Risk Factor | Unit | Univariate Analysis | | Adjusted for Bone Mineral Density | |
|---|---|---|---|---|---|
| | | OR | 95% CI | OR | 95% CI |
| Age | 7.7 years | 1.41 | 1.29–1.55 | 1.16 | 1.04–1.31 |
| Femoral neck BMD | 0.12 g/cm$^2$ | 0.72 | 0.63–0.82 | — | — |
| Quadriceps strength | 10 kg | 0.81 | 0.71–0.91 | 0.88 | 0.75–0.99 |
| Body sway | 515 mm$^2$ | 1.16 | 1.04–1.29 | 1.13 | 1.01–1.27 |
| Previous falls | Yes/no | 1.10 | 1.0–1.29 | 1.19 | 1.07–1.33 |
| Previous fractures | Yes/no | 1.19 | 1.10–1.30 | 1.35 | 1.23–1.50 |
| Weight | 12.7 kg | 0.81 | 0.72–0.92 | 0.90 | 0.79–1.04 |
| Height | 6.9 cm | 0.81 | 0.71–0.90 | 0.87 | 0.77–0.99 |
| Alcohol use | Yes/no | 0.73 | 0.66–0.81 | 0.93 | 0.83–1.05 |
| Activity index | 7.0 | 0.71 | 0.55–0.91 | 0.86 | 0.72–1.02 |
| Thiazide use | Yes/no | 0.89 | 0.81–1.00 | 0.97 | 0.86–1.10 |

**FIGURE 4-17.** Risk factors for osteoporotic fracture in elderly men. Risk factors for total fractures as analyzed individually and adjusted for femoral neck bone mineral density (BMD) were: advancing age, fracture within previous 5 years, falls within previous 12 months, higher body sway, and shorter height. Risks of atraumatic fractures in elderly men, expressed as standardized odds ratios (OR) and 95% confidence intervals (CI) for 1 standard deviation change were estimated by Cox's proportional hazards model. Data from the Dubbo Osteoporosis Epidemiology Study, Australia, 1989–1994. Adjustment for femoral BMD in height, body sway, previous falls, previous fractures, and quadriceps strength as the only significant predictors of fractures. (*Reprinted from* Nguyen et al. [24]; with permission.)

## MULTIVARIATE ANALYSIS OF RISK FACTORS FOR HIP FRACTURES IN BLACK WOMEN

| Variable | Adjusted Odds Ratio* (95% CI) |
|---|---|
| Body mass index[†] | |
| ≤ 22.6 | 13.5 (4.3–43.3) |
| 22.7–24.4 | 4.2 (1.3–14.0) |
| 24.5–27.2 | 3.5 (1.2–10.3) |
| 27.3–31.5 | 1.5 (0.4–5.3) |
| ≥ 31.6 | 1.0 |
| Estrogen therapy lasting ≥ 1 y | |
| Women < 75 | 0.1 (<0.1–0.5) |
| Women ≥ 75 | 1.1 (0.2–6.3) |
| Alcohol consumed past year (drinks/per week[‡]) | |
| ≤ 1 | 1.0 |
| 2–6 | 2.0 (0.8–5.0) |
| > 7 | 4.6 (1.5–4.1) |
| History of stroke (vs. none) | 3.1 (1.2–8.1) |
| Use of ambulatory aids (vs. none) | 5.6 (2.7–11.5) |
| Chronic illnesses (number) | |
| 0 | 1.0 |
| 1 | 1.8 (0.9–3.7) |
| 2–6 | 0.9 (0.3–2.4) |

*Ratios based on conditional logistic regression models, with control for age category, zip code or telephone exchange, age as a continuous variable, and all other variables shown in the table.
†Expressed in quintiles based on the distribution of community controls.
‡Based on the assumption that one bottle of beer, one glass of wine, and one drink of spirits each contain 30 mL (1 oz) of alcohol.
§Includes women who used a cane, walker, wheelchair, artificial leg, or leg brace or who were confined to bed.
¶Expressed as a categorical variable and including the following six conditions: diabetes mellitus, coronary heart disease, epilepsy, kidney disease, Parkinson's disease, and cancer.

**FIGURE 4-18.** Multivariate analysis of risk factors for hip fractures in black women. (*Reprinted from* Grisso *et al.* [25]; with permission.)

## OSTEOPOROSIS ATTRIBUTION PROBABILITIES BY FRACTURE TYPE, GENDER, AND AGE: WHITE POPULATION

| Site | Age Group (y) 45–64 Median Attribution Probability (Range)* | 65–84 Median Attribution Probability (Range) | ≥85 years Median Attribution Probability (Range) |
|---|---|---|---|
| Women | | | |
| Hip | 0.80 (0.25–0.80) | 0.90 (0.80–0.95) | 0.95 (0.90–1.0) |
| Spine | 0.80 (0.50–0.85) | 0.90 (0.70–0.95) | 0.95 (0.80–1.0) |
| Forearm | 0.70 (0.10–0.70) | 0.70 (0.50–0.80) | 0.80 (0.70–0.95) |
| Other sites | 0.45 (0.05–0.55) | 0.50 (0.25–0.65) | 0.60 (0.45–0.80) |
| Men | | | |
| Hip | 0.60 (0.10–0.70) | 0.80 (0.60–0.95) | 0.85 (0.80–0.95) |
| Spine | 0.70 (0.50–0.90) | 0.90 (0.50–0.95) | 0.90 (0.60–0.95) |
| Forearm | 0.40 (0.05–0.50) | 0.45 (0.15–0.60) | 0.45 (0.30–0.60) |
| Other sites | 0.15 (0.05–0.30) | 0.30 (0.20–0.40) | 0.45 (0.30–0.50) |

*Probability can range from 0.00 (no attribution) to 1.00 (100% attribution).

**FIGURE 4-19.** Osteoporosis attribution probabilities by fracture type, gender, and age: white population. It is estimated that 90% of proximal femur fractures in white women aged 65 to 84 years are related to osteoporosis, whereas about 80% of hip fractures among white men are attributed to osteoporosis. The attribution probabilities were consistently less for white men than for white women. Using a three-round Delphi process [25], a panel of expert clinicians estimated the probability that each of 72 categories, consisting of four fracture types (hip, spine, forearm, all other sites combined), three age groups (45–64, 65–84, 85 years and older), three racial groups (white, black, all others [not shown]), and both genders (female, male) are associated with osteoporosis. (*Reprinted from* Melton *et al.* [26]; with permission.)

## OSTEOPOROSIS ATTRIBUTION PROBABILITIES BY FRACTURE TYPE, GENDER, AND AGE: BLACK POPULATION

| Site | 45–64 Median Attribution Probability (Range)* | 65–84 Median Attribution Probability (Range) | ≥85 years Median Attribution Probability (Range) |
|---|---|---|---|
| Women | | | |
| Hip | 0.65 (0.15–0.75) | 0.80 (0.50–0.95) | 0.95 (0.60–0.95) |
| Spine | 0.65 (0.40–0.75) | 0.80 (0.50–0.90) | 0.90 (0.60–0.95) |
| Forearm | 0.55 (0.05–0.60) | 0.60 (0.30–0.75) | 0.70 (0.40–0.85) |
| Other sites | 0.35 (0.05–0.40) | 0.40 (0.15–0.50) | 0.45 (0.20–0.70) |
| Men | | | |
| Hip | 0.30 (0.05–0.65) | 0.65 (0.10–0.85) | 0.75 (0.25–0.90) |
| Spine | 0.55 (0.30–0.80) | 0.75 (0.30–0.90) | 0.85 (0.30–0.95) |
| Forearm | 0.20 (0.05–0.40) | 0.30 (0.10–0.50) | 0.35 (0.20–0.50) |
| Other sites | 0.15 (0.05–0.20) | 0.15 (0.05–0.30) | 0.25 (0.15–0.40) |

*Probability can range from 0.00 (no attribution) to 1.00 (100% attribution).

**FIGURE 4-20.** Osteoporosis attribution probabilities by fracture type, gender, and age: black population. It is estimated that 80% of proximal femur fractures in black women aged 65–84 years are related to osteoporosis, whereas about 65% of hip fractures among black men are attributed to osteoporosis. The attribution probabilities were consistently less for black than white women and men. (*Reprinted from* Melton et al. [26]; with permission.)

# Role of Falls

## ORIENTATION OF THE FALL, POINT OF IMPACT, AND RISK OF HIP FRACTURE AND WRIST FRACTURE (VERSUS NO FRACTURE) AMONG THOSE WHO FELL

| Variable (units) | Odds Ratio (95% Confidence Limits) for Risk of Fracture in Those Who Fell* | |
|---|---|---|
| Hip | | |
| Age (+ 5 years) | 1.3 (1.1, 1.7) | 1.4 (1.1, 1.8) |
| Walking speed (-0.23 m/s)† | 1.1 | 1.0 |
| Fall during stand/turn/transfer (0, 1 = yes) | 1.8 (1.1, 3.0) | 1.4 |
| Fall while descending steps (0, 1 = yes) | 1.1 | 0.9 |
| Fall sideways, straight down (0, 1=yes) | | 3.3 (2.0, 5.6) |
| Fall on hip/side of leg/buttocks (0, 1 = yes) | | 32.5 (9.9, 10) |
| Wrist‡ | | |
| Age (+ 5 years) 1.0 | 1.0 | 1.1 |
| Walking speed (-0.23 m/s)† | 1.0 | 1.0 |
| Fall while walking/running (0, 1 = yes) | 1.3 | 1.4 |
| Fall backward vs sideways (0, 1 = yes) | | 2.2 (1.3, 3.8) |
| Fall forward vs sideways (0, 1 = yes) | | 0.5 (0.3, 0.8) |
| Fall on hand/wrist (0, 1 = yes) | | 20.4 (11.5, 36.0) |

*Comparison of subjects who fell and fractured a hip with those who fell without a fracture. Odds ratios are adjusted for all the other variables in each column plus calcaneus bone density. Confidence limits shown only for significant odds ratios.

†Odds ratios are for 1-standard deviation decrease.

‡Comparison of subjects who fell and fractured a wrist and those who fell without a fracture. Odds ratios are adjusted for all the other variables in each column plus distal radius bone density.

**FIGURE 4-21.** Orientation of the fall, point of impact, and risk of hip fracture and wrist fracture (versus no fracture) among those who fell. Nonblack women age 65 and older living in the community who suffered hip fractures (n = 130) as a result of a fall and a consecutive sample of women who fell without a fracture (n = 467) were interviewed about their falls. These results are based on a case-control analysis nested in a prospective cohort study—the Study of Osteoporotic Fractures. (*Reprinted from* Nevitt et al. [27]; with permission.)

## RISK FACTORS ASSOCIATED WITH HIP FRACTURE FROM A FALL

| Factor | Adjusted Odds Ratio | 95% Confidence Intervals |
|---|---|---|
| Fall to side | 5.7 | 2.3–14.0 |
| Femoral neck BMD, $g/cm^2$* | 2.7 | 1.6–4.6 |
| Fall energy, $j$† | 2.8 | 1.5–5.2 |
| Body mass index, $kg/m^2$ | 2.2 | 1.2–3.8 |

*Calculated for a decrease of one SD.
†Calculated for an increase of one SD.

**FIGURE 4-22.** Risk factors associated with hip fracture from a fall. (*Data from* Greenspan et al. [28] and Melton [29].)

# Economic Impact of Osteoporotic Fractures

## HEALTH CARE EXPENDITURES ATTRIBUTABLE TO OSTEOPOROTIC FRACTURES IN THE UNITED STATES, BY TYPE OF SERVICE, AGE, RACE AND TYPE OF FRACTURE, 1995

| Covariates | Expenditure for Women (in Millions) | % of Total | Expenditure for Men (in Millions) | % of Total | Total Expenditure (in Millions) | % of Total |
|---|---|---|---|---|---|---|
| Hospital | 6805 | 49.4 | 1788 | 13.0 | 8594 | 62.4 |
| Nursing home | 3252 | 23.6 | 623 | 4.5 | 3875 | 28.2 |
| Outpatient | 1007 | 7/3 | 289 | 2.1 | 1296 | 9.4 |
| 45–64 y | 1134 | 8.2 | 569 | 4.1 | 1704 | 12.4 |
| 65–04 y | 5896 | 42.8 | 1376 | 10.0 | 7271 | 52.8 |
| 85+ y | 4034 | 29.3 | 755 | 5.5 | 4789 | 34.8 |
| White | 10,338 | 75.1 | 2526 | 18.4 | 12,863 | 93.5 |
| Non-white | 727 | 5.3 | 174 | 1.3 | 901 | 6.5 |
| Hip | 6720 | 48.8 | 1962 | 14.3 | 8682 | 63.1 |
| Other sites | 4345 | 31.6 | 737 | 5.4 | 5082 | 36.9 |
| Total | 11,065 | 80.4 | 2700 | 19.6 | 13,764 | 100.0 |

**FIGURE 4-23.** Health care expenditures attributable to osteoporotic fractures in the United States, 1995.

In 1995, health care expenditures attributable to osteoporotic fractures were estimated at $13.76 billion, of which $10.34 billion (75.1%) was for the treatment of white women, $2.53 billion (18.4%) was for the treatment of white men, $0.73 billion (5.3%) was for the treatment of nonwhite women, and $0.17 billion (1.3%) was for the treatment of nonwhite men. (*Reprinted from* Ray et al. [30]; with permission.)

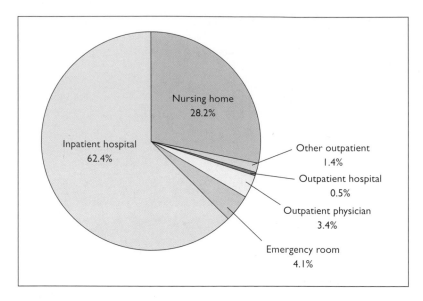

**FIGURE 4-24.** Health care expenditures attributable to osteoporotic fracture In the United States by type of service, 1995. Other outpatient includes home health care, ambulance services, and medical equipment. (*Data from* Ray *et al.* [30].)

# References

1. Consensus Development Conference. Diagnosis, prophylaxis, and treatment of osteoporosis. *Am J Med* 1993, 94:646–650).

2. Melton LJ III, Chrischilles EA, Cooper C, *et al.*: Perspective: How many women have osteoporosis? *J Bone Miner Res* 1992, 7:1005–1010.

3. Melton LJ III. How many women have osteoporosis now? *J Bone Miner Res.*: 1995, 10:175–177.

4. Jones G, Nguyen T, Sambrook PN, *et al.*: Symptomatic fracture incidence in elderly men and women: the Dubbo Osteoporosis Epidemiology Study. *Osteoporosis Int* 1994, 4:277–282

5. Center J, Eisman J: The epidemiology and prevention of osteoporosis. *Bailliere's Clin Endocrinol Metab* 1997, 11:23–62.

6. Nguyen T, Sambrook P, Kelly P, *et al.*: Prediction of osteoporotic fractures by postural instability and bone density. *BMJ* 1993, 307:1111–1115.

7. Miller PD, Bonnick SL, Rosen CJ: Consensus of an international panel on the clinical utility of bone mass measurements in the detection of low bone mass in the adult population. *Calcif Tiss Intl* 1996, 58:207–214.

8. Cooper C, Melton U III: Magnitude and impact of osteoporosis and fractures. In *Osteoporosis* Edited by Marcus R. San Diego: Academic Press. 1996:419–434.

9. Seeley DG, Browner WS, Nevitt MC, Genant HK, Scott JC, Cummings SR and the Study of Osteoporotic Fractures Group: Which fractures are associated with low appendicular bone mass in elderly women. *Ann Intern Med* 1991, 115:837–842.

10. Kanis JA, Melton LJ III, Christiansen C *et al.*: The diagnosis of osteoporosis. *J Bone Miner Res.*: 1994, 9:113 7–1141.

11. Wasnish RD: Epidemiology of Osteoporosis. In *Primer on the Metabolic Bone Diseases and Disorders of Mineral Metabolism*, edn 3. Edited by Favus MJ. Philadelphia: Lippincott-Raven, 1996:249–251.

12. Looker AC, Orwoll ES, Johnston CC Jr, *et al.*: Prevalence of low femoral bone density in older U.S. adults from NHANES III. *J Bone Miner Res* 1997, 12:1761–1768.

13. Looker AC, Johnston CC Jr, Wahner HW, *et al.*: Prevalence for low femoral bone density in older U.S. women from NHANES III. *J Boner Miner Res* 1995, 10:796–802.

14. National Osteoporosis Foundation: 1996 and 2015 osteoporosis prevalence figures. State-by-state report. January 1997.

15. Cooper CC, Campion G, Melton LJ III: Hip fractures in the elderly: A worldwide projection. *Osteoporosis Int* 1992, 2:285–289.

16. Gullberg B, Johnell 0, Kanis JA: World-wide projections for hip fracture. *Osteoporosis Int* 1997, 7:407–413.

17. Cummings SR, Black DM, Nevitt MC, *et al.*: Bone density at various sites for the prediction of hip fractures. *Lancet* 1993, 341:72–75.

18. Cooper C and Melton LJ III: Epidemiology of osteoporosis. *Trends Endocninol Metab* 1992, 3:224–29.

19. Ensrud KE, Lipschutz RC, Cauley JA, *et al.*: Body size and hip fracture risk in older women: a prospective study. Study of Osteoporotic Research Group. *Am J Med* 1997, 103:274–280.

20. Leske MC, Ederer F, Podgor M: Estimating incidence from age-specific prevalence in glaucoma. *Am J Epidemiol* 1981, 113:606–613.

21. Melton LJ, Lane AW, Cooper C, *et al.*: Prevalence and incidence of vertebral deformities. *Osteoporosis Int* 1993, 3:113–119.

22. Kanis JA, McCloskey EV. Evaluation of the risk of hip fracture. *Bone* 1996, 18:127S–132S.

23. Cummings SR, Nevitt MC, Browner WS, *et al.*: Risk factors for hip fracture in white women. *N Engl J Med* 1995, 332:767–773.

24. Nguyen TV, Elsman JA, Kelly PJ, Sambrook PN: Risk factors for osteoporotic fractures in elderly men. *Am J Epidemiol* 1996, 144:255–263.

25. Grisso JA, Kelsey JL, Strom BL, *et al.*: Risk factors for hip fracture in black women. *N Engl J Med* 1994, 330:1555–1559.

26. Melton LJ III, Thamer M, Ray NF, *et al.*: Fractures attributable to osteoporosis: report from the National Osteoporosis Foundation. *J Bone Miner Res* 1997, 12:16–23.

27. Nevitt MC, Cummings SR, and the Study of Osteoporotic Fractures Research Group: Type of fall and risk of hip and wrist fractures: The Study of Osteoporotic Fractures. *J Am Geriatr Soc* 1993, 41:1226–1234.

28. Greenspan SL, Myers ER, Maitlans LA, *et al.*: Fall severity and bone mineral density as risk factors for hip fracture in ambulatory elderly. *JAMA* 1994, 271:128–133.

29. Melton LJ III: Epidemiology of hip fractures: Implications of the exponential increase with age. *Bone* 1996, 18:121S–125S.

30. Ray NF, Chan J, Thamer M, Melton JL III: Medical expenditures for the treatment of osteoporotic fractures in the United States in 1995: Report from the National Osteoporosis Foundation *J Bone Miner Res.*: 1997, 12:24–35.

# RADIOLOGY OF OSTEOPOROTIC FRACTURE

## Jan E. Vandevenne, Gabrielle Bergman, and Philipp Lang

Osteoporosis is characterized by a decrease in bone mineral density of structurally normal bone: the dynamic equilibrium between bone resorption and bone formation is perturbed in favor of bone resorption resulting in osteopenia. Decreased bone mineral density undermines the structural integrity of bone. Quantitative bone densitometry may predict fracture risk [1]. The elastic range of osteopenic bone is decreased and deformative stress on these bones more readily results in microfractures. Continued and progressive stress on osteoporotic bone may lead to structural failure [2, 3]. For this reason, insufficiency fractures as well as fractures after minor trauma occur more frequently in the osteopenic skeleton of the patient suffering from osteoporosis. Osteoporotic fractures are mainly seen in older white women, but osteoporosis induced by any other condition, *eg,* hyperparathyroidism, cortisone treatment, and pregnancy, can lead to fractures [4]. Healing of osteoporotic fractures may be slow and difficult and nonunion of fractures can result.

Insufficiency fractures due to osteoporosis and fractures from minor traumatic events tend to involve certain locations of the axial and appendicular skeleton. Typically, the thoracic and lumbar vertebrae and the hip, wrist, and proximal humerus are the areas involved. Thoracic and lumbar vertebrae may show collapse, and spontaneous fractures frequently occur in the pelvic girdle, especially in the sacral wings, the pubic symphysis, and the supra-acetabular region [5]. Femoral neck insufficiency fractures may occur spontaneously but are more often related to trauma. A fall on the outstretched hand is the most frequent cause for fracture of the distal radius and the proximal humerus. Less frequently, osteoporotic fractures are seen in the calcaneus, talus, proximal tibia, and ribs. This chapter provides an overview of osteoporotic fractures and their characteristic locations.

## Vertebral Compression Fractures

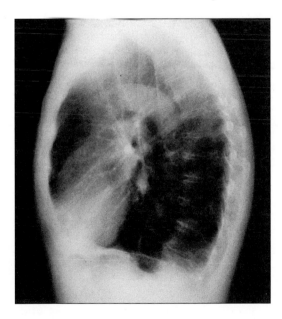

**FIGURE 5-1.** Radiograph showing osteopenia of the thoracic spine, seen on a lateral view of the chest in a 71-year-old man. A generalized decrease in density is noted in the thoracic vertebrae, which represents bone demineralization and thinning of both the bony trabeculae and the cortical bone. Although clearly osteopenic, the vertebrae of the thoracic spine of this patient have a normal shape with parallel endplates and a normal height. In some cases of early osteopenia, the relatively more pronounced decrease in density of the trabecular bone compared to the cortical and subchondral bone may give the erroneous impression of increased bone density in the cortical and subchondral bone. In this patient, no vertebral fractures are present.

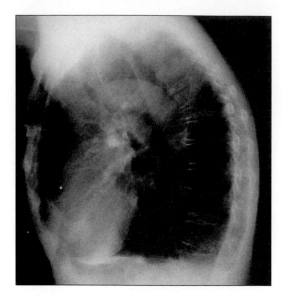

**FIGURE 5-2.** Wedge-shaped compression fracture of a mid-thoracic vertebra as seen on a lateral view of the chest of the same patient shown in Figure 5-1, one year later. As a result of loading and weight-bearing forces that overmatch the strength of the demineralized bone, a mid-thoracic vertebra has collapsed. The loss of height is more pronounced anteriorly than posteriorly and a wedge-shaped deformity of the vertebra is seen. Note the increased kyphosis compared to Figure 5-1, due to the wedge-shaped vertebral collapse. The thoracic kyphosis often increases with age.

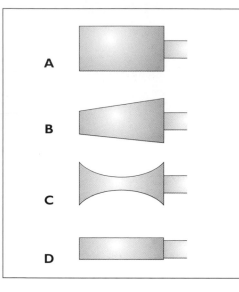

**FIGURE 5-3.** Vertebral deformity after vertebral fracture can be classified into three groups. Normal vertebrae have parallel endplates (**A**). On the lateral view, most collapsed vertebrae are wedge-shaped or biconcave. Wedge-shaped deformity is most frequently seen in thoracic vertebrae that sustain more compression anteriorly than posteriorly (**B**). Biconcave or "fish" vertebrae have concave depressions of the upper and sometimes also the lower endplates and are more common in the lumbar spine (**C**). The completely collapsed vertebra demonstrates a flattened or pancake appearance (**D**).

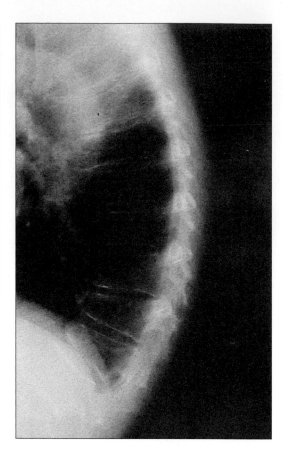

**FIGURE 5-4.** Two compression fractures of the vertebrae in the lower thoracic and upper lumbar spine as seen on the lateral chest view of a 91-year-old woman. General osteopenia of the spine is evident, with decreased density of the vertebrae and thinning of the cortical and subchondral bone. Weight-bearing forces have overmatched the structural integrity of the osteopenic vertebral bodies at the thoracico-lumbar level of the spine, which resulted in anterior collapse of the twelfth thoracic and the first lumbar vertebral body. Vertebral collapse is frequently seen at the point of transition between the thoracic kyphosis and the lumbar lordosis.

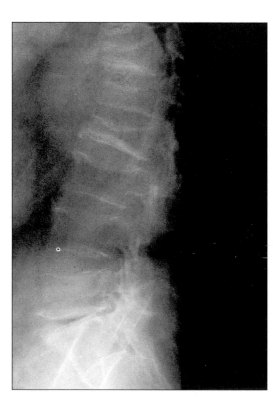

**FIGURE 5-5.** Multiple compression fractures of the lumbar spine in a 55-year-old man who received prolonged cortisone treatment. Decreased density of the vertebrae results from drug induced demineralization of the vertebrae. Compression fractures with decreased vertebral height are seen in the twelfth lumbar vertebra, and the first, second, and third lumbar vertebrae. Biconcave collapse of the fourth lumbar vertebra is seen. Note that the disk spaces are not narrowed, and even appear to be enlarged due to the collapse of the vertebrae. Prolonged cortisone treatment may induce pronounced osteopenia and lead to multiple compression fractures of the spine.

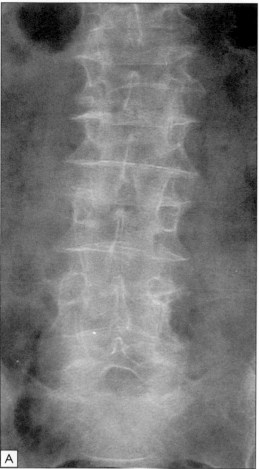

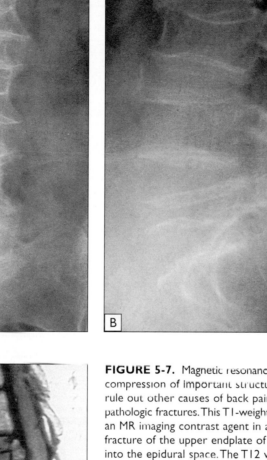

A

B

**FIGURE 5-6.** Multiple compression fractures, as seen on the anteroposterior (**A**) and lateral (**B**) view of the lumbar spine in a 76-year-old woman. Note generalized osteopenia with increased translucency of the vertebral bodies and thinning of the cortical and subchondral bone. Vertebral collapse has occurred at multiple levels. Severe compression of the fifth lumbar vertebra has resulted in a flattened vertebra. Partial collapse with loss of height and biconcave deformity is seen in the twelfth thoracic and the first three lumbar vertebrae. The height of the fourth lumbar vertebra is unchanged.

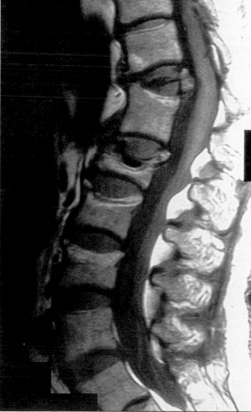

**FIGURE 5-7.** Magnetic resonance (MR) imaging of compression fractures in the spine is useful to demonstrate compression of important structures such as spinal nerves and the spinal cord. MR imaging is also used to rule out other causes of back pain, and may help to differentiate osteoporotic compression fractures from pathologic fractures. This T1-weighted MR image was obtained after intravenous injection of gadolinium-DTPA, an MR imaging contrast agent in a 48-year-old woman. It confirms the presence of a concave compression fracture of the upper endplate of the first lumbar vertebra. A bone fragment is seen to extend posteriorly into the epidural space. The T12 vertebral body is completely collapsed demonstrating low signal intensity on this sequence. There is a second, larger bone fragment in the epidural space posteriorly at this level. Also seen is depression of the superior endplates of the second and third lumbar vertebrae. The spinal cord compression by the collapsed vertebral bodies represents clinically important information in this patient.

MR imaging can be used to rule out the presence of a neoplastic process as the underlying cause for compression fractures, eg, by absence of a mass lesion. Specific sequences or injection of gadolinium contrast agent can be used to demonstrate a neoplastic mass within the collapsed vertebra [6, 7, 8]. When malignancy is suspected for clinical reasons and magnetic resonance can not rule out a neoplastic process, biopsy should be performed.

# Hip Fractures

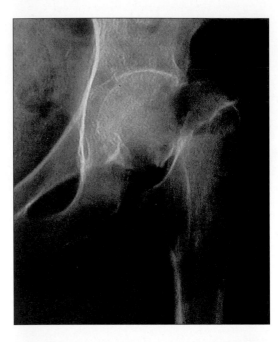

**FIGURE 5-8.** Femoral neck fracture of the left hip in a 66-year-old woman. Note the presence of a fracture of the femoral neck at the transition between the neck and the femoral head. The distal fracture fragment (femoral shaft) is displaced in a superior direction and rotated externally. Overall decreased density of the hip is indicative of osteopenia. In the normal hip, specifically arranged groups of bony trabeculae, vertically directed (compressive) and horizontally directed (tensile) groups, run through the obliquely oriented femoral neck and connect the femoral shaft with the femoral head. Bone demineralization secondary to osteoporosis decreases the loading capacity of the obliquely oriented femoral neck; as a result fractures may occur after minor trauma. In this patient, a fall with the leg externally rotated caused the femoral neck fracture. Fractures that occur as a consequence of osteopenia in patients suffering from osteoporosis are most frequently seen in the spine, followed by the hip (proximal portion of the femur). However, hip fractures are clinically more significant and may lead to permanent disability or death, eg, from pulmonary embolism.

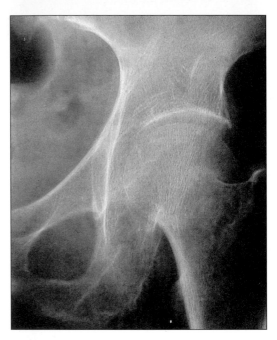

**FIGURE 5-9.** Cervical fracture of the left hip in a 73-year-old woman. Note the decreased bone mineral density in the hip and the pelvic bones. No definite fracture line can be seen, and no displacement of fracture fragments is present. However, the foreshortening of the femoral neck and the presence of a linear area of increased density perpendicular to the normal direction of the bone trabeculae indicate an impaction fracture. Classification of hip fractures by anatomic location includes subcapital, cervical, basicervical, intertrochanteric, and subtrochanteric types. Intracapsular fractures (subcapital and cervical fractures) are often classified according to the degree of displacement, as described in the Garden system [9]. Type I fractures are incomplete or impacted in nature; type II fractures are complete without osseous displacement; type III fractures are complete with partial displacement of the fracture fragments; and type IV fractures are complete with total displacement of the fracture fragments. Intracapsular hip fractures with displacement of the fracture fragments often cause avascular necrosis of the femoral head because the disrupted capsule contains the most important vessels that supply blood to the femoral head. The cervical fracture in this patient was classified as a type I according to the Garden system.

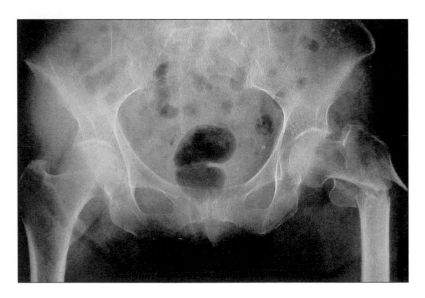

**FIGURE 5-10.** Combined subtrochanteric and intertrochanteric fracture of the left hip in a 74-year-old woman after a fall. A transverse fracture line is present inferior to the lesser and the greater trochanter which both have been avulsed. Note varus position of the proximal fracture fragment (femoral neck) and proximal shift of the distal fracture fragment (femoral shaft). Generalized osteopenia is seen in all pelvic bones, related to osteoporosis.

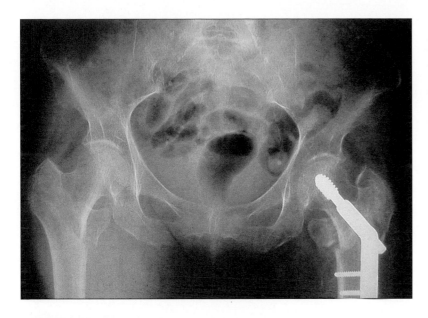

**FIGURE 5 -11.** Intertrochanteric fracture of the right hip in the same patient as in Fig 5-9, six weeks later. Note the presence of a complete fracture through the lesser and the greater trochanters of the right hip without displacement of the fracture fragments. The fracture of the left hip has been treated surgically using a dynamic hip screw and plate device to fixate the femoral neck to the femoral shaft. Three weeks after release from the hospital, the patient fell again and fractured the right hip. Elderly patients tend to fall more often for a variety of reasons, which can contribute substantially to their increased incidence of hip fractures.

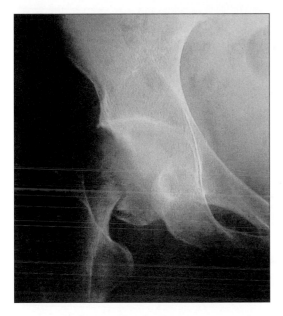

**FIGURE 5-12.** Subcapital fracture of the right hip in a patient, a few weeks after delivery of her second child. Thinning and obscuration of the subchondral cortex and decreased density of the bony trabeculae in the femoral head suggest extensive bone demineralization in the femoral head whereas bone mineralization remains normal in the adjacent acetabulum. This radiological image in a young woman in the postpartum period strongly suggests presence of "transient osteoporosis of the hip." Although this does not usually lead to fracture, it has resulted in a subcapital fracture in this patient. The etiology of pregnancy related transient osteoporosis is unknown and other joints and bones may be affected [ 10, 11 ]. Pregnancy-related osteoporotic fractures are rare, but may be seen in the hip and the thoracic spine. Transient osteoporosis of the hip occurs in young and middle-aged adults and more frequently in men. It starts with spontaneous hip pain without previous trauma that progresses in a few weeks and usually subsides in two to six months. Radiographically progressive marked osteoporosis of the femoral head is seen several weeks after the onset of the hip pain, and restoration of the normal bone density follows clinical recovery. Magnetic resonance (MR) imaging is currently the most sensitive technique for early detection of the bone marrow edema that may indicate transient osteoporosis of the hip: extensive diffuse increased signal intensity of the femoral neck and head is seen on fat-suppressed T2-weighted MR images.

# Pelvic Insufficiency Fractures

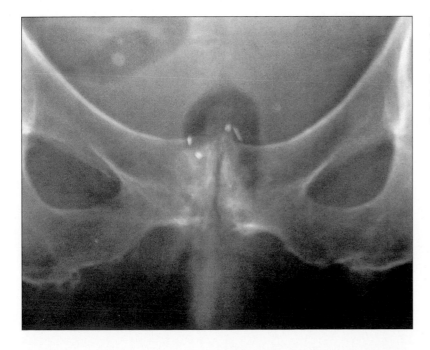

**FIGURE 5-13.** Insufficiency fracture of the symphysis pubis in a 69-year-old woman. The pubic bones are poorly outlined at the symphysis and irregular areas of increased and decreased density are seen in the trabecular bone. These bilateral areas of mixed osteosclerosis and osteolysis are typically seen in insufficiency fractures of the symphysis pubis and may represent areas of microfractures and areas of bone regrowth. In some cases, bone tumors such as chondrosarcoma can mimic this radiologic presentation, in particular when the pathology is unilateral [12, 13].

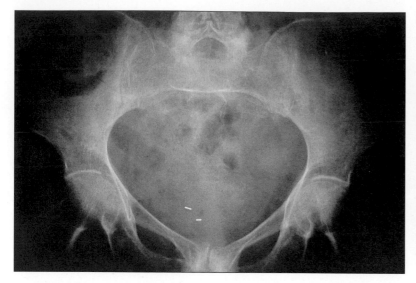

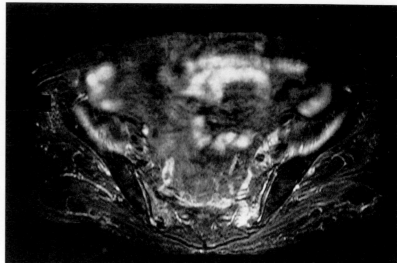

**FIGURE 5-14.** Pelvic insufficiency fractures in a 72-year-old woman. Note the overall osteopenic aspect of the pelvic bones. As in the previous example, the pubic bones have a mixed sclerotic and lytic appearance and the cortical bone at the symphysis is not well defined. This is indicative of insufficiency fracture of the symphysis pubis. The sacrum appears very osteopenic and the arcuate lines outlining the sacral neuroforamina are indistinct. This radiologic appearance together with the patient's clinical complaints of pain posteriorly at the pelvic girdle raises the suspicion for sacral pathology eg, sacral insufficiency fracture (see Fig. 5-15). Additionally, a step-off is noted at the inferior aspect of the left sacrum adjacent to the sacroiliac joint.

**FIGURE 5-15.** MR imaging of sacral insufficiency fracture in the same patient as shown in Figure 5-14. In this axial fat-saturated T2-weighted MR image, all structures with high water content have a bright signal. For example, the small intestines superiorly in the image are filled with fluid and have a bright (white) signal. Note the normal low signal (black) of the bone marrow in the iliac bones. However, increased signal (white) is seen in the sacrum bilaterally, which indicates increased water content of the bone marrow (*bottom center of image*). This pattern of bone marrow edema in elderly osteopenic patients is highly suggestive of bilateral sacral insufficiency fractures [14]. Bone tumors and metastases can simulate this condition, but tend to be unilateral and asymmetric, while the bone marrow edema of insufficiency fractures is usually bilateral and decreases with adequate treatment. Also, a fracture line with low signal intensity on both T1- and T2-weighted images may be visualized.

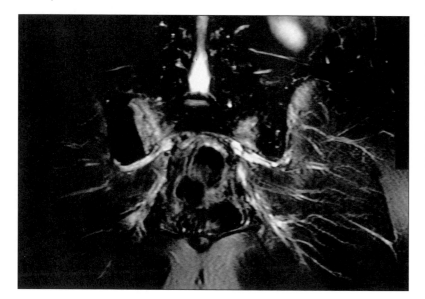

**FIGURE 5-16.** Coronal T2-weighted MR image of insufficiency fracture of the sacrum in a 67-year-old woman. This patient was previously treated with radiotherapy for ovarian carcinoma. No metastatic lesions were diagnosed at the time of treatment. Recently, the patient complained of pain at the sacrum and bone metastasis of ovarian carcinoma was suspected on clinical grounds. The MR examination however demonstrates the presence of bilateral sacral insufficiency fractures. The bone marrow edema associated with sacral insufficiency fractures is characterized by increased (white) signal in the normal dark bone marrow of the sacral wings on fat-saturated T2-weighted MR images. No definite tumoral lesion is seen. Note the thin irregular black line in the middle of the bone marrow edema (on the *left* in the image), which represents the fracture line.

# Wrist Fractures

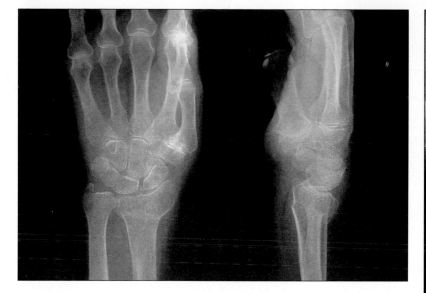

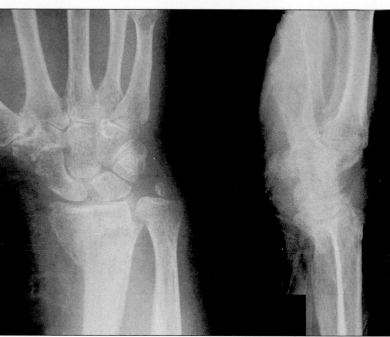

**FIGURE 5-17.** Colles' fracture as seen on the posteroanterior and lateral view of the left wrist in a 83-year-old woman. The Colles' fracture usually occurs in older individuals after a fall on the outstretched hand. Note the decreased bone mineralization. Clinically, a characteristic "dinner fork" or "bayonet" deformity is seen due to the dorsal angulation and shift of the distal fracture fragment and wrist. The fracture of the distal radius and the dorsal angulation are confirmed on the conventional radiographs. Additional findings commonly may include impaction and displacement of the fracture fragments of the radius and avulsion of the styloid process of the ulna. In this patient, widening of the normal space between the lunate and the scaphoid may represent scapholunar dissociation caused by axial stress of the capitate at this articulation at the time of trauma. Treatment for uncomplicated Colles' fractures mainly consists of (closed) reduction of the fracture fragments to reestablish the normal volar tilt of the radial articular surface and stabilization of the fracture fragments by casting. Note extensive osteoarthritic changes at the first carpometacarpal joint.

**FIGURE 5-18.** Smith's fracture of the wrist in a 84-year-old woman. On the posteroanterior view on the left, a fracture of the distal radius is seen. Volar angulation or displacement is characteristic of Smith's fracture as seen on the right. Smith's fracture is much less common than the Colles' fracture, and is called a Barton's fracture when the fracture involves the articular surface of the distal radius, Smith's fracture may result from a (backward) fall on the wrist in dorsiflexion and the forearm supinated. Note the concomitant avulsion of the styloid process of the ulna and the osteoarthritic changes at the first carpometacarpal joint.

# Fractures of the Proximal Humerus

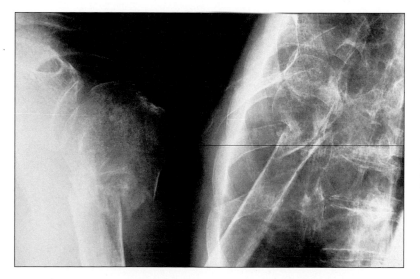

**FIGURE 5-19.** Fracture of the left proximal humerus in a 66-year-old man, as seen on the anteroposterior view (*left*) and on the transthoracic view (*right*). Note the overall decreased bone mineralization. A fracture is present at the level of the surgical neck of the humerus. The humeral head is well centered over the glenoid (see transthoracic view) and is therefore not dislocated. The distal fracture fragment (humeral shaft) is displaced anteriorly and medially as a result of traction of the pectoralis major muscle. Fracture of the greater or lesser tuberosities are not seen, and the fracture of this patient may be classified as a two-part fracture of the proximal humerus according to the Neer classification [9]. Rotator cuff tears may be associated with fractures of the greater tuberosity. Fractures of the proximal humerus in patients having osteoporosis are less common than vertebral, hip, and wrist fractures and most often result from a fall of the outstretched hand. Closed and rarely open reduction of the fracture may sometimes be required.

# Other Insufficiency Fractures

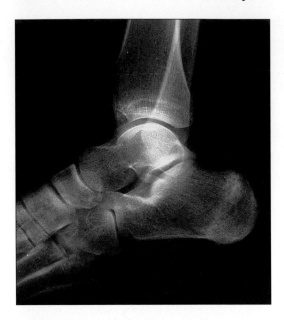

**FIGURE 5-20.** Insufficiency fracture of the right calcaneus in a 62-year-old woman. A linear area of radio-density in the posterior part of the calcaneus is present, and aligned perpendicular to the direction of the bony trabeculae. This represents bone sclerosis and healing of a cancellous bone insufficiency fracture of the calcaneus. Calcaneal stress fractures may also be seen in healthy runners or in patients with diabetes. Decreased bone mineralization as in patients with osteoporosis results in a decreased elastic capacity of the bones and microfractures occur more easily. Although these fractures occur less frequently in patients with osteoporosis, a predilection for certain anatomical locations is known and include the posterior third of the calcaneus, the medial portion of the proximal tibia, and the third and fourth metatarsal bones [15, 16, 17]. Cancellous bone stress fractures such as in the calcaneus may not be visible on initial radiographs, but if a radiograph is repeated two weeks later a linear area of bone sclerosis is often readily visible. Early diagnosis of insufficiency fractures may be enhanced using radionuclide scanning or magnetic resonance imaging.

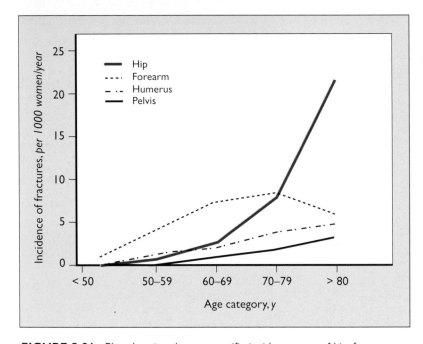

**FIGURE 5-21.** Plot showing the age-specific incidence rate of hip, forearm, humerus and pelvic fracture per 1000 women per year in the United States [18]. The incidence of fractures in the appendicular skeleton increases with age above 50 years. Pelvic and humerus fracture incidences gradually increase to 3 and 4 respectively per 1000 women who are 80 years or older. Forearm fracture incidence increases relatively quickly above the age of 50 years and reaches a plateau of 8 per 1000 women who are between the ages of 60 and 80 years old. Above the age of 80, there is a decrease of forearm fracture incidence. On the other hand, hip fractures are not frequent under the age of 60 years. Above the age of 60 years, there is a very steep increase in hip fractures, reaching over 20 per 1000 in women older than 80 years. High mortality and morbidity is associated with hip fractures in the elderly. Maintaining body weight, walking for exercise, avoiding long-acting benzodiazepines, minimizing caffeine intake, and treating impaired visual function to prevent falls are among the steps that may decrease the risk for hip fracture in white women [19].

Most fractures above the age of 50 years are related to low bone density (osteoporosis). Other factors such as severe trauma or specific pathologic processes (eg, metastatic malignancies) causing fracture are less common. The National Osteoporosis Foundation reported on the contribution of osteoporosis to specific types of fractures among different populations residing in the United States [20]. They estimated that 90% of hip fractures in white women between 65 and 84 years old were related to osteoporosis. The estimate for spine fractures (vertebral compression fractures) was 90% and for wrist fractures was 70%. White women in general have the highest risk for osteoporotic fractures. Men are less at risk than women of the same race. Black races have the lowest risk and Asian races intermediate risks.

The chance for fracture has been calculated in numerous studies and includes estimations on lifetime risk, cumulative risk, and actuarial risk. Cumulative risk is the probability that a person of an exact age (eg, 65 years) will sustain a fracture at a later exact age (eg, 90 years). The actuarial risk takes into account the chance that a person can die from another disease during this period. Therefore, actuarial risks are lower than cumulative risks. In a study using data from a 5% sample of US Medicare recipients the reported actuarial risk for a 65-year-old white woman sustaining a fracture by age 90 to be 16% for the hip, 9% for the distal forearm, and 5% for the proximal humerus [21]. (*From* Cummings, *et al.* [18].)

# References

1. Lang P, Steiger P, Faulkner K, *et al.*: Osteoporosis. Current techniques and recent developments in quantitative bone densitometry. *Radiol Clin North Am* 1991, 29(l): 49–76.

2. Resnick D: Diagnosis of Bone and Joint Disorders. Philadelphia: WB Saunders; 1997.

3. Brunelli MP, Einhorn TA: Medical management of osteoporosis. Fracture prevention. *Clin Orthop* 1998;Mar (348):15–21.

4. Lafforgue P, Daumen-Legre V, Clairet D, *et al.*: Insufficiency fractures of the medial femoral condyle. *Rev Rhum Engl Ed* 1996, 63(4): 262–269.

5. Otte MT, Helms CA, Fritz RC: MR imaging of supra-acetabular insufficiency fractures. *Skeletal Radiol* 1997, 26(5): 279–283.

6. Baur A, Stabler A, Bruning R, *et al.*: Diffusion-weighted MR imaging of bone marrow: differentiation of benign versus pathologic compression fractures [see comments]. *Radiology* 1998, 207(2):349–356.

7. Cuenod CA, Laredo JD, Chevret S, *et al.*: Acute vertebral collapse due to osteoporosis or malignancy: appearance on unenhanced and gadolinium-enhanced MR images. *Radiology* 1996, 199(2):541–549.

8. Rupp RE, Ebraheim NA, Coombs RJ: Magnetic resonance imaging differentiation of compression spine fractures or vertebral lesions caused by osteoporosis or tumor. *Spine* 1995, 20(23):2499–2504.

9. Weissman BN, Sledge CB: Orthopedic Radiology. Philadelphia: WB Saunders; 1986.

10. Blanch J, Pacifici R, Chines A: Pregnancy-associated osteoporosis: report of two cases with long-term bone density follow-up. *Br J Rheumatol* 1994; 33 (3):269–272.

11. Breuil V, Brocq 0, Euller-Zlegler L, Grimaud A: Insufficiency fracture of the sacrum revealing a pregnancy associated osteoporosis. First case report [letter]. *Ann Rheum Dis* 1997, 56(4):278–279.

12. Hosono M, Kobayashi H, Fujimoto R, *et al.*: MR appearance of para-symphyseal insufficiency fractures of the os pubis. *Skeletal Radiol* 1997, 26(9):525–528.

13. Peh WC, Khong PL, Yin Y, *et al.*: Imaging of pelvic insufficiency fractures. *Radiographics* 1996, 16(2):335–348.

14. Grangier C, Garcia J, Howarth NR, *et al.*: Role of MRI in the diagnosis of insufficiency fractures of the sacrum and acetabular roof. *Skeletal Radiol* 1997, 26(9):517–524.

15. Lafforgue P, Pham T, Denizot A, *et al.*: Bone insufficiency fractures as an inaugural manifestation of primary hyperparathyroidism. *Rev Rhum Engl Ed* 1996, 63(7–8):475–479.

16. Lechevalier D, Fournier B, Leleu T, *et al.*: Stress fractures of the heads of the metatarsals. A new cause of metatarsal pain. *Rev Rhum Engl Ed* 1995, 62(4): 255–259.

17. Umans H, Pavlov H: Insufficiency fracture of the talus: diagnosis with MR imaging. *Radiology* 1995, 197(2):439–442.

18. Cummings SR, Kelsey JL, Nevitt CN, O'Dowd KJ. Epidemiology of osteoporosis and osteoporotic fractures. *Epidemiol Rev* 1985, 7:178–208.

19. Cummings SR, Nevitt MC, Browner WS, *et al.*: Risk factors for hip fracture in white women. *N Engl J Med* 1995, 332:767–773.

20. Melton LJ II, Thamer M, *et al.*: Fractures attributable to osteoporosis: report from the National Osteoporosis Foundation. *J Bone Miner Res* 1998, 13:1915–1923.

21. Barret JA, Baron JA, Karagas MR, Beach ML: Fracture risk in the U.S. Medicare population. *J Clin Epidemiol* 1999, 52:243–249.

# SKELETAL ASSESSMENT

## *Alan Burshell and Sonia Victores*

Osteoporosis is a common preventable and treatable disease that is influenced by both heredity and environment. The morbidity and excess mortality due to osteoporosis are the consequence of low-trauma fractures. Although such fractures occur most often in older women and men, the loss of bone leading to skeletal fragility begins decades earlier. Hip fractures are associated with an increased mortality of 12% to 20% within the first year after the fracture, and often result in major disability and nursing home placement. Compression fractures of the vertebral bodies are under-appreciated as a source of pain and disability in older people. This chapter discusses the skeletal assessment of patients who have, or are suspected of having, osteoporosis. Emphasis is given to aspects of patient history, physical examination, and laboratory studies as well as to the primary noninvasive technique for measuring bone, photon absorptiometry.

## History and Physical Examination

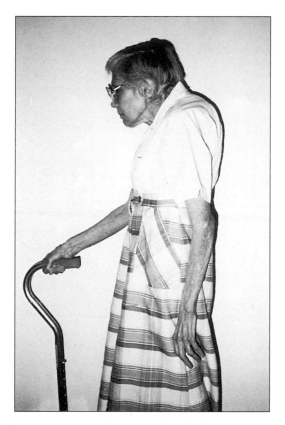

**FIGURE 6-1.** Osteoporosis phenotype. This woman exemplifies many of the characteristic manifestations of osteoporosis. She is elderly, shows a dowager hump (kyphosis), and has thin friable skin. She carries a cane, suggesting problems with balance and a propensity to fall. Both of these factors are associated with an increased risk for future fractures (*Courtesy of* Novartis Pharmaceuticals Inc.)

## A. HEALTH HISTORY FOR OSTEOPOROSIS ASSESSMENT

Basic history

Demographic features: age, sex, race

Fracture history: age at time of fracture, site, relation to trauma

Family history of osteoporosis, fracture, skeletal deformity

Changes in height, posture, dentition

Reproductive history

Women: age at menarche, menstrual history, pregnancies, interruptions of menses (number and duration), gynecologic surgery

Men: age at puberty, androgen use, sexual history

Past medical history (contributory disorders): History of diabetes, eating disorder, hyperparathyroidism, liver, biliary or kidney disease, malignancy, arthritis, thyroid disease

Tobacco and alcohol use

Medication history

Calcium supplements

Glucocorticosteroids

Anticoagulants

Anticonvulsants

Estrogen, progestins

Thiazide diuretics

Thyroid hormones

Vitamins A and D

Aluminum-containing antacids

Anti-estrogens

Exercise history

Amount and kind of exercise during childhood and adolescence

Habitual exercise patterns as an adult

Current exercise program

History of immobilization (causes, duration)

## B. PHYSICAL EXAMINATION OF PATIENTS WITH OSTEOPOROSIS

Basic examination

Height, weight, overall nutritional status

Deformities: kyphosis, scoliosis, lordosis, bone tenderness

Back tenderness, paraspinous muscle spasm

Dentition, particularly periodontitis

Skin thickness, premature graying of hair

Muscle strength, particularly limb girdle muscles

Range of motion of limbs

Testicular or pelvic examination

Gait and balance (need for assistance)

Evidence for other systemic disease

Physical findings suggestive of secondary causes of osteoporosis

Cushing syndrome: "Buffalo hump," supraclavicular fullness, bruises, proximal muscle atrophy

Marfan syndrome: arachnodactyly, lens displacement

Mastocytosis: dermatographia

Osteogenesis imperfecta, Ehlers-Danlos syndrome: hyperelasticity cutis

Rheumatoid arthritis: joint subluxation, ulnar deviation

Hyperthyroidism: tachycardia, goiter, skin changes, thinning of hair, stare, lid-lag

**FIGURE 6-2.** Screening for and diagnosis of osteoporosis. The term *screening* implies searching for affected individuals within a healthy population. The role of screening for osteoporosis remains highly controversial, and actually is a misnomer. In screening, bone mass is assessed, with the goal of identifying individuals who are at risk for fractures by virtue having a low bone mineral density, and who would benefit from an intervention aimed at protecting the skeleton against further bone loss. By contrast, the *diagnosis* of osteoporosis requires some evidence of skeletal fragility, such as a low-trauma fracture. Bone mass measurements can give substantial evidence that a patient is highly likely to have osteoporosis, or to develop it in the future, but no value of bone mineral density is sufficiently sensitive or specific to provide a "gold-standard" for this diagnosis. One reason for this lack of diagnostic rigor is the fact that various age-related qualitative features of bone fragility are not detected by measuring bone density (see Chapter 1).

**A,** Health history for osteoporosis assessment. The first step in making a diagnosis of osteoporosis is to take a careful health history. This provides information on important risk factors for low bone mass and bone loss, as well as pointing toward other secondary causes of skeletal fragility, such as malignancy or osteomalacia. The history helps to identify individuals at higher risk for osteoporosis who are particularly suitable candidates for bone mass measurement, and provides an opportunity to suggest interventions that can be undertaken, such as smoking cessation, provision of adequate calcium and vitamin D intake, or initiating an exercise program. It is also important to focus on areas that often are overlooked in a general medical practice, including events during adolescence (eating disorders, low body weight, menstrual irregularities, growth hormone deficiency, delayed puberty, and Turner's syndrome), because it is a critical period for acquisition of peak bone mass; fracture history; episodes of systemic illness or immobilization; and exposure to medications that are deleterious to bone.

**B,** Physical examination for osteoporosis. The physical examination should include an accurate measurement of standing height, abnormalities of posture and gait, and spasm of paraspinous muscles, as well as other elements listed in the figure. Several physical findings are suggestive of secondary causes of osteoporosis, including "buffalo hump," arachnodactyly, joint subluxation, and goiter, among others.

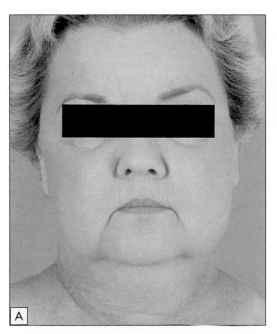

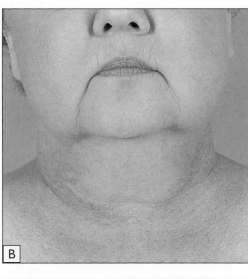

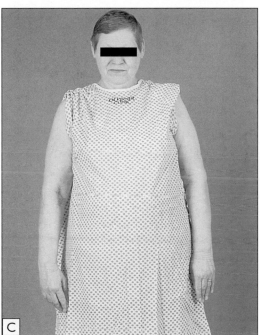

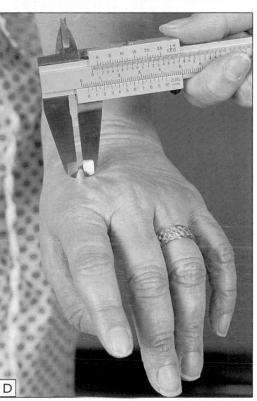

**FIGURE 6-3.** Cushing syndrome (**A** and **B**) and insulin resistance (**C** and **D**) with or without diabetes have many similarities. Both can be associated with obesity and round facies and an increased waist-to-hip ratio. Whereas Cushing syndrome is associated with thin skin and osteoporosis, insulin resistance, particularly with the polycystic ovary syndrome, is associated with thick skin and a normal or high bone mineral density.

# Laboratory Assessment

## LABORATORY TESTS FOR OSTEOPOROSIS DIAGNOSIS

Core tests for most patients with osteoporosis
  Complete blood count
  Serum chemistries: calcium, inorganic phosphorus, albumin, total protein, urea nitrogen and creatinine
  Serum alkaline phosphatase activity
  Serum free thyroxine and TSH concentrations
Special tests when clinically indicated
  24-hour urine for calcium, creatinine
  24-hour urine free cortisol determination
  Serum concentrations of 25-hydroxyvitamin D, intact PTH (IRMA)
  Serum concentrations of LH/FSH, estradiol, testosterone
  Serum concentrations of anti-endomysial and anti-gliaden antibodies (to rule out non-tropical sprue)

**FIGURE 6-4.** Laboratory tests for osteoporosis. These tests cannot establish the diagnosis of osteoporosis, but they do help to identify its underlying causes. Routine chemistry values that should be obtained are listed in the top portion of this figure. Other tests section should be performed if symptoms, physical findings, or features in the patient's history indicate that they are necessary. FSH—follicle-stimulating hormone; IRMA—immunoradiometric assay; LH—luteinizing hormone; PTH—parathyroid hormone; TSH—thyrotropin.

## BIOCHEMICAL MARKERS OF BONE TURNOVER

Bone resorption markers
  Classic tests
    Urinary hydroxyproline: classic test, now clinically obsolete
    Urine calcium/creatinine ratio: not specific for bone resorption
    Serum tartrate-resistant acid phosphatase: highly variable, rarely done
      Specific tests for bone collagen breakdown
    Urinary pyridinoline and deoxypyridinolines: cross-linked collagen telopeptides; kits available for both carboxy- and amino terminal peptides
Bone formation markers
  Classic test: serum alkaline phosphatase activity; still robust for Paget's disease of bone; generally normal in osteoporosis
  Specific tests of osteoblast function
  Osteocalcin
  Bone-specific alkaline phosphatase
  Type I procollagen carboxyterminal extension peptide

**FIGURE 6-5.** Biochemical markers of bone turnover. The rate at which bone is formed or degraded can be assessed either by measuring an enzymatic activity of the bone-forming (osteoblasts) or bone-resorbing (osteoclasts) cells, such as alkaline and acid phosphatase, or by measuring bone matrix constituents released into the circulation during the process of bone remodeling [1]. Bone markers do not discriminate changes in turnover in specific regions of the skeleton, but reflect whole body net changes. In general, bone resorption and formation activities are coupled (see Chapter 1), so all of the markers can be used as a rough guide to the rate of whole body bone turnover. The appropriate clinical role for bone turnover markers has not yet been determined. Patients who are placed on antiresorptive treatment show significant suppression of marker activity, but the response of individual patients is less reliable for predicting therapeutic response. Markers appear to be of help in deciding whether low bone mass in an individual patient is associated with high or low rates of bone turnover.

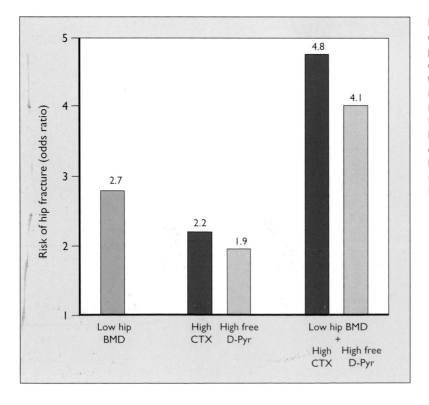

**FIGURE 6-6.** Use of bone turnover markers to predict hip fracture risk in elderly women. Evidence suggests that the rate of bone turnover plays an independent role in determining the likelihood of fracture. One mechanism for this observation could be that individuals with higher rates of bone turnover have focal areas of weakness in the bone that is undergoing a remodeling event. That is, increased resorption cavities that are being created or have been partially filled in may constitute regions of lower resistance to fracture. A large, multinational European study of fracture (EPIDOS) found that both low hip bone density and high bone turnover rate, reflected by an increase in urinary resorption marker concentrations, doubled the risk for hip fracture. The combination of low hip bone mineral density (BMD) and high urinary resorption marker increased the risk of fracture more than four-fold. CTX—type I procollagen carboxy terminal; D-Pyr—deoxypyridinolines. (*From* Garnero *et al.* [2]; with permission.)

## SECONDARY CAUSES OF OSTEOPOROSIS

| | | |
|---|---|---|
| **Genetic disorders** | **Malignant disorders** | **Miscellaneous disorders** |
| Cystic fibrosis | Multiple myeloma and other hematologic malignancies | Anorexia nervosa |
| Galactosemia | Humoral hypercalcemia of malignancy (PTHrP-mediated) | Immobilization |
| Glycogen storage diseases | Malignancy cachexia | Inflammatory bowel disease |
| Hemochromatosis | Chemotherapy- and radiation-related bone loss | Celiac disease |
| Homocystinuria | **Endocrine and metabolic disorders** | Hepatic disorders (eg, primary biliary cirrhosis) |
| Hypophosphatasia | Cushing syndrome | Rheumatologic disorders |
| Marfan and Ehlers-Danlos syndromes | Diabetes mellitus (type 1) | **Medications** |
| Osteogenesis imperfecta and its variants | Hyperthyroidism, thyroid hormone excess | Anticonvulsant medications |
| | Primary hyperparathyroidism | Cyclosporine |
| | | Glucocorticosteroids |
| | | Heparin (subcutaneous, long-term) |
| | | Hypervitaminosis A and D |

**FIGURE 6-7.** Secondary causes of osteoporosis. There are a number of specific, so-called secondary causes of decreased bone mineral density (BMD) and fracture. It is important to identify patients in whom these factors are present, because management may differ. Identification of secondary causes of osteoporosis alters the management strategy because effective treatment requires correcting the underlying cause, eg, treatment of hyperthyroidism or Cushing syndrome. Osteoporosis associated with gonadal failure generally is considered to be "primary" and is not listed among these examples of secondary osteoporosis.

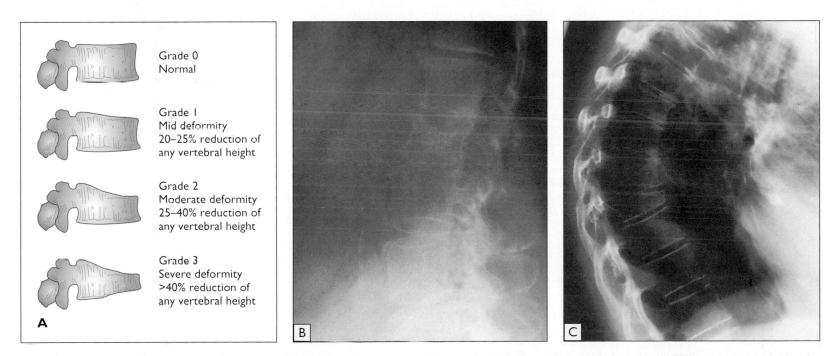

**FIGURE 6-8.** Lateral spine radiograph of a patient with osteoporosis. Assessment of spine deformity is best accomplished with a lateral view of the thoracic and lumbar spines. Although many spinal compression fractures are obvious even to an untrained examiner, some degrees of spinal deformity are subtle and require accurate measurements. No gold standard exists for the definition of a spinal deformity, but one reasonable approach is to measure the anterior, middle, and posterior heights of a vertebral body. A fracture is diagnosed if any single measurement is reduced by 20% or more compared to the other measurements. Compression of 20% to 25% is said to be mild, and 25% or greater is considered "moderate." Occasional fractures involve the entire vertebral body, so that reductions in all three measurements are observed. Vertebral body height increases progressively as one proceeds down the spine from high thoracic to low lumbar, so that any single vertebral body that measures relatively low for its position must be suspected of having been fractured. **A,** Varying degrees of compression deformity. **B,** Lumbar vertebral compression in a patient with degenerative joint disease and aortic calcifications. **C,** Thoracic wedge deformity.

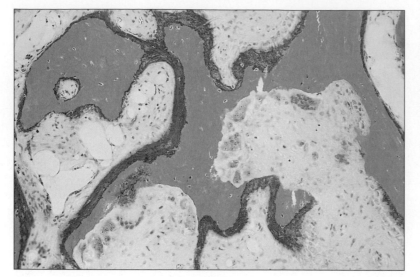

**FIGURE 6-9.** (*see* Color Plate) The role of bone biopsy. Iliac crest biopsy with assessment of both static and dynamic components of bone turnover is a standardized approach to determine what is taking place at the bone tissue level in individuals with osteoporosis. Special stains applied to non-demineralized specimens distinguish between mineralized (shown in green) and non-mineralized (shown in red) bone. This histologic section from an iliac bone biopsy is from a patient with renal osteodystrophy and illustrates the important point that fractures from bone disease may be secondary not only to osteoporosis but also to other conditions—in this case, to aluminum-related renal osteodystrophy. Most patients with osteoporosis do not require iliac crest biopsy, but occasional patients in whom diagnostic dilemmas occur may benefit from such a biopsy. Occasionally, biopsy suggests a diagnosis that could not otherwise have been established, such as systemic mastocytosis or occult forms of osteomalacia.

# Bone Densitometry

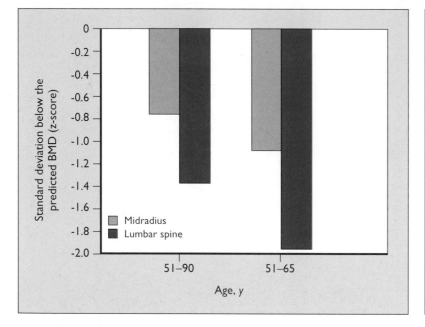

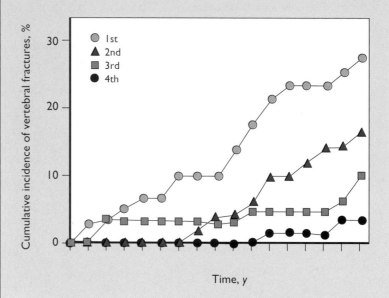

**FIGURE 6-10.** BMD variability in women with vertebral fractures *vs* women without fractures. Women with vertebral fractures have a lower BMD than age-matched controls. The BMD is a better predictor of vertebral fractures in the 51–65 age group than in the elderly. The lumbar BMD decreases with age, and thus the BMD difference between women with and without fractures is reduced. The lumbar spine BMD is a better predictor of lumbar fractures than the radius measurement or other sites (data not shown). (*From* Riggs, *et al.* [3].)

**FIGURE 6-11.** Relationship between cumulative incidences of vertebral fractures vs. lumbar spine BMD. The fracture prevalence at eight years is six times greater in women with the lowest BMD (*i.e.,* 1st quartile) compared with those with the highest BMD (4th quartile). For every one standard deviation below age-predicted mean values that an individual's BMD falls, there is at least a doubling of fracture rate. Fractures are very uncommon at BMD values above 1.20 g/cm$^2$, but this should not be construed as evidence for a "fracture threshold." Whether a person fractures or not will always reflect a composite effect of the bone itself (as reflected in BMD) and the force that is applied to it (such as a fall). (*From* Melton, *et al.* [4].)

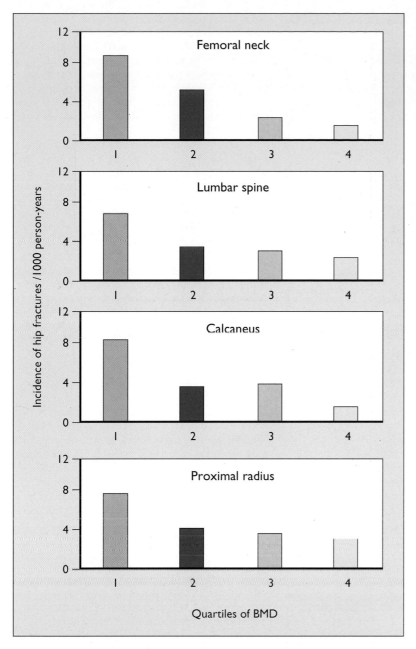

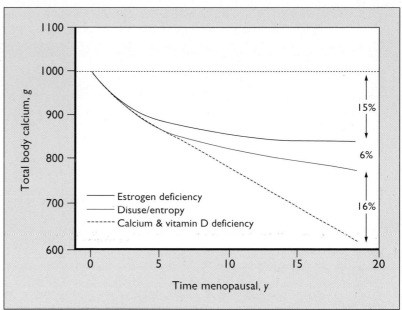

**FIGURE 6-13.** Which skeletal site should be measured? The bone mineral density (BMD) predicts fracture risk, and serial measurements indicate bone loss or accretion. Hip BMD (see Fig. 6-12) best reflects the risk of hip fractures, which are associated with significant morbidity and mortality.

Trabecular bone is more responsive than cortical tissue to many hormonal changes and therapeutic interventions. Bone loss at menopause is greater for the lumbar spine than for the total hip, and the BMD response to estrogen or alendronate is greater at the lumbar spine than at the hip. The vertebral BMD often is the preferred measurement site for follow-up evaluations. Unfortunately, osteophytes and calcifications of the aorta may affect the lumbar BMD.

The total body calcium measures the skeleton in grams. This measurement addresses primarily cortical bone. The cortical bone is affected by deficiencies of calcium and vitamin D.

The BMD site to be measured should be selected based on the age of the patient, anatomy (eg, scoliosis), underlying disease process (eg, vitamin D or estrogen deficiency), purpose of the study (ie, quantitation of fracture risk vs. evaluation of therapeutic intervention), evaluation of future fracture risk, or follow-up of therapy. Peripheral BMD measurements using ultrasound are available, and their use is increasing, but there are few data regarding the usefulness of this technology vs. dual x-ray absorptiometry (DXA). It is likely that one measurement is better than none, but the relative advantages and disadvantages of the various technologies are debatable. (*Adapted from* Heany [6].)

**FIGURE 6-12.** Relationship of bone mineral density (BMD) to risk of hip fracture. As with vertebral fracture, BMD is an independent predictor of hip fracture. This graph, taken from a large observational epidemiologic study, shows that the quantifiable relationship between BMD and hip fracture is greatest for BMD values at the femoral neck. It appears that when BMD at any site is used to predict an individual's general risk of experiencing a fracture (without specifying a site), the risk increases two-fold for each standard deviation that BMD drops below age-matched norms. However, when BMD at a specific site is used to predict the risk of fracture at that same site (eg, femoral neck BMD and hip fracture), then the relationship between BMD and fracture is greater, approximately three-fold for each decrease below the standard deviation. (*From* Cummings *et al.* [5]; with permission.)

## COMPARISON OF BONE MASS MEASUREMENT TECHNIQUES

| Technique | Sites | Scan time, *min* | Errors, % Precision | Errors, % Accuracy | Radiation exposure, *mrem* |
|-----------|-------|------------------|---------------------|--------------------|----------------------------|
| SPA | Radius | 5–15 | 2–5 | 3–8 | 2–5 |
|  | Calcaneus |  |  |  |  |
| DPA | Spine | > 20 | 2–5 | 3–10 | 5–10 |
|  | Proximal femur |  |  |  |  |
|  | Whole body |  |  |  |  |
| DXA | Spine | 3–6 | 0.5–3 | 3–8 | < 5 |
|  | Proximal femur |  |  |  |  |
|  | Whole body |  |  |  |  |
| QCT | Spine | 5–30 | 2–6 | 5–15 | 100–1000 |
|  | Proximal femur |  |  |  |  |

*research basis only

**FIGURE 6-14.** Comparison of bone mass measurement techniques. Several different methods to assess bone mineral density (BMD) have been introduced since the late 1970s. This table presents those methods achieving at least moderate research and clinical use. Single photon absorptiometry (SPA) is restricted to estimating BMD in appendicular sites such as the forearm or calcaneus. Dual photon absorptiometry (DPA) was the first method to permit estimation of BMD in central regions. DPA is now obsolete and has been virtually replaced by dual x-ray absorptiometry (DXA) (formerly known as dual *energy* x-ray absorptiometry [DEXA]). DXA, by virtue of its very low radiation exposure and reasonable precision and accuracy, has emerged as the dominant technique for clinical purposes. DXA values are reported as an "areal" BMD (g/cm$^2$) and do not fully account for differences in bone thickness. Thus, very large- and very small-boned individuals will have artifactually high and low BMD values by this technique (see also Chapter 1). Quantitative computed tomography (QCT) is unique in one respect: it offers the ability to assess bone mass specifically in vertebral trabecular bone, in contrast to DXA or DPA, which are projection methods and therefore include vertebral spinous processes and cortical shells in the BMD reading. However, as generally used, QCT is far less precise and exposes patients to greater radiation than does DXA. Radiographic absorptiometry (RA) requires nothing more than taking an x-ray film of the hand. An aluminum wedge of known mineral density is included in the x-ray, and the density of the meta-carpal bones is compared to that of the wedge with the use of a special densitometer. RA has been used for many years in research, but is still under development as a clinical tool.

One difficulty with standard DXA and QCT as clinical tools is lack of availability. It is necessary for patients to come to densitometry facilities, which are in short supply in many parts of the United States. Thus, there has been great interest in development of smaller, less expensive instruments that could be positioned in physician's offices. Peripheral QCT and DXA instruments have been introduced to serve this function. The final role of these "peripheral" measurements has not yet been determined. It may be that patients identified as having low bone mass on the basis of a peripheral measurement could be referred to a standard DXA facility for more comprehensive measurements.

Another recently approved technique for assessing skeletal risk is the use of quantitative ultrasound transmission through bone. The speed at which sound travels through a bone directly reflects its mineral density. Thus, machines to measure ultrasound transmission were introduced as surrogates for isotope-based methods. It appears, however, that ultrasound properties of bone may provide additional predictive value for fracture risk, even once the effect of BMD has been accounted for. The ultimate value of ultrasound remains to be established, but in the United States ultrasound devices have received FDA approval for clinical purposes. (Adapted from Erlich and Holohan [7].)

## COEFFICIENTS FOR CALCULATING SCORE

| Variable | Score | For women |
|----------|-------|-----------|
| Race | 5 | is *not* black |
| Rheumatoid arthritis | 4 | *has* rheumatoid arthritis |
| History of fractures | 4 | for *each type* (wrist, rib, hip) of nontraumatic fracture after age 45 (maximum score = 12) |
| Age | 3 | × first digit of age in years |
| Estrogen | 1 | if *ever* received estrogen therapy |
| Weight | -1 | × weight divided by 10, to nearest integer |

**FIGURE 6-15.** Use of risk factors as a surrogate for bone mass measurements. In response to problems with accessibility of bone densitometry, a number of attempts have been made to construct validated questionnaires designed to identify patients with low bone mass who would benefit from pharmacologic interventions. One such formula, SCORE (simple calculated osteoporosis risk estimation), is shown here. A numerical score is developed on the basis of the listed factors.

For example, a 67-year-old Caucasian woman weighs 126 pounds and has a history of rheumatoid arthritis. She has not sustained a fracture, and she has taken replacement estrogen since menopause. Her SCORE would be as follows:

5 (race) + 4 (rheumatoid disease) + 0 (no fracture) + 18 (age) + 0 (estrogen exposure) - 12 (weight) = 15. Because 15 exceeds the threshold score of 6, this woman would be referred for a bone density measurement. The SCORE instrument has undergone formal evaluation. Although it has been shown to be very sensitive, serious problems with specificity remain. (*From* Lydick *et al.* [8]; with permission.)

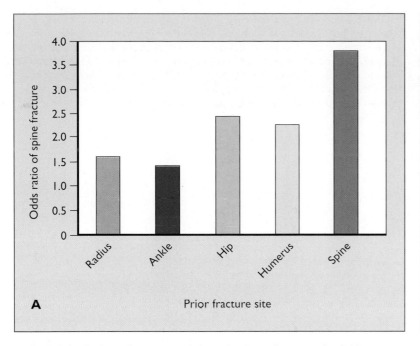

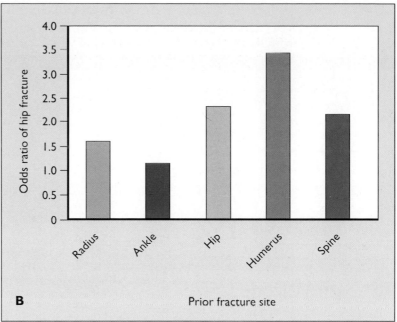

**FIGURE 6-16.** Prior fractures and the risk of new fractures. **A,** Odds ratio (95% confidence interval) of a spine fracture if fractures have occurred within previous 10 years. **B,** Odds ratio of a hip fracture if a fracture occurred within the preceding 10 years.

The fracture history is a critical component of the decision process concerning osteoporosis. A history of a previous fracture of the hip, vertebrae, humerus, ankle, or radius increases the risk of a hip or vertebral fracture [9–12]. Individuals with a trochanteric fracture are more likely to have a similar fracture on the

contralateral side than to fracture the ipsilateral hip or the femoral neck. The greater the number of prior fractures, the higher the risk of future fractures.

Prior vertebral fractures are a better predictor of future vertebral fractures than is a vertebral BMD that is 2 SD below the average BMD of a 25-year-old woman [13]. Antiresorptive agents (calcium, vitamin D, calcitonin, estrogen alendronate, or raloxifene) should be considered for individuals with a history of hip and multiple vertebral fractures independently of the bone mineral density (BMD). (*From* Lauritzen and Lund [14]; with permission.)

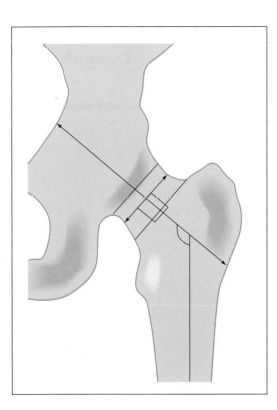

**FIGURE 6-17.** Bone geometry. Dual x-ray absorptiometry (DXA) measures the "areal" bone mineral density (BMD) in g/cm$^2$ and is affected by bone size and density; it also correlates with bone strength. Stiffness is proportional to bone strength. The greater the distance from the periosteum to the center of a long bone, the greater the bending forces required to induce a fracture. The areal BMD of a tall, heavy football player is likely to be greater than that of a petite marathon runner, and the former is less likely to develop a Colles' fracture. Hip fractures are influenced by the femoral and pelvic geometry. The hip axis length (HAL) is defined as the distance from the inner edge of the pelvic brim to the outer edge of the trochanter along the axis of the femoral neck. A 0.5-cm increase in the HAL is associated with a twofold increase in the risk of trochanteric and femoral neck fractures. (*From* Faulkner *et al.* [15] and Faulkner *et al.* [16].)

## CONDITIONS FOR WHICH MEDICARE COVERS BONE MASS MEASUREMENTS

Estrogen-deficient patient at risk for osteoporosis

Radiologic evidence of osteoporosis, osteopenia, or vertebral fracture

Glucocorticoid therapy anticipated to exceed 3 months at a daily dose equivalent to 7.5 mg

Hyperparathyroidism

Monitor response to FDA-approved drug

Follow-up measurement at 2 year interval

**FIGURE 6-18.** Medicare coverage for bone mass measurements. Medicare reimburses beneficiaries with appropriate indications for bone mass measurement once every 2 years. However, if it is determined to be medically necessary, Medicare may cover a bone mass measurement more frequently than every 2 years in the following situations: 1) long-term glucocorticoid therapy of more than 2 months, or 2) confirmatory baseline bone mass measurement to permit monitoring in the future if the initial test was performed with a technique that is different from the proposed monitoring method.

# References

1. Delmas PD, Garnero P: Utility of biochemical markers of bone turnover in osteoporosis. In: *Osteoporosis.* Edited by Marcus R, Feldman D, Kelsey J. San Diego: Academic Press, 1996:1075–1088.

2. Garnero P, Hausherr E, Chapuy M-C, *et al.*: Markers of bone resorption predict hip fracture in elderly women: the EPIDOS prospective study. *J Bone Miner Res* 1996, 11:1531–1538.

3. Riggs JL, Wahner E, Seeman K, *et al.*: Changes in bone mineral density of the proximal femur and spine with aging. *J Clin Invest* 1982, 70:716–723.

4. Melton LF, Atkinson EJ, O'Fallon M, *et al.*: Long-term fracture prediction by bone mineral assessed at different skeletal sites. *J Bone Min Res* 1993, 8:1227–1233.

5. Cummings SR, Black DM, Nevitt MC, *et al.*: Bone density at various sites for prediction of hip fractures. *Lancet* 1993, 341: 72–75.

6. Heany RP: Osteoporosis, Nutrition and Risk for Osteoporosis. Edited by R. Marcus, D. Feldman, J. Kelsy. San Diego: Academic Press; 1996: 483–509.

7. Erlichman M, Holohan T: Nuclear Medicine Diagnosis and Therapy, Bone Densitometry. Edited by J. Harbert, W. Eckelman, R. Neumann. New York: Thieme Medical Publishers; 1996: 865-878.

8. Lydick E, Cook K, Turpin J, *et al.*: Development and validation of a simple questionnaire to facilitate identification of women likely to have low bone density. *Am J Managed Care* 1998, 4:37–48.

9. Schroder HM, Petersen KK, Erlandsen M: Occurrence and incidence of the second hip fracture. *Clin Orthop Rel Res* 1993, 289:166–169.

10. Gunnes M, Mellstrom D, Johnell O: How well can a previous fracture indicate a new fracture? *Acta Orthopaedica Scandinavica* 1998, 69:508–512.

11. Silman AJ: The patient with fracture: the risk of subsequent fractures. *Am J Med* 1995, 98 (2A) 12S–16S.

12. Finsen V, Benum P. Past fractures indicate increased risk of hip fractures. *Acta Orthopaedics Scandinavica* 1986, 57:337–339.

13. Ross PD, Genant HK, Davis JW, Miller PD, Wasnich RD: Predicting vertebral fracture incidence from prevalent fractures and bone density among non-black, osteoporotic women. *Osteoporosis Int* 1993, 3:120–6.

14. Lauritzen B, Lund B: Risk of hip fracture after osteoporosis fractures. *Acta Orthopaedica Scandinavica* 1993, 64:297–300.

15. Faulkner KG, Cummings DB, Black D, *et al.*: Simple measurement of femoral geometry predicts hip fracture: the study of osteoporotic fractures. *J Bone Miner Res* 1993, 8:1211–1217.

16. Faulkner KG, McClung M, Cummings SR: Automated evaluation of hip axis length for predicting hip fractures. *J Bone Miner Res* 1994, 9:1065–1070.

# ESTROGEN-DEPENDENT BONE LOSS AND OSTEOPOROSIS

## Robert Marcus and Nelson B. Watts

The relationship between estrogen deficiency and osteoporosis was first called to attention by Fuller Albright in the 1940s. Only recently, however, has it been demonstrated formally that estrogen replacement therapy (ERT) offers skeletal protection. The decade-long hiatus between these two events reflects that approval of ERT for treatment of menopausal women was granted in 1942 by the Food and Drug Administration without regard for proof of efficacy of skeletal protection. Consequently, no incentive existed for the pharmaceutical industry to demonstrate prospectively the effect of ERT on fracture protection in the same way that must be done for other classes of pharmaceuticals. Thus, much of the literature supporting such an effect has been epidemiologic in nature, rather than having come from controlled clinical trials. The current knowledge about the skeletal effects of estrogen is reviewed here.

## Bone Mass Protection and Reduction of Fracture Risk

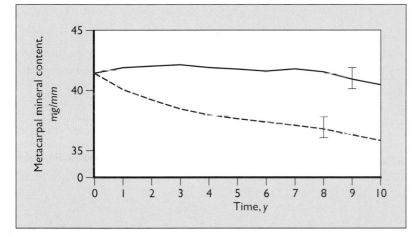

**FIGURE 7-1.** Effect of estrogen replacement therapy (ERT) on bone mass. Timely administration of ERT at or near menopause conserves bone mass. In this study, Lindsay and colleagues [1] randomly assigned recently menopausal women to receive ERT or placebo and followed up these women for bone mineral density (BMD) for 10 years. It can be seen that placebo treatment was associated with sustained bone loss, whereas women receiving ERT maintained BMD. Two features of this study cannot be replicated today. Because of this study and subsequent studies, it is not ethical to maintain a group of estrogen-deficient women on placebo for 10 years. In addition, mestranol, the estrogen used in this study, is not available in the United States as a single prescription drug. Mestranol is a component of several oral contraceptive preparations but cannot be prescribed alone. It is important to remember that bone is fairly promiscuous in its response to estrogen and that at the proper dosage any active estrogen offers skeletal conservation [1]. Currently approved estrogens for replacement therapy used for skeletal protection include the following: conjugated equine estrogens, 0.625 mg/d (Premarin; Wyeth-Ayerst Laboratories, Philadelphia, PA); piperazine estrone sulfate, 0.625 mg/d (Ogen; Abbott Laboratories, Inc., Lake Forest, IL); micronized 17 β estradiol, 0.5 mg/d (Estrace; Bristol-Myers Squibb, Princeton, NJ); and transdermal 17 β estradiol, 0.05-mg patch (Estraderm Transdermal; Novartis; Summit, NJ). (*Courtesy of* R. Lindsay, MD.)

| ESTIMATED RELATIVE RISK OF HIP OR WRIST FRACTURE IN WOMEN ACCORDING TO POSTMENOPAUSAL ESTROGEN USE | | | |
| --- | --- | --- | --- |
| **Reference** | **No. of Cases** | **Duration of Use** | **RR** |
| Hutchinson [2] | 157 | 6 mo | 0.68 |
| Kreiger [3] | 98 | 6 mo | 0.4–.5 |
| Paganini-Hill [4] | 91 | 1–60 mo | 0.97 |
| | | > 61 mo | 0.42 |
| Weiss [5] | 320 | 1–2 y | 0.84 |
| | | 3–5 y | 0.89 |
| | | 6–9 y | 0.38 |
| | | ≥ 10 y | 0.46 |

**FIGURE 7-2.** Estrogen replacement therapy (ERT) confers protection against forearm and hip fracture on postmenopausal women. The epidemiologic evidence that ERT reduces the risk of fracture is shown. Continuous ERT for 5 years or longer was associated with a reduction in fracture by about 60%. RR—relative risk.(*From* Weiss *et al.* [5]; with permission.)

## BONE MINERAL DENSITIES OF ATHLETES WITH AMENORRHEA AND EUMENORRHEA (MEANS ±SD)

| Site | Amenorrheic, g/cm² | Eumenorrheic, g/cm² |
|---|---|---|
| Midradius | 0.672 ± 0.043 | 0.711 ± 0.060 |
| Lumbar spine (L2–L4) | 0.928 ± 0.056 | 1.050 ± 0.110* |
| Proximal femur | | |
| Neck | 0.737 ± 0.048 | 0.871 ± 0.85† |
| Trochanter | 0.621 ± 0.051 | 0.737 ± 0.061† |
| Intertrochanter | 0.964 ± 0.075 | 1.127 ± 0.130‡ |
| Ward's triangle | 0.610 ± 0.054 | 0.739 ± 0.12‡ |
| Whole body | 1.032 ± 0.050 | 1.090 ± 0.059§ |
| Arm | 0.751 ± 0.029 | 0.812 ± 0.07§ |
| Leg | 1.083 ± 0.086 | 1.171 ± 0.066§ |
| Femoral shaft (1/3) | 1.295 ± 0.111 | 1.440 ± 0.07‡ |
| Femoral shaft (1/9) | 1.333 ± 0.109 | 1.491 ± 0.08‡ |
| Tibial midshaft ¶ | 1.073 ± 0.075 | 1.110 ± 0.075 |

*P = 0.01
†P - 0.001
‡P = <0.005
§P = <0.05
¶Tibial midshaft data represent five patients with amenorrhea and six with eumenorrhea.

**FIGURE 7-3.** The effect of interrupting estrogen status during young adult life is shown. For optimal bone health, adequate provision must be made for regular mechanical loading (exercise), nutrient intake (diet), and reproductive hormone status. Attention to any two of these factors at the expense of the third places the skeleton in jeopardy. Young women who exercise to the point of disrupting menstrual cycles lose bone and experience increased incidence of both fatigue and traumatic fracture. Shown is a comparison of bone mineral density of women athletes who are either oligo-amenorrheic (defined in this study as three or less menstrual cycles per year) or eumenorrheic (more than 10 cycles per year). Bone mineral deficits occur throughout the skeleton in the oligo-amenorrheic women [6]. Subtle degrees of menstrual abnormality alone, such as the presence of short luteal phase cycles, do not lead to bone loss [7].

## MECHANISMS OF ESTROGEN ACTION ON BONE

Binds to estrogen receptors in bone cells
  Activates responsive gene elements in osteoclasts and osteoblasts
  Alters cytokine and growth factor production
  Sensitizes bone response to mechanical forces
Modulates calcium balance
  Alters production of calcitropic hormones
  Alters response to calcitropic hormones

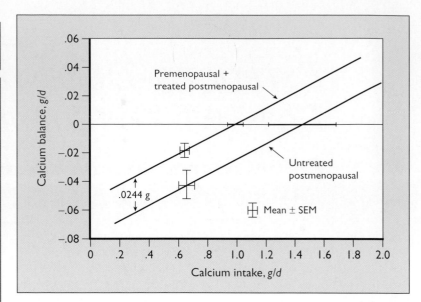

**FIGURE 7-4.** Effect of estrogen loss at menopause on calcium balance. The linear relationship between calcium intake and balance in women is illustrated. The upper curve reflects data obtained in premenopausal and postmenopausal women treated with estrogen replacement therapy (ERT). An intake of approximately 900 mg/d of calcium establishes the level at which neutral calcium balance is achieved (ie, where intake and loss are equal). In contrast, the lower line shows data from postmenopausal estrogen-deficient women. Here, an average calcium intake of over 1400 mg/d is required for neutral balance, representing a deterioration in calcium balance of several hundred milligrams. Another representation of the same phenomenon is seen in the vertical distance between these two curves at any given calcium intake. By this calculation it is seen that going through menopause causes a decrease in the average calcium balance of approximately 24 mg/d. Over a 1-year period this added deficit amounts to an additional calcium loss of over 8 g. SEM—standard error of the mean. (*From* Heaney *et al.* [8]; with permission.)

**FIGURE 7-5.** Estrogens bind to receptors in the nuclei of target cells and activate responsive genes, suppressing bone resorption, likely through multiple pathways. Estrogen has important effects on cytokine and growth factor production and action in both osteoclasts and osteoblasts. It appears that estrogen sensitizes remodeling units to respond to electrical and mechanical forces by altering the so-called mechanistat. Calcium homeostasis also is affected by estrogen through actions on bone, kidney, and bowel. Estrogen may affect calcitropic hormones and tissue responsiveness to these hormones.

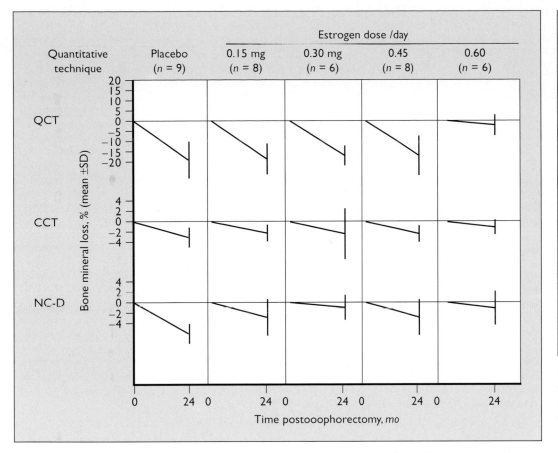

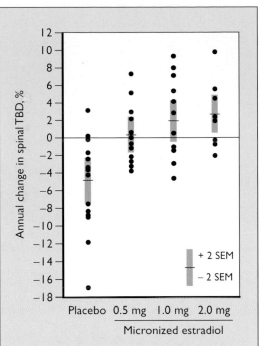

**FIGURE 7-6.** Effect of estrogen replacement therapy (ERT) on bone mass. In this study, premenopausal women who recently underwent oophorectomy were randomly assigned to placebo or various dosages of conjugated equine estrogens (Premarin®; Wyeth-Ayerst Laboratories, Philadelphia, PA). Bone status was monitored by three separate techniques: quantitative computed tomography (QCT), a method specific for trabecular bone of the lumbar spine; combined cortical thickness (CCT), a radiographic measurement of bone cortices; and Norland-Cameron densitometry (NC-D), an old term for single-photon absorptiometry, the earliest densitometric approach to measure bone mass. By all measurements, women assigned to placebo and to dosages of estrogen below 0.6 mg/d lost bone. Women assigned to the highest dosage maintained bone for 2 years. This study was too small to permit valid conclusions about the minimum dosage of estrogen required for skeletal protection of most menopausal women. SD—standard deviation. (From Genant et al. [9]; with permission.)

**FIGURE 7-7.** Effect of estrogen replacement therapy (ERT) on bone mass. In this study, recently menopausal women were administered placebo or one of several dosages of micronized estradiol (Estrace; Bristol-Myers Squibb, Princeton, NJ) for 1 year, and bone mineral density (BMD) of the lumbar spine was monitored. Women assigned to placebo lost bone, whereas groups of women assigned to each dosage of estradiol maintained BMD. Individual results, indicated by dots, show that some women lost bone on active treatment although their treatment group as a whole did not. TBD—trabecular bone density; SEM—standard error of the mean. (From Ettinger et al. [10]; with permission.)

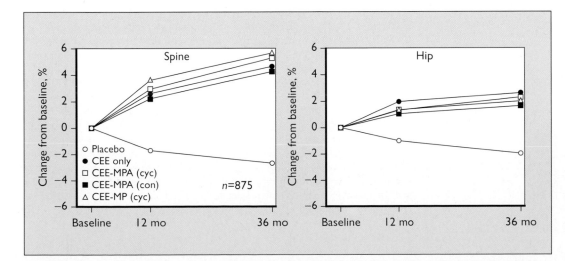

**FIGURE 7-8.** Effect of estrogen replacement therapy (ERT) on bone mass. The Post-menopausal Estrogen/Progestin Interventions (PEPI) Trial is the largest clinical trial to date comparing the effects of unopposed estrogen to those of various combinations of estrogen and progestins. The 875 women who participated were up to 10 years beyond menopause and randomly assigned to one of the following groups for 3 years of treatment: (1) placebo; (2) conjugated equine estrogen (CEE) (Premarin; Wyeth-Ayerst Laboratories, Philadelphia, PA), 0.625 mg/d; (3) Premarin plus medroxyprogesterone acetate (MPA) (Provera; Upjohn Co., Kalamazoo, MI), 10 mg/d, for 12 days each month; (4) Premarin plus Provera, 2.5 mg/d, continuously; and (5) Premarin plus micronized progesterone (MP), 200 mg/d, for 12 days each month.

The primary endpoints of PEPI were cardiovascular risk factors; bone mineral densities at the lumbar spine and proximal femur were secondary endpoints. Shown are the lumbar spine and proximal femur bone mineral density (BMD) results for women who complied with over 80% of their assigned medication. Placebo treatment was associated with bone loss at both spine and hip, whereas all active treatment groups showed increased BMD at both sites. No significant difference in BMD changes among the progestin groups was observed, and in no case did addition of progestin modify the response to estrogen [8]. Women in the PEPI Trial assigned to therapy with continuous unopposed estrogen experienced endometrial hyperplasia at a rate of approximately 20% per year. Thus, endometrial protection with progesterone or other progestin is mandated. The standard progestins used for this purpose in the United States, MPA and MP, do not influence the skeletal response to estrogen. Use of 19-nor testosterone derivatives (such as norethindrone) appears to augment the BMD response to estrogen alone, probably because these compounds also exert independent actions on the androgen receptor. cyc—cyclic administration (days 1–12 of each month); con—continuous administration (daily throughout the month). (From The Writing Group for the PEPI Trial [11]; with permission.)

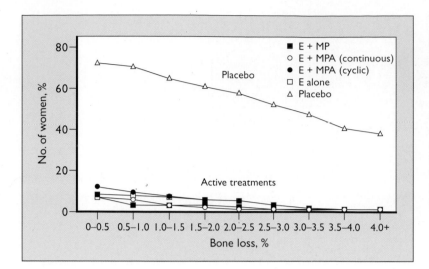

**FIGURE 7-9.** Bone mineral density (BMD) responder analysis in The Post-menopausal Estrogen/Progestin Interventions (PEPI) Trial: lumbar spine. Plotted here are the percentage of women who experienced given changes in spinal BMD over 3 years. Because the precision error of the dual energy x-ray absorptiometry (DXA) measurement is 1.5%, an apparent loss of approximately 3% would be required to state with 80% confidence that bone had been lost. Using that criterion, most women treated with placebo but only about 4% treated with estrogen lost bone. Results at the proximal femur were similar, except that 6% of women treated with estrogen lost bone. It may be concluded that over 90% of women who comply with a dosage of Premarin® (Wyeth-Ayerst Laboratories, Philadelphia, PA), 0.625 mg/d, have very low BMD failure rates and that significant bone loss when this dosage has been prescribed most likely represents patient noncompliance. E—estrogen; MPA—medroxyprogesterone acetate; MP—micronized progesterone. (*From* R. Marcus, unpublished data.)

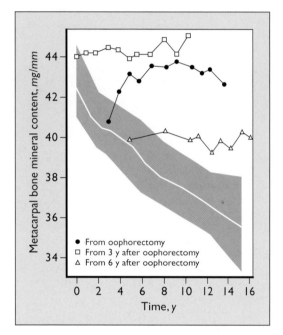

**FIGURE 7-10.** Effect of age on skeletal response to estrogen replacement therapy (ERT). It frequently has been stated that ERT provides skeletal protection only if it is begun within a few years of menopause. This report [12] and others clearly show that ERT constrains bone loss at any age, even decades after menopause. When ERT is begun immediately on termination of menses the remodeling space has not yet expanded fully; therefore, the bone mineral density (BMD) response reflects maintenance of baseline values rather than an increase. Over the next few years, the remodeling space increases substantially. ERT given at that time constricts the remodeling space, thereby promoting an increase in BMD of several percentage points. *Screened area* represents normal range of bone mineral changes for oophorectomized women not treated with estrogen. (*From* Lindsay [12]; with permission.)

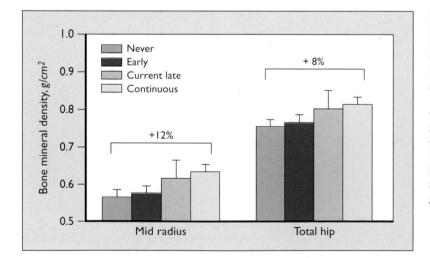

**FIGURE 7-11.** Timing of postmenopausal estrogen replacement therapy (ERT). To be effective in reducing the risk of fracture, ERT must be taken for a long time. Data from the Rancho Bernardo retirement community [13] shows the following in women by 75 years of age: *continuous users*, those who took ERT faithfully from menopause on, had bone mineral density about 10% higher at all skeletal sites than did nonusers; *early users*, women who took ERT for 5 to 10 years beginning at menopause, were almost no better off than were women who never had taken ERT; and *current late users*, women who began taking ERT at aged 60 or later, were almost as well off as were women who never had taken ERT. Thus, it seems wise to begin ERT at menopause and continue taking it lifelong. Even when not begun at menopause, substantial benefit is obtained by beginning ERT at almost any age. One group of women began ERT at menopause and then discontinued it. Their results fall in the middle of those of the other groups. (*From* Schneider *et al.* [13]; with permission.)

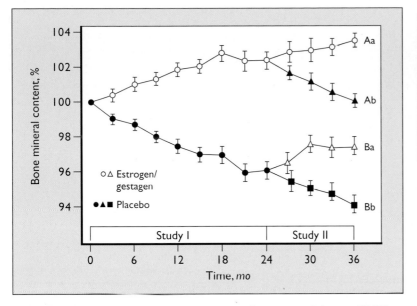

**FIGURE 7-12.** Effect of estrogen cessation on bone mineral density (BMD). In this study, recently menopausal women were assigned to placebo or estrogen replacement therapy (ERT) for 2 years. Placebo was associated with bone loss, and ERT produced bone gain. After 2 years, these women were re-randomized to placebo or ERT and were followed up for another year. For women who were treated with ERT originally, reassignment to placebo rapidly led to bone loss, so that BMD gains achieved during the first 2 years were lost. These data indicate that once ERT is initiated, it must be sustained to maintain skeletal benefits. Aa—estrogen-gestagen (Studies I and II); Ab—estrogen-gestagen (Study I), placebo (Study II); Bb—placebo (Study I), estrogen-gestagen (Study II); Bb—placebo (Studies I and II). (*From* Christiansen *et al.* [14]; with permission.)

### ESTROGEN AND FRACTURE PROTECTION

| Fracture | Current | Past |
|----------|---------|------|
| Hip | 0.27 | 1.67 |
| Wrist | 0.25 | 0.90 |
| Nonspinal | 0.60 | 1.00 |

**FIGURE 7-13.** One of the largest observational epidemiologic study of fractures in older women is the Study of Osteoporotic Fractures (SOF), which involves long-term surveillance of about 9700 elderly white women. In this analysis, fracture incidence was compared in two groups of women. Each group had received estrogen replacement therapy (ERT) for at least 10 years (average, 14 years). Women in one group still were receiving ERT, whereas women in the other group had stopped ERT during the previous few years. Shown are the relative risks (RR) for various fractures. (An RR of 0.25 indicates a fracture incidence only 25% of that seen in women who never received ERT, *ie,* a 75% reduction in risk). Substantial reductions in fracture risk were observed in women who continued ERT, whereas those who had stopped taking ERT had relative risks equal to those who had never received it. Thus, the antifracture benefits of ERT require long-term, essentially lifelong adherence to treatment. (*From* Cauley *et al.* [15]; with permission.)

# Nonskeletal Consequences of Estrogen Administration

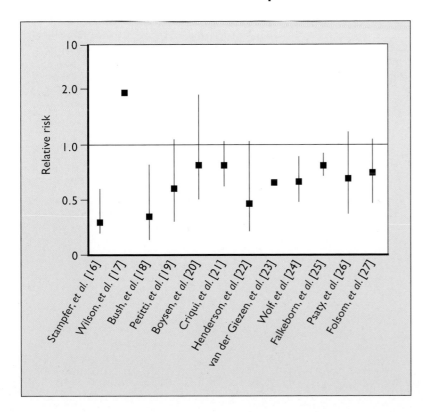

**FIGURE 7-14.** Impact of estrogen on cardiovascular disease [16–27]. In deciding whether to prescribe estrogen replacement therapy (ERT), the physician must consider other factors along with its skeletal benefits. In making this decision, the physician must assess the individual risks for several major aspects of morbidity and mortality in older women. Summarized are recent studies showing the relationship between estrogen (ERT) or estrogen plus progestin (*ie,* hormone replacement therapy [HRT]) and cardiovascular endpoints. These studies are retrospective epidemiologic reports and do not represent the results of randomized controlled trials. Nonetheless, the weight of evidence points toward an overall protective effect of ERT, corresponding to a relative risk of about 0.5. The single exception is the report of Wilson and colleagues [17], representing data from the Framingham study. In a second report using more rigorous definitions of coronary events, these authors found a lower risk of fatal cardiovascular disease among women who took ERT in their 50s and no significant relationship for older women [28].

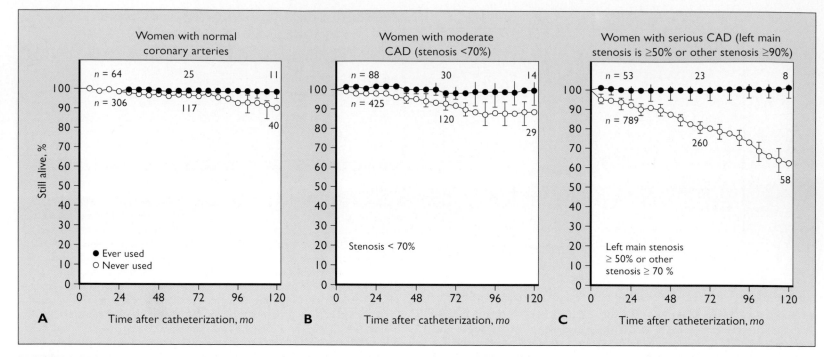

**FIGURE 7-15.** Impact of estrogen replacement therapy (ERT) on survival by severity of coronary artery disease (CAD). In this study, women who underwent cardiac catheterization were stratified by the extent of CAD. The results clearly show that improved survival for women who had taken ERT is directly related to the extent of disease [29]. This study confirms other evidence that the more risk factors a woman has for heart disease the more likely she is to benefit from ERT [15]. (*From* Sullivan *et al.* [29]; with permission.)

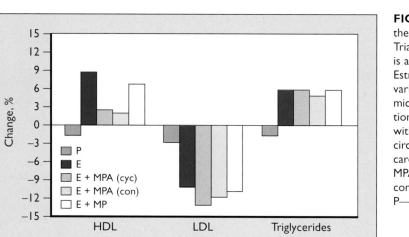

**FIGURE 7-16.** Impact of estrogen and progestins on blood lipids. Shown are the results from the Post-menopausal Estrogen/Progestin Interventions (PEPI) Trial (*see* Fig. 7-8) [30]. Circulating high-density lipoprotein (HDL) cholesterol is a powerful independent risk factor for coronary heart disease in women. Estrogen alone significantly increased HDL-cholesterol, whereas addition of various progestins diminished this response. The least inhibitory progestin was micronized progesterone. In contrast, all active therapies decreased concentrations of low-density lipoprotein (LDL) cholesterol. Estrogen also was associated with a modest increase in circulating triglycerides. Estrogen-induced changes in circulating lipoproteins are thought to account for approximately 40% of the cardioprotective effect of hormone replacement therapy. E—estrogen; E + MPA(cyc)—estrogen plus cyclic progestin; E + MPA(con)—estrogen plus continuous progestin; E + MP—estrogen plus cyclic micronized progestin; P—placebo. (*From* the Writing Group for the PEPI Trial [30]; with permission.)

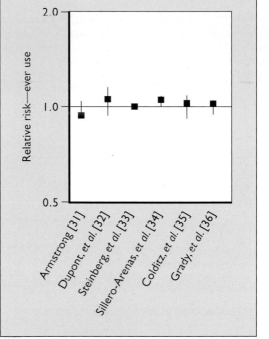

**FIGURE 7-17.** Impact of estrogen replacement therapy (ERT) on breast cancer. The possibility that ERT may be associated with an increased risk for breast cancer is an issue of powerful importance to many women when deciding whether to take either ERT or hormone replacement therapy. Although short-term ERT (< 5 years) carries no added risk for breast cancer, long-term use may be associated with a small but significant added risk. Summarized here are several meta-analyses. In composite it appears that a modest added risk may occur, with a relative risk of 1.14 for "ever" use and 1.35 for "current" use.

## RELATIVE RISK OF BREAST CANCER MORTALITY AMONG EVER USERS OF HORMONE REPLACEMENT THERAPY OR ESTROGEN REPLACEMENT THERAPY

| Reference | Year | N | RR (95% CI) |
|---|---|---|---|
| Bergkvist et al. [37] | 1989 | 6878 | 0.7 (0.5–0.9) |
| Hunt et al. [38] | 1990 | 4544 | 0.6 (0.3–1.0) |
| Henderson et al. [39] | 1991 | 8881 | 0.8 (0.7–1.0) |
| Colditz et al. [40] | 1995 | 69,586 | 1.1 (0.9–1.5) |
| Willis et al. [41] | 1996 | 422,373 | 1.2 0.8 (0.8–0.9) |

**FIGURE 7-18.** The impact of estrogen replacement therapy (ERT) on breast cancer mortality is shown. Long-term ERT appears to convey a small increase in the incidence of breast cancer. However, several reports indicate that breast cancer associated with ERT carries a lower mortality rate than does breast cancer among nonusers of ERT. Shown are the relative risk (RR) values and 95% confidence intervals (CI) for five such studies.

## HORMONE REPLACEMENT THERAPY AND ALZHEIMER'S DISEASE

| Reference | Design | RR | 95% CI |
|---|---|---|---|
| Brenner et al. [42] | Case/Cont | 1.1 | 0.6–1.8 |
| Paganini et al. [43} | Case/Cont | 0.65 | 0.49–0.88 |
| Lerner et al. [44] | Case/Cont | 0.58 | 0.25–0.91 |
| Tang et al. [45] | Cohort | 0.40 | 0.22–0.85 |
| Kawas et al. [46] | Cohort | 0.46 | 0.21–1.00 |

**FIGURE 7-19.** The impact of estrogen replacement therapy (ERT) on Alzheimer's disease is shown. Although the results must be viewed as preliminary, it seems highly likely that ERT is protective of cognitive function and against the onset of Alzheimer's disease. This summary of recent epidemiologic studies indicates that use of ERT or hormone replacement therapy may provide as much as a 50% reduction in risk for Alzheimer's disease. Shown are the relative risk (RR) values and 95% confidence intervals (CI) for five such studies. Cont—control.

## RELATIVE RISK OF ENDOMETRIAL CANCER ASSOCIATED WITH HORMONE REPLACEMENT THERAPY (WOMEN WITH INTACT UTERI)

| | RR | 95% CI |
|---|---|---|
| No HRT | 1.0 | — |
| Estrogen only | 5.0 | 1.6–5.9 |
| Estrogen plus Progestin | 0.9 | 0.7–1.2 |

**FIGURE 7-20.** The impact of estrogen on endometrial cancer is shown [47–49]. Continuous use of estrogen without opposition by progestin clearly is associated with the development of endometrial hyperplasia (approximately 20% of patients per year of continued use) and has been associated with increased risk for endometrial carcinoma. A long-term follow-up of a large Swedish cohort shows that the addition of progestin to estrogen therapy greatly ameliorates the added uterine risk seen with estrogen alone. CI—confidence interval; HRT—hormone replacement therapy; RR—relative risk. (*From* Persson et al. [49]; with permission.)

### ESTIMATED CHANGES IN MORTALITY INDUCED BY 0.625 MG OF CONJUGATED ESTROGENS

| Condition | RR | Cumulative change/100,000 |
|---|---|---|
| Fractures | 0.4 | -563 |
| Gallbladder | 1.5 | +2 |
| Uterine cancer | 2.0 | +63 |
| Breast cancer | 1.1 | +187 |
| Ischemic heart disease | 0.5 | -5250 |
| Net change | | -5561 |
| Net percent change | | -41% |

RR—relative risk.

**FIGURE 7-21.** The impact of estrogen replacement therapy on long-term survival in women aged 50 to 75 years is shown. This table represents a model in which 100,000 women are treated with 0.625 mg/d of conjugated estrogens for 25 years. The third column shows the number of lives predicted to be saved (-) or lost (+) for each category of event. Estimates for endometrial cancer were made without the use of progestins, because the impact of progestin on the other categories listed is uncertain. It can be seen that cardiovascular protection is the overwhelming factor determining the overall outcome for this population. RR—relative risk. (*Courtesy of* R. Ross, MD.)

## Alternatives to Estrogen Replacement Therapy

### LONG-TERM COMPLIANCE WITH ESTROGEN

Facts

　30%–50% of prescriptions for estrogen are never filled.

　Only 20% of those who begin long-term HRT are still taking it 5 years later.

　In the United States, only about 15% of women who might benefit from HRT are taking it.

Problems

　HRT is not recommended by physicians.

　Patients do not understand the need for long-term HRT.

　Patients find that the side effects (eg, bleeding and breast tenderness) are unacceptable.

　Patients have unresolved concerns about HRT and breast cancer.

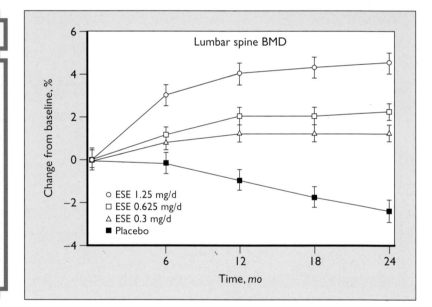

**FIGURE 7-22.** Compliance issues with estrogen. Of every 100 first prescriptions for estrogen, approximately 30 are never filled. Even among women who agree to estrogen replacement therapy (ERT), half have stopped taking it before 1 year. Reasons for low adherence to ERT include dissatisfaction with periodic uterine bleeding and the perceived long-term risk of breast cancer. Thus, long-term compliance remains an important challenge if the potential cardiovascular and skeletal benefits of ERT are to be realized.

**FIGURE 7-23.** One approach to noncompliance has been to design treatments using lower dosages of estrogen (presumably to minimize toxicity while maintaining beneficial effects) or using estrogens with differing tissue effects. Shown here is the bone mineral density (BMD) response to various dosages of esterified estrogens (ESE) in menopausal women who also were given supplemental calcium. Although the changes in BMD were greater at high dosages, low dosage (0.3 mg/d) resulted in a modest increase in BMD [46]. However, a relatively high number of women failed to maintain BMD on this low-dose regimen. Thus, the use of estrogen at dosages below those with established efficacy must be accompanied by adequate BMD surveillance to determine whether the patient has not lost bone while on treatment. (*From* Genant *et al.* [50]; with permission.)

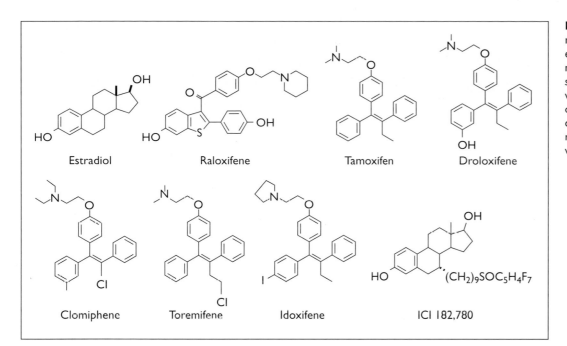

**FIGURE 7-24.** Alternatives to standard estrogen replacement therapy. Shown are the structures of estradiol and a group of selective estrogen-receptor modulators (SERMs), which also are called *tissue-specific estrogens*. Recent engineering of molecules with estrogen-like actions has led to the development of molecules that bind to the estradiol receptor but confer changes in the tertiary structure of the ligand-receptor complex that differ from those achieved with estradiol.

## SELECTIVE ESTROGEN-RECEPTOR MODULATORS: ANTI-ESTROGENS WITH SOME PROPERTIES OF ESTROGEN

| Target | Tamoxifen | Raloxifene |
|---|---|---|
| Breast | Antagonist | Antagonist |
| Bone | Agonist | Agonist |
| Lipids | | |
| High-density lipoprotein | Neutral | Neutral |
| Low-density lipoprotein | Agonist | Agonist |
| Endometrium | Agonist | Antagonist |

**FIGURE 7-25.** Tamoxifen, the first selective estrogen-receptor modulator (SERM), has been in clinical use for several decades. It is an effective estrogen at the bone, liver, and endometrium. Tamoxifen is an effective estrogen antagonist at the breast and hypothalamus, and its antagonism of estrogen action at the breast underlies its extensive use as adjunctive treatment of patients with breast cancer. Raloxifene (Evista; Eli Lilly Co, Indianapolis, IN) was approved in 1998 for the prevention of bone loss in menopausal women. It is a tissue-specific estrogen that differs from tamoxifen in its spectrum of tissue actions. Raloxifene has no important estrogenic effect on the uterus, making it unnecessary to provide routine uterine protection with progestins. It is an estrogen agonist on bone. Treatment with raloxifene, 60 mg/d, increases bone mineral density and lowers fracture risk. Like estradiol, raloxifene lowers circulating low-density lipoprotein cholesterol; however, unlike estradiol, raloxifene does not increase either circulating high-density lipoprotein cholesterol or triglycerides. Raloxifene is a potent anti-estrogen at the breast. Other SERMs in this table remain in various stages of development.

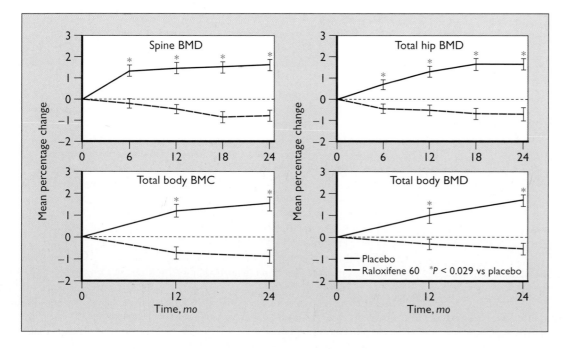

**FIGURE 7-26.** Effect of raloxifene on bone mineral density (BMD). In a 2-year clinical trial in postmenopausal women, when compared with placebo, raloxifene, 60 mg/d, significantly increased BMD at the spine, hip, and total body. (*From* Delmas et al. [51]; with permission.)

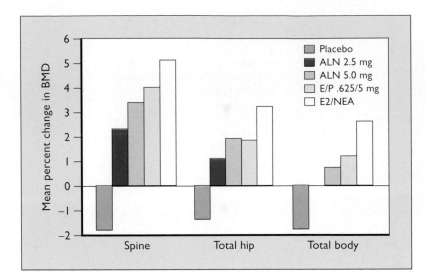

**FIGURE 7-27.** Alendronate (ALN) (Fosamax; Merck, West Point, PA) as an alternative to estrogen. This potent bisphosphonate is approved for prevention of bone loss in menopausal women and for treatment of established osteoporosis. An interim report from the Early Post-Menopausal Intervention Cohort (EPIC) Trial (Merck Research Laboratories) is shown comparing the skeletal effects of alendronate, 5 mg/d, on bone mineral density (BMD) with those of placebo and two different hormone replacement therapy (HRT) regimens. The HRT regimen used in North American centers included Premarin (Wyeth-Ayerst Laboratories, Philadelphia, PA), 0.625 mg/d, and Provera (Upjohn Co., Kalamazoo, MI), 5 mg/d (E/P). European centers used estradiol as the estrogen with norethindrone acetate as the progestin (E2/NEA). All three active treatments prevented bone loss and increased BMD compared with placebo. However, both HRT strategies achieved significantly greater effects on BMD than did the bisphosphonate. Thus, despite important developments in hormonal and nonhormonal antiresorptive drugs, standard HRT remains the most effective strategy for skeletal protection of menopausal women. (*From* Merck Research Laboratories EPIC results [52]; with permission.)

## The Decision to Take Hormone Replacement Therapy

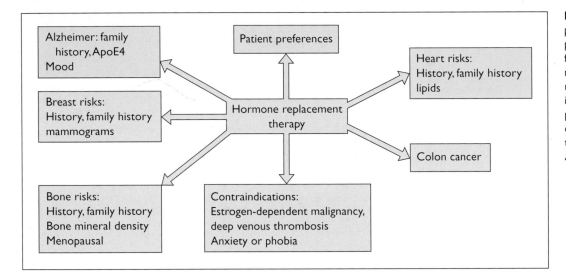

**FIGURE 7-28.** Each woman should undertake this process based on the objective data concerning her personal history, family history, and individual risk factors. The latter include measurements of bone mass and fasting lipoproteins and mammography results. The literature is not yet compelling for inclusion of some health issues for which estrogen protection is likely, such as Alzheimer's disease and colon cancer. Definitive information concerning these issues, however, should soon be available. ApoE4—Apolipoprotein E4.

## References

1. Lindsay R, Hart DM, Aitken JM, *et al.*: Long-term prevention of postmenopausal osteoporosis by oestrogen. Evidence for an increased bone mass after delayed onset of oestrogen treatment. *Lancet* 1976 I:1038–1040.

2. Hutchinson TA, Polansky SM, Feinstein AR: Post-menopausal oestrogens protect against fractures of the hip and distal radius. *Lancet* 1979, 2:705–709.

3. Kreiger N, Kelsey JL, Holford TR, O'Connor T: An epidemiologic study of hip fracture in postmenopausal women. *Am J Epidemiol* 1982, 116:141–148.

4. Paganini-Hill A, Ross RK, Gerkins VR, *et al.*: Menopausal estrogen therapy and hip fractures. *Ann Int Med* 1981, 95:28–31.

5. Weiss NS, Ure CL, Ballard JH, *et al.*: Decreased risk of fractures of the hip and lower forearm with postmenopausal use of estrogen. *N Engl J Med* 1980, 303:1195–1198.

6. Myburgh KH, Bachrach LK, Lewis B, *et al.*: Low bone mineral density at axial and appendicular sites in amenorrheic athletes. *Med Sci Sports Exerc* 1993, 25:1197–1202.

7. Waller K, Reim J, Fenster L, *et al.*: Bone mass and subtle abnormalities in ovulatory function in healthy women. *J Clin Endocrinol Metab* 1996, 81:669–676.

8. Heaney RP, Recker RR, Saville P: Menopausal changes in calcium balance performance. *J Lab Clin Med* 1978, 92:953–963.

9. Genant HK, Christopher CE, Ettinger B, Gordan GS: Quantitative computed tomography of vertebral spongiosa: a sensitive method for detecting early bone loss after oophorectomy. *Ann Intern Med* 1982, 97:699–705.

10. Ettinger B, Genant HK, Steiger P, Madvig P: Low-dosage micronized 17-estradiol prevents bone loss in postmenopausal women. *Am J Obstet Gynecol* 1992, 166:479–488.

11. The Writing Group for the PEPI Trial: Effects of hormone therapy on bone mineral density. Results from the Postmenopausal Estrogen/Progestin Interventions (PEPI) Trial. *JAMA* 1996, 276:1389–1396.

12. Lindsay R: The menopause: sex steroids and osteoporosis. *Clin Obstet Gynecol* 1987, 30:847–859.

13. Schneider DL, Barrett-Connor EL, Morton DJ: Timing of postmenopausal estrogen for optimal bone mineral density. The Rancho Bernardo Study. *JAMA* 1987, 277:543–547.

14. Christiansen C, Christensen MS, Transbøl I: Bone mass in postmenopausal women after withdrawal of oestrogen/gestagen replacement therapy. *Lancet* 1981, 1:459–461.

15. Cauley JA, Seeley DG, Enstrud K, *et al.*: for the Study of Osteoporotic Fractures Research Group. Estrogen replacement therapy and fractures in older women. *Ann Intern Med* 1995, 122:9–16.

16. Stampfer MJ, Willett WC, Colditz GA, et al.: A prospective study of postmenopausal estrogen therapy and coronary heart disease. N Engl J Med 1985, 313:1044–1049.

17. Wilson PWF, Garrison RJ, Castelli WP: Post-menopausal estrogen use, cigarette smoking, and cardiovascular morbidity in women over 50. N Engl J Med 1985, 313:1038–1043.

18. Bush TL, Barrett-Connor E, Cowan LD, et al.: Cardiovascular mortality and noncontraceptive use of estrogen in women: results from the Lipid Research Clinics Program Follow-up Study. Circulation 1987, 75:1102–1109.

19. Petitti DB, Perlman JA, Sidney S: Noncontraceptive estrogens and mortality: long-term follow-up of women in the Walnut Creek Study. Obstet Gynecol 1987, 70, 289–293.

20. Boysen G, Nyboe J, Appleyard M, et al.: Stroke incidence and risk factors for stroke in Copenhagen, Denmark. Stroke 1988, 19:1345–1353.

21. Criqui MH, Suarez L, Barrett-Connor E, et al.: Postmenopausal estrogen use and mortality. Am J Epidemiol 1988, 128:606–614.

22. Henderson BE, Paganini-Hill A, Ross RK: Estrogen replacement therapy and protection from acute myocardial infarction. Am J Obstet Gynecol 1988, 159:312–317

23. Van der Giezen AM, Schopman-Geurts van Kessel JG, Schouten EG, et al.: Systolic blood pressure and cardiovascular mortality among 13,740 Dutch women. Prev Med 1990, 19:456–465.

24. Wolf PH, Madans JH, Finucane FF, et al.: Reduction of cardiovascular disease-related mortality among postmenopausal women who use hormones: evidence from a national cohort. Am J Obstet Gynecol 1991, 164:489–494.

25. Falkeborn M, Persson I, Adami HO, et al.: The risk of acute myocardial infarction after oestrogen and oestrogen-progestogen replacement. Br J Obstet Gynaecol 1992, 99:821–828.

26. Psaty BM, Heckbert SR, Atkins D, et al.: The risk of myocardial infarction associated with the combined use of estrogens and progestins in postmenopausal women. Arch Intern Med 1994, 154:1333–1339.

27. Folsom AR, Mink PJ, Sellers TA, et al.: Hormonal replacement therapy and morbidity and mortality in a prospective study of postmenopausal women. Am J Public Health 1995, 85:1128–1132.

28. Eaker ED, et al.: Coronary Disease in Women. New York, NY; Haymarket Doyma; 1987, 122–130.

29. Sullivan JM, Vander Zwaag R, et al.: Estrogen replacement and coronary heart disease. Effect on survival in postmenopausal women. Arch Intern Med 1990, 150:2557–2562.

30. The Writing Group for the PEPI Trial: Effects of estrogen or estrogen/ progestin regimens on heart disease risk factors in postmenopausal women. JAMA 1995, 273:199–208.

31. Armstrong BK: Oestrogen therapy after the menopause: boon or bane? Med J Austr 1988, 148:213–214.

32. DuPont WD, Page DL: Menopausal estrogen replacement therapy and breast cancer. Arch Int Med 1991, 67–72.

33. Steinberg KK, Thacker SB, Smith SJ, et al.: A meta-analysis of the effect of estrogen replacement therapy on the risk of breast cancer. JAMA 1991, 265:1985–1990.

34. Sillero-Arenas M, Delgado-Rodriguez M, Rodrigues-Canteras R, et al.: Menopausal hormone replacement therapy and breast cancer: a meta-analysis. Obstet Gynecol 1992, 79:286–294.

35. Colditz GA, Egan KM, Stampfer MJ: Hormone replacement therapy and risk of breast cancer: results from epidemiologic studies. Am J Obstet Gynecol 1993, 168:1473–1478.

36. Grady D, Rubin SM, Petitti DB, et al.: Hormone therapy to prevent disease and prolong life in postmenopausal women. Ann Intern Med 1992, 117:1016–1037.

37. Bergkvist L, Adami HO, Persson I, et al.: Prognosis after breast cancer diagnosis in women exposed to estrogen and estrogen-progestogen replacement therapy. Am J Epidemiol 1992, 130:221–228.

38. Hunt K, Vessey M, McPherson K: Mortality in a cohort of long-term users of hormone replacement therapy: an updated analysis. Br J Obstet Gynaecol 1990, 97:1080–1086.

39. Henderson BE, Paganini-Hill A, Ross RK: Decreased mortality in users of estrogen replacement therapy. Arch Intern Med 1991, 151:75–78.

40. Colditz GA, Hankinson SE, Hunter DJ, et al.: The use of estrogens and progestins and the risk of breast cancer in postmenopausal women. N Engl J Med 1995, 332:1589–1593.

41. Willis DB, Calle EE, Miracle-McMahill HL, et al.: Estrogen replacement therapy and risk of fatal breast cancer in a prospective cohort of postmenopausal women in the United States. Cancer Causes Control 1996, 7:449–457.

42. Brenner DE, Kukull WA, Stergachis A, et al.: Postmenopausal estrogen replacement therapy and the risk of Alzheimer's disease: a population-based case-control study. Am J Epidemiol 1994, 140:262–267.

43. Paganini-Hill A, Henderson VW. Estrogen replacement therapy and risk of Alzheimer disease. Arch Intern Med 1996, 156:2213–2217.

44. Lerner AJ, et al.: 26th Annual Meeting of the Society of Neuroscience, Washington DC, 1996.

45. Tang MX, et al.: Effect of estrogen during menopause on risk and age of onset of Alzeimer's disease. Lancet 1996, 348:429-432.

46. Kawas C, Resnick S, Morrison A, et al.: A prospective study of estrogen replacement therapy and the risk of developing Alzheimer's disease: the Baltimore Longitudinal Study of Aging. Neurology 1997, 48:1517–1521.

47. Ziel HK, Finkel WD. Increased risk of endometrial carcinoma among users of conjugated estrogens. N Engl J Med 1975, 293:1165–1170.

48. Smith DC, Prentice R, Thompson DJ, et al.: Association of exogenous estrogen and endometrial carcinoma. N Engl J Med 1975, 293:1164–1167.

49. Persson I, Yuen J, Bergkvist L, et al.: Cancer incidence and mortality in women receiving estrogen and estrogen-progestin replacement therapy: long-term follow-up of a Swedish cohort. Int J Cancer 1996, 67:327-332.

50. Genant HK, Lucas J, Weiss S, et al.: Low-dose esterified estrogen therapy. Effects on bone, plasma estradiol concentrations, endometrium, and lipid levels. Arch Intern Med 1997, 157:2609–2615.

51. Delmas PD, Bjarnason NH, Mitlak BH, et al.: Effects of raloxifene on bone mineral density, serum cholesterol concentrations, and uterine endometrium in postmenopausal women. N Engl J Med 1997, 337:1641–1647.

52. Merck Research Laboratories: Early Post-menopausal Intervention Cohort (EPIC) results presented to Food and Drug Administration.

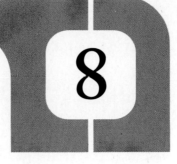

# OSTEOPOROSIS IN MEN

## *Robert F. Klein*

Although long recognized as a disease of women, osteoporosis also has an important impact on men. Only recently has the magnitude of the problem of osteoporosis in men been recognized, and few data exist concerning the character and cause of osteoporosis. Epidemiologic data indicate that one in seven 50-year-old white men will experience an osteoporotic fracture during his remaining lifetime. As such, osteoporosis in men represents a serious public health problem. Osteoporosis is similar in many ways to that in women but exhibits unique features and clinical challenges.

Bone mass decreases with advancing age regardless of gender, leading to an increased risk of skeletal fracture. In many ways the skeletal changes in men parallel those in women; however, it is likely that several differences influence the presentation of this disorder in men. During puberty diverging growth trends result in obvious gender differences in peak skeletal development. Most skeletal dimensions in men are larger than those in women. As a result, total body bone mineral is approximately 20% greater in men than in women. The larger size of the bones of men adds greatly to their strength, and the gender differences in peak bone mass and size in part underlie the differences in fracture patterns between men and women that emerge later in life. Changes in bone mineral density (BMD) are not particularly different between men and women. Differences in the nature of structural changes with aging between men and women, however, may have important biomechanical consequences because the load bearing of bone specimens appears to be better-preserved in men.

The incidence of skeletal fractures is biphasic in men. Early in life fracture occurrence is actually higher in men than women, probably as a result of serious trauma. Between the ages of 40 to 50 years the trend reverses and fractures become more common in women. Later, the incidence of fractures increases in men over the age of 60 years, reflecting an increasing prevalence of skeletal fragility. The cause of age-related bone loss in men is unclear. Both increased osteoclastic and reduced osteoblastic activities have been postulated to occur; however, the relative participation of each is unknown. Dietary calcium insufficiency, alterations in vitamin D metabolism, an age-related decrease in sex steroid levels, and relative inactivity may all play a role. Additional conditions may secondarily accelerate bone loss in men, including alcohol and tobacco abuse, glucocorticoid therapy, hypogonadism, and hypercalciuria. The prevalence of these conditions in men with osteoporosis is unclear. Various biochemical markers of bone remodeling have been related to BMD in both healthy men and those with osteoporosis; however, use of these markers as diagnostic tools requires further investigation.

In men who exhibit findings suggestive of the presence of reduced bone mass (*ie*, low-trauma fractures, radiographic criteria of osteopenia, or conditions associated with bone loss), measurement of bone mass (or density) should be strongly considered. Bone mass determinations in men can be used to confirm the diagnosis of low bone mass, gauge its severity, and serve as a baseline from which to judge the progression or improvement of disease. If a man is found to be osteopenic, an evaluation should be performed to determine the cause of the disorder with reasonable certainty. The history, physical examination, and routine laboratory studies can be helpful in directing the focus of the evaluation of a man with low bone mass. It is appropriate to be aggressive diagnostically when no clear pathophysiology is identified, primarily because the potential for occult secondary causes of osteoporosis may be higher in men.

Therapy for osteoporotic disorders in men is virtually unexplored and, in the United States, no approved pharmacologic therapies exist for osteoporosis in men. Recommendations therefore must come from assumptions based on the much larger knowledge base in women. Treatment options for men with osteoporosis include agents to slow bone resorption and augment bone formation. Any of the medical conditions associated with excessive bone loss should be specifically addressed to prevent and treat osteoporosis.

In summary, osteoporosis in men is a common disorder and its incidence is increasing. Despite the considerable public health burden attributable to this disease, our understanding of its pathogenesis is incomplete and no established treatment exists for osteoporosis in men. Many clinical decisions must be based on extrapolations from the more complete understanding of osteoporosis in women. Within these constraints, however, it is possible to formulate an approach that is effective in men with osteoporosis. Osteoporosis in men presents a unique array of scientific challenges and opportunities and deserves the same vigorous evaluation as that applied to postmenopausal osteoporosis.

# Incidence and Risk

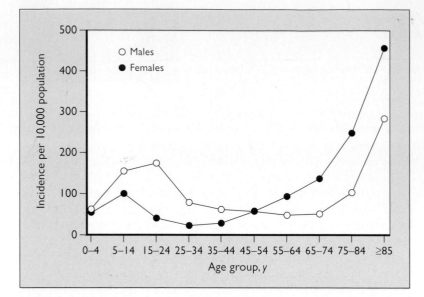

**FIGURE 8-1.** Fracture incidence rate by age group and gender. In women, the relationships between fractures and bone mass, propensity for falls, and other risk factors have become increasingly well defined. In men, less information is available regarding the causation of fracture; hence, the current understanding of osteoporosis epidemiology is limited primarily to fracture patterns [1]. From adolescence through midlife the incidence of all fractures is higher in men than in women, and the personal and economic impact (in terms of hospitalizations and lost work days) of these early-life fractures is enormous. Despite the importance of early-life fractures in men, little has been done to understand their cause. Many result from serious trauma; however, to some extent, relative bone fragility also may contribute to fracture risk during this period. For instance, men who have sustained traumatic tibial or forearm fractures in early midlife are at much greater risk for hip fracture later in life [2,3]. A reversal of this trend occurs between 40 and 50 years of age, with fractures in general and those of the pelvis, humerus, forearm, and femur in particular becoming much more common in women. However, the incidence of fractures resulting from minimal to moderate trauma (particularly the hip and spine) also increases rapidly with aging in men and reflects an increasing prevalence of skeletal fragility.

## ESTIMATED LIFETIME FRACTURE RISK* IN WHITE WOMEN AND MEN AGED 50 YEARS

| Fracture Site | Women | Men |
|---|---|---|
| Proximal femur | 17.5 (16.8–18.2) | 6.0 (5.6–6.5) |
| Vertebra† | 15.6 (14.8–16.3) | 5.0 (4.6–5.4) |
| Distal forearm | 16.0 (15.7–16.7) | 2.5 (2.2–3.1) |
| Any of the above | 39.7 (38.7–40.6) | 13.1 (12.4–13.7) |

*95% confidence intervals
†clinically diagnosed fractures

**FIGURE 8-2.** Risk of an osteoporotic fracture from aged 50 years. The lifetime risk of sustaining an osteoporotic fracture of the hip, spine, or wrist for a 50 year-old man is about one third of that in women (13% *vs* 39%) [4]. The incidence of hip fracture increases exponentially in men with aging, as it does in women. However, the age at which the increase begins is slightly older (approximately 5–10 years) in men. Because there are fewer older men than women, the absolute number of hip fractures tends to be proportionately less in men. However, it is estimated that about 30% of the two million hip fractures worldwide occur in men. Vertebral fracture also is an important sequel of osteoporosis in men. As in women, the presence of vertebral fracture in men is associated with loss of height, kyphosis, increased risk of other fractures, and increased disability. Previously considered uncommon in men in the United States, recent information suggests that the incidence of osteoporotic vertebral fracture in men is about half that in women [5]. Vertebral bone mineral density values are reduced in men with vertebral fractures compared with those in the control group without fracture. This fact indicates that vertebral fracture in men is not merely the result of a higher rate of trauma but also is related to the presence of low bone mass. Fractures occur primarily in low thoracic vertebrae in men but are found at all levels. Most fractures are anterior compression in type, with vertebral crush fractures occurring less frequently than is reported in women. Vertebral epiphysitis (Scheuermann disease) is an uncommon cause of significant vertebral deformity in men. The incidence of forearm fractures increases markedly in aging women but remains relatively stable throughout life in men. (*From* Melton, *et al.* [4]; with permission.)

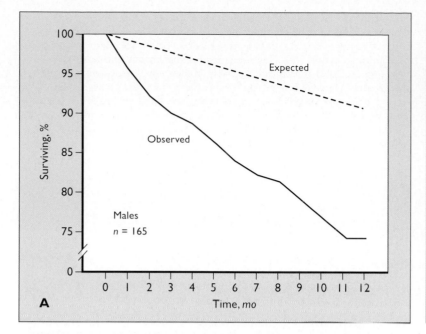

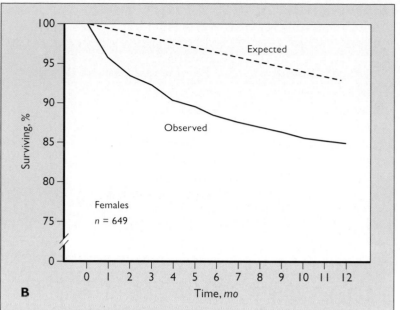

**FIGURE 8-3.** Survival of women and men after hip fracture. Men who present with hip fracture usually are elderly and fragile and have multiple pre-existing medical conditions [6]. In men (**A**), hip fracture results in significant functional decline and a threefold higher postfracture mortality rate compared with aged-matched women (**B**) [7]. These facts highlight the need to identify men with osteoporosis in the community and find effective strategies for preventing hip fracture. (*From* Diamond, *et al.* [6] and Magaziner, *et al.* [7].)

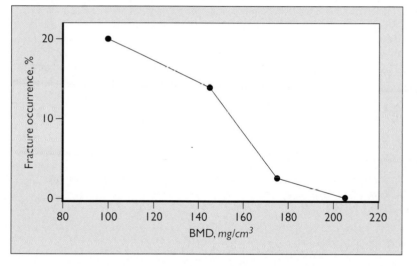

**FIGURE 8-4.** Fracture occurrence in men with different bone densities. Substantial evidence exists that in a postmenopausal elderly white woman, low bone mass is associated with increased risk of fracture. A single bone density measurement at any commonly assessed appendicular or axial site predicts the overall risk of fractures in white women. Although data are scant in men, accumulating evidence suggests a similar inverse relationship of bone mass to fracture. Shown here are the results of a 5-year study investigating the predictive value of baseline calcaneal bone mineral density (BMD) on fracture occurrence at any skeletal site in a cohort of elderly men [8]. As in women the gradient of increasing fracture risk with decreasing bone mass in men appears to be continuous. Based on available data the fracture risk increases about twofold for every one standard deviation below the young normal mean BMD, which is similar to the risk increase in women. (*From* Cheng, *et al.* [8].)

## FACTORS ASSOCIATED WITH HIP FRACTURES IN MEN

| Metabolic Disorders | Movement and Balance Disorders |
|---|---|
| Thyroidectomy | Alcoholism |
| Gastrectomy | Anemia |
| Pernicious anemia | Blindness |
| Chronic respiratory diseases | Neurologic diseases: |
| Lean body mass | Hemiparesis |
| | Hemiplegia |
| | Parkinsonism dementia |
| | Other |
| | Use of cane or walker |
| | Vertigo |

**FIGURE 8-5.** Factors associated with hip fractures in men. As in women, there is overlap of bone density in men with fractures and the control group without fracture, indicating that bone density is not the sole determinant of osteoporotic fracture risk. Fracture is a somewhat chance event, and the propensity to fall is an important variable. In men, few prospective data exist that directly relate fall propensity to subsequent fractures; however, a variety of factors indirectly related to the risk of falling have been related to hip fracture. Many of these differences suggest a body habitus and lifestyle more conducive to falls and injury and the possibility of other interacting risk factors such as nutritional deficiencies and comorbidities.

# Bone Mass Density and Structure

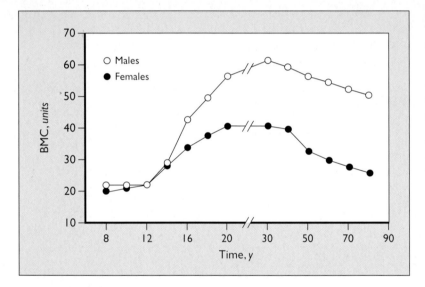

**FIGURE 8-6.** Changes in bone mass with growth and aging in men and women. Both men and women exhibit a dramatic increase in bone mass that begins during adolescence and is almost complete when puberty ends. A lifetime peak is reached in both men and women at about 20 to 30 years. By the fourth or fifth decade, men and women begin an age-related process of gradual bone loss that continues throughout the remainder of life. This age-related decrease in bone mass results from an excess of bone resorption over bone formation, the causes of which are not well understood. Women experience an accelerated phase of bone loss lasting 5 to 15 years that is a result of the relatively abrupt decline in gonadal function occurring with menopause. In contrast to the clearly demarcated event of menopause in women, the reproductive changes that take place in men as they age are more subtle. Acceleration occurs in the rate of bone loss in elderly men (>50 years), which most likely also is a result of reductions in sex steroid levels. At any given time, bone mass depends on the peak bone mass achieved in adolescence and subsequent bone loss. BMC—bone mineral content. (*Adapted from* Nevitt [9].)

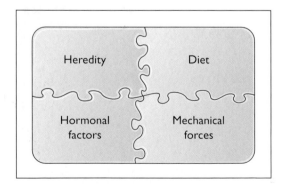

**FIGURE 8-7.** Determinants of peak bone mass in men. Peak bone mass is the major determinant of osteoporotic fracture risk up to the age of approximately 65 years, when factors such as age-related bone loss become relatively more important. Hence, the failure to achieve optimal peak bone mass is an important pathogenetic mechanism in osteoporosis in both men and women. Although comparatively little attention has been paid over the years to the determinants of peak bone mass in men, heredity, dietary components (calcium and protein), endocrine factors (sex steroids, calcitriol, and insulin-like growth factor-I), and mechanical forces (physical activity and body weight) all have been shown to have an influence. As in women, the most prominent determinant appears to be genetically related; however, the precise genes involved remain to be elucidated.

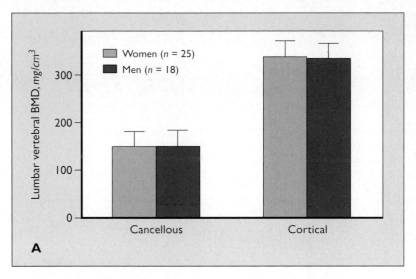

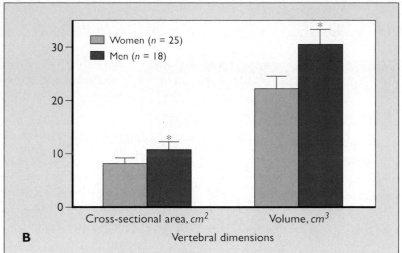

**FIGURE 8-8.** Gender differences in bone size and density. In early childhood, few discernible differences can be observed between the skeletons of boys and girls; however, as the skeleton matures during puberty, obvious sexual differences in bone morphology emerge [10–12]. Most skeletal dimensions in men are larger than are those in women. As a result, total body bone mineral is greater in men (2300–2700 g in young women *vs* 3100–3500 g in young men). Although maximal adult bone mineral density (BMD) also is frequently reported to be greater in men, this result is primarily an artefact of the measurement methods used. For instance, adult vertebral BMD determined by quantitative computed tomography (QCT), which is a true volumetric assessment, is alike in men and women (**A**). Whereas vertebral density by measures of area (eg, dual photon absorptiometry [DPA] or dual-energy X-ray absorptiometry [DXA]) appears to reach slightly higher levels in men, this apparent advantage disappears (or is even slightly reversed) once those values are corrected for differences in vertebral dimensions. The adolescent development of adult bone mass depends on changes in both density and size, with increases in size being quantitatively much more important. From the time of puberty on, mean vertebral cross-sectional area is 15% to 25% greater in men and tubular bones exhibit greater total and cortical widths in early adulthood (**B**). The larger size of bones in men adds greatly to their strength, and the sex differences in peak bone mass and partly size underlie the differences in fracture patterns that emerge later in life. *$P < 0.0001$. (*Adapted from* Gilsanz et al. [11].)

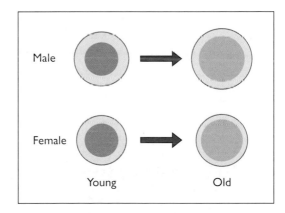

**FIGURE 8-9.** Gender differences in age-related changes in cortical bone. Bone loss occurs with aging in men as it does in women; however, gender differences in the pattern of age-related bone loss affect eventual fracture risk. Both men and women experience an increase in porosity, although the rate is somewhat slower in men. This increase results in a reduction in density and mechanical strength, thereby increasing fracture risk. However, the decrease in mass to some extent is compensated by changes in cortical dimensions. An age-related increase in total cortical width exists in men and women. This change is beneficial because fracture resistance is dependent on geometry. The rate of cortical loss is very similar in both men and women; however, periosteal apposition is somewhat greater in men and endocortical loss somewhat less, mitigating the loss of thickness and overall mass [13,14]. The typical pattern of age-related change observed in cross sections of long bones is depicted. Men and women experience cortical thinning; however, men undergo compensatory increases in section breadth to a greater degree than do women. Because the tensile resistance of a long bone to fracture is exponentially related to its diameter, the morphologic changes are in accord with the fracture patterns observed in the elderly, in whom the rate of appendicular fractures is less in men than women. (*Adapted from* Beck et al. [13].)

# Causes

## DIFFERENTIAL DIAGNOSIS OF OSTEOPOROSIS IN MEN

Primary
  Idiopathic cause
  Senility
Secondary
  Alcoholism
  Anticonvulsants
  Gastrointestinal disorders
  Glucocorticoid excess
  Homocystinuria
  Hypercalciuria
  Hypogonadism
  Immobilization
  Neoplastic diseases
  Osteogenesis imperfecta
  Rheumatoid arthritis
  Smoking
  Systemic mastocytosis
  Thyrotoxicosis

**FIGURE 8-10.**  Osteoporosis in men is a heterogeneous condition, encompassing a wide variety of causes and clinical presentations. In practice, it is not uncommon to identify several potential explanations for bone loss and fractures in a single patient. The principal conditions found in men with reduced bone mass are presented. Prominent are glucocorticoid excess, hypogonadism, alcoholism, gastrectomy and other gastro-intestinal disorders, and hypercalciuria. Similar attempts to examine the contributing factors in women with osteoporosis suggest that the spectrum of disorders is somewhat different; however, glucocorticoid excess, premature hypogonadism, and gastrointestinal disorders are prominent in women as well. It has been suggested that the number of men with "secondary" osteoporosis is higher than in women. However, in other objective evaluations the proportion of women with major illnesses contributing to the development of bone disease is very similar to that observed in men with osteoporosis.

## REPRESENTATIVE CAUSES OF HYPOGONADISM IN MEN

| Primary | Secondary |
|---|---|
| Alcohol consumption | Alcohol consumption |
| Castration | Craniopharyngioma |
| Cryptorchidism | Glucocorticoids |
| Hyperprolactinemia | Gonadotropin-releasing hormone agonists |
| Klinefelter syndrome | Hemochromatosis |
| Orchitis: | Kallman syndrome |
|   Infiltrative diseases | Pituitary tumor |
|   Leprosy | Specific genetic syndromes: |
|   Mumps |   Laurence-Moon-Biedl syndrome |
|   Radiation exposure |   Prader-Willi syndrome |
| Chemotherapy |   Other rarer disorders |
| Trauma | |

**FIGURE 8-11.**  Sex steroids have major influences on the regulation of bone metabolism. The obvious importance of menopause to osteoporosis drew early attention to the role of estrogen. More recently, both clinical and basic observations have also highlighted the importance of androgens in bone physiology. Androgens influence osteoblast proliferation, growth factor and cytokine production, and bone-matrix protein production by way of skeletal androgen receptors. The causes of primary (testicular failure) and secondary (defective gonadotrophin elaboration and secretion) hypergonadism are shown.

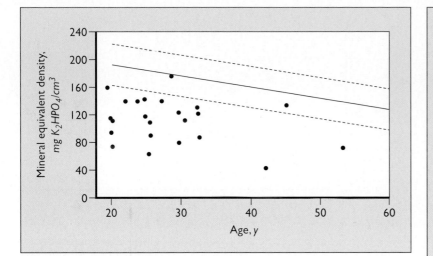

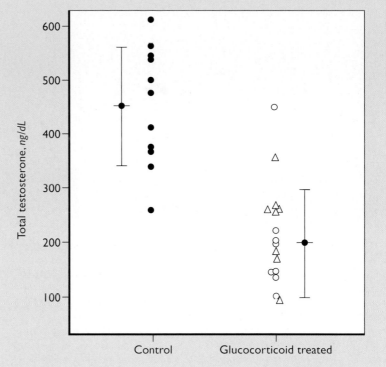

**FIGURE 8-12.** Hypogonadism and osteopenia in men. Because puberty is very important in skeletal maturation, disorders of puberty have the potential to impair peak bone mass development and thus influence fracture risk throughout adulthood. Supporting the importance of androgen action in the achievement of peak bone mass in men is the fact that genetic males with complete androgen insensitivity (testicular feminization) experience increased pubertal growth but achieve a bone mass typical of genetic women [15]. Reduced bone mass is found in men who experienced an abnormal puberty (Klinefelter and Kallmann syndromes), and even constitutionally delayed puberty is associated with permanent reductions in bone density. The results of a study by Finkelstein and colleagues [16] are shown, who examined spinal trabecular bone mineral density in 23 men with idiopathic hypogonadotrophic hypogonadism. Androgens also appear to be essential for the maintenance of bone mass in adult men because the development of hypogonadism in mature men is associated with low bone mass. Hypogonadism is present in up to one third of men evaluated for vertebral fractures and osteoporosis, and hip fractures in elderly men apparently occur more commonly in the setting of hypogonadism. Reduced bone mass and fractures are associated with many forms of hypogonadism, including castration, hyperprolactinemia, anorexia, and hemochromatosis. The degree of reduction in bone density has been correlated with levels of serum testosterone in some series; however, in other studies no association between the two variables is apparent. A threshold level of serum testosterone may exist below which skeletal health is impaired. At present, however, it is not possible to establish that hypothesis. (*From* Finkelstein, *et al.* [16]; with permission.)

**FIGURE 8-13.** Glucocorticoid-induced hypogonadism. In addition to the link between primary testicular dysfunction and low bone mass, reduction in gonadal function secondary to several other medical conditions (*eg*, glucocorticoid excess and renal insufficiency) is now postulated to contribute to the development of bone loss. The pathologic mechanisms responsible for the markedly reduced testosterone levels observed in men with these conditions have not been fully defined. These mechanisms may include central inhibition of release of gonadotropin-releasing hormone (Gn-RH), suppression of pituitary sensitivity to Gn-RH, and direct antagonism of testicular steroidogenesis. In men, impotence and loss of libido frequently occur in these clinical settings and are attributed to the effects of the chronic illness. However, these symptoms may actually be due to the disease-related hypogonadism, which in turn may contribute substantially to the resulting low bone mass. Clinicians who care for men with osteoporosis should be aware of this phenomenon and recognize it as an important cause of a low serum testosterone level. Reproduced here are the results from a study by MacAdams and colleagues [17] in which total testosterone levels were determined in 11 men with chronic obstructive pulmonary disease used as controls and 16 age- and disease-matched men receiving chronic glucocorticoid therapy. (*From* MacAdams, *et al.* [17]; with permission.)

## CHANGES IN BONE METABOLISM AFTER CASTRATION IN MEN

| Parameter | Normal | Orchidectomy |
|---|---|---|
| Serum testosterone, *nmol/L* | 19.4 ± 7.6 | 1.6 ± 1.1* |
| Bone formation: | | |
| Serum osteocalcin, *mg/L* | 5.0 ± 1.6 | 12.1 ± 2.8* |
| Bone-specific alkaline phosphatase, *U/L* | 10.2 ± 2.3 | 20.4 ± 3.2* |
| Bone resorption: | | |
| Serum tartrate–resistant acid phosphatase, *U/L* | 4.33 ± 0.7 | 6.51 ± 1.0* |
| Urine hydroxyproline/creatinine, *mmol/mol* | 16.2 ± 2.8 | 27.7 ± 5.8* |
| Bone mineral density, $g/cm^2$ | 0.94 ± 0.14 | 0.83 ± 0.15* |

**FIGURE 8-14.** Effects of hypogonadism on male skeletal physiology. The histologic pattern of hypogonadal bone loss in adult men is inadequately described. A single report examines skeletal metabolism in the period immediately after gonadal failure. Stepan and colleagues [18] studied a small group of men in the years immediately after castration. These men were found to lose bone rapidly (approximately 7% per year) and to have clear biochemical indications of increased bone remodeling (increased serum osteocalcin levels and urinary hydroxyproline excretion). Unfortunately, no direct histomorphometric analyses were reported. Thus, no firm conclusions can be drawn concerning the remodeling defect induced by hypogonadism in men. The early increase in remodeling after androgen withdrawal, however, is consistent with recent reports of the biochemical and cellular events associated with androgen action (a suppression of cytokine production and osteoclast formation) [19]. *Significantly different from normal (*P* < 0.01). (*Adapted from* Stepan, *et al.* [18]; with permission.)

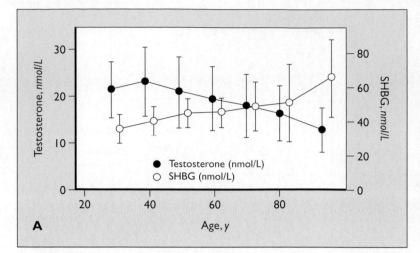

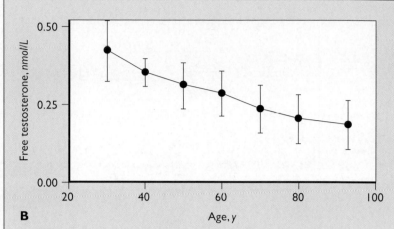

**FIGURE 8-15.** Testosterone levels decrease in aging men. The reproductive changes that take place in men as they age occur over a long period of time. These changes are more gradual than are the profound changes in gonadal function that occur in women at menopause. A decrease in total testosterone levels with aging has been reported in many but not all studies of normal healthy men (**A**). Most studies have reported a greater decrease in bioavailable testosterone rather than in total testosterone concentrations with age in men [20] (**B**). This fact is explained mainly by an age-related increase in the binding capacity of sex hormone–binding globulin (SHBG). The increase in SHBG is likely multifactorial in origin. Hepatic SHBG production is stimulated by estrogen and inhibited by insulin. Increased SHBG levels therefore may be a result of reduced insulin secretion and peripheral insulin sensitivity commonly observed in the elderly or a consequence of increased aromatization of androstenedione to estrone in peripheral (principally adipose) tissue known to occur in older men. Although great interindividual variability is observed in free testosterone levels with advancing age, it is estimated that nearly half of men over the age of 50 years have a free testosterone level below the lowest level seen in men under aged 40.

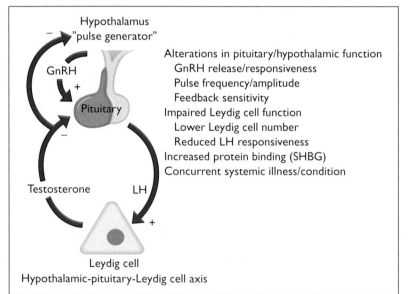

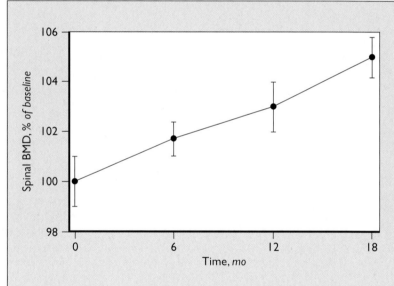

**FIGURE 8-16.** Causes of the decrease in testosterone concentrations in aging men. Primary testicular factors (*eg*, impaired testicular perfusion and decreased Leydig cell number) undoubtedly play a major role in the age-dependent decrease in plasma testosterone levels. However, perturbations in central mechanisms also contribute. In elderly men with clinical and biologic signs of hypoandrogenism, the expected increase in luteinizing hormone (LH) levels is much less pronounced than that observed in younger men with hypogonadism. The mechanism for the blunted response to diminished androgen feedback inhibition in older men is unknown; however, alterations at the hypothalamic or pituitary level are presumed. *Plus signs* indicate positive influence; *minus signs* indicate negative influence. GNRH—gonadotropin-releasing hormone.

**FIGURE 8-17.** Impact of testosterone replacement therapy on bone density. The effectiveness of androgen replacement therapy in men with hypogonadism is unclear. Several reports have suggested that androgen replacement therapy may have beneficial effects on bone mass, at least in the short term. For example, in the study shown here, mean spinal bone mineral density (BMD) increased by 5% ($P < 0.001$) in a group of 36 men with acquired hypogonadism [21]. However, it is not certain that all men respond or whether other factors (*eg*, age and duration of hypogonadism) influence the success of treatment. Moreover, all studies that suggest a beneficial effect of androgen therapy are of short duration (1–5 y), and it is uncertain whether a sustained increase in bone mass occurs with therapy or whether bone mass ever reaches eugonadal levels. In addition, the minimal effective dose of androgen is not known. Of great importance is that the potential risks of androgen replacement therapy, particularly in the elderly, are uncertain in relation to the possible skeletal benefits to be gained. Nevertheless, the concern of bone loss and fractures should represent one of the indications for androgen therapy in gonadal failure.

## TESTOSTERONE DELIVERY SYSTEMS

Parenteral:

17β-esters: cypionate, enanthate, and proprionate

Transdermal:

Scrotal (Testoderm; Alza Corp., Palo Alto, CA)

Nongenital (AndroDerm, SmithKline Beecham, Philadelphia, PA; Testoderm)

**FIGURE 8-18.** Androgen replacement therapy is available in injectable, oral, and transdermal dosage forms. Knowledge of the individual merits and drawbacks of currently available testosterone preparations is necessary when treating patients with hypogonadism. For oral administration, testosterone is alkylated at the 17α-position to prevent metabolism in the gastrointestinal tract and to prolong its duration of action once it is absorbed. Unfortunately, because of erratic absorption and well-recognized hepatic toxicity (cholestatic hepatitis and hepatocellular carcinoma), oral testosterone is used infrequently. Injectable forms of testosterone are esterified at the 17β-hydroxyl position to prolong their *in vivo* activity. Injectable preparations (testosterone cypionate, enanthate, or proprionate) generally are well tolerated and remain the gold standard for effectiveness. Disadvantages of this form of testosterone delivery include the need for periodic intramuscular administration and supraphysiologic activity in the first few days after administration that is followed by a noticeable decrease toward the end of the cycle. More recently, skin-patch formulations have been developed that enable transdermal delivery of native unmodified testosterone. Transdermal delivery circumvents the wide fluctuations in testosterone concentrations produced by intramuscular administration and more closely mimics the normal circadian rhythm of testosterone concentrations.

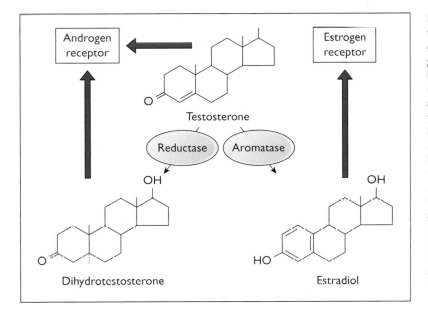

**FIGURE 8-19.** Metabolic conversion of testosterone. Once synthesized, testosterone can be converted either to dihydrotestosterone by 5α-reductase or to estrogen by aromatase, a member of the microsomal cytochrome P450 group of enzymes. Both testosterone and dihydrotestosterone are capable of binding to and activating androgen receptors in osteoblasts. However, estrogen receptors are at least equally abundant in these cell lines and aromatase activity also is present in these cells. These observations raise the intriguing possibility that, in addition to androgens, estrogens are also of major importance for skeletal health in men. Recent case reports of osteoporosis in men with genetic disorders resulting in either defective aromatase activity or nonfunctioning estrogen receptors have called attention to the importance of estrogens in skeletal growth [22–25]. Convincing evidence that estrogen is essential for the establishment of peak bone mass in growing boys comes from the demonstration that although testosterone therapy produces no benefit, replacement of estrogen in men with inactivating aromatase genes mutations (and consequently lifelong estrogen deficiency) results in skeletal maturation with increased bone mass and epiphyseal closure [23,24]. Estrogens also may play an important role in the maintenance of bone mass in adult men. A number of epidemiologic studies have shown that the slow age-related decrease in bone mass in men is more directly related to declining estrogen concentrations than to declining androgen concentrations [26–28].

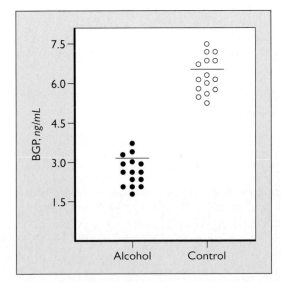

**FIGURE 8-20.** Alcohol consumption inhibits osteoblast function. Reduced bone mass is evident on routine radiographs in a significant percentage (25%–50%) of persons whose drinking habits have prompted them to seek medical help. The degree to which bone disease is present in the entire population of alcoholics remains uncertain, and determination of the true incidence of alcohol-induced reductions in bone mass in men must await a survey of a large number of cases. The habitual consumption of alcoholic beverages, however, clearly is recognized as a significant negative determinant of bone mass in epidemiologic surveys and in longitudinal studies has been shown to be associated with increased rates of bone loss [29]. Although a definite relationship exists between alcohol abuse and bone disease, the mechanisms by which alcohol induces bone disease remain unclear. Microscopic examination of bone (bone histomorphometry) from patients who are alcoholics reveals considerable suppression of osteoblastic bone formation, whereas indices of osteoclastic bone resorption activity for the most part do not differ substantially from that observed in a control group [30]. Further evidence implicating a direct effect of ethanol on osteoblast activity comes from studies examining the effects of ethanol on circulating osteocalcin levels. Osteocalcin is a small peptide synthesized by active osteoblasts. As depicted, patients who are chronic alcoholics exhibit significantly lower osteocalcin levels than do age-matched controls, and alcohol consumption acutely depresses circulating osteocalcin levels [31]. These biochemical and histomorphometric findings argue strongly that a primary target of the adverse effects of ethanol on the skeleton is the osteoblast. Because bone remodeling and mineralization are dependent on osteoblasts, it follows that a deleterious effect of alcohol on these cells will ultimately lead to reduced bone mass and fractures. BGP—bone Gla protein (osteocalcin).

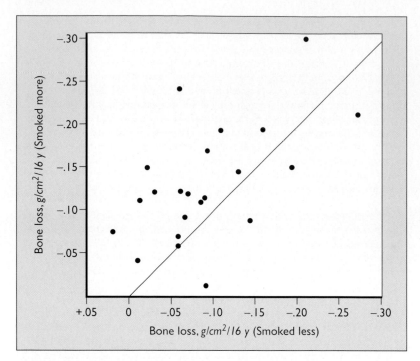

**FIGURE 8-21.** Accelerated bone loss in cigarette smokers. Tobacco use is associated with lowered bone mass and fractures in women. Tobacco use also is linked to an increased prevalence of vertebral and hip fractures in men. In support of this observation, Slemenda and colleagues [29] have examined the adverse effects of smoking on bone health in men by measuring rates of bone loss over 16 years in members of twin pairs who differed in cigarette-smoking behavior. As depicted here, the smokers lost more bone than did their nonsmoking twins. The mechanism by which smoking affects bone in men is unclear. In women, tobacco use has been associated with lower weight, lower calcium absorption, and lower estrogen levels, all of which are negatively associated with bone mass. Alternatively, smoking may either impair respiratory function, and hence bone metabolism, or exert a direct toxic effect on bone metabolism. No data are available concerning the effects of tobacco use in other forms (chewing and snuff). Whether smoking adversely affects sex steroid levels or other potential effectors of bone remodeling in men is unknown.

## CAUSES OF GASTROINTESTINAL BONE DISEASE

Decreased intake of vitamin D or calcium

Inadequate contact between nutrients and their absorptive sites:

　Altered anatomy

　Rapid transit

Inadequate sunlight exposure

Malabsorption of vitamin D or calcium

**FIGURE 8-22.** In men and women, disorders of gastrointestinal function have been associated with skeletal disease, frequently as a result of malabsorption of calcium, vitamin D, or other nutrients. In men, a particularly striking relationship has been observed between gastrectomy and vertebral osteoporosis. Similarly, bone disease commonly results from a variety of small bowel disorders. Large bowel disorders rarely are associated with low bone mass. The cause of gastro-intestinal bone disease remains unclear. Proposed causes are listed. A single functional lesion that results in bone disease in most patients has not been convincingly demonstrated, although classic vitamin D deficiency and osteomalacia are most commonly associated with frank malabsorption.

## RENAL DISORDERS AND OSTEOPOROSIS IN MEN

Dent disease

Hypercalciuria

　Absorptive

　Renal

Medullary sponge kidney disease

Phosphate leak

Renal tubular acidosis

**FIGURE 8-23.** Hypercalciuric disorders have been linked to a reduction in bone mineral density in men. It is not clear whether this apparent increase in bone disease in men is a result of a greater impact of hypercalciuria or merely reflects the fact that hypercalciuria is more than twice as common in men than women. The cause of the low bone mass observed in persons with hypercalciuria is unclear but has been postulated to involve an alteration in mineral metabolism. Somewhat surprisingly, osteopenia has been reported in patients with absorptive hypercalciuria. In this setting, it is likely that increased 1,25-dihydroxy vitamin D levels increase bone resorption. Both absorptive and resorptive hypercalciuria are associated with an absolute increase in vitamin D bioactivity, leading to more pronounced trabecular rather than cortical bone loss. In contrast, renal hypercalciuria is associated with a negative calcium balance and secondary hyperparathyroidism (including increased 1,25-dihydroxyvitamin D levels), leading to more cortical rather than trabecular bone loss. This hypothesis is supported by the finding that lower dietary calcium intakes in men with renal hypercalciuria are associated with further reductions in bone mass. However, in some patients, hypercalciuria may be only part of a more diffuse metabolic abnormality that affects bone metabolism in other ways. For instance, renal tubular acidosis may be present with hypercalciuria and low bone mass in the presence of complex abnormalities of mineral and bone metabolism. Hypercalciuria also has been linked to phosphate-wasting disorders causing low bone mass, and medullary sponge kidney is not uncommonly associated with increased urinary calcium excretion and disordered parathyroid function.

# Diagnosis and Evaluation

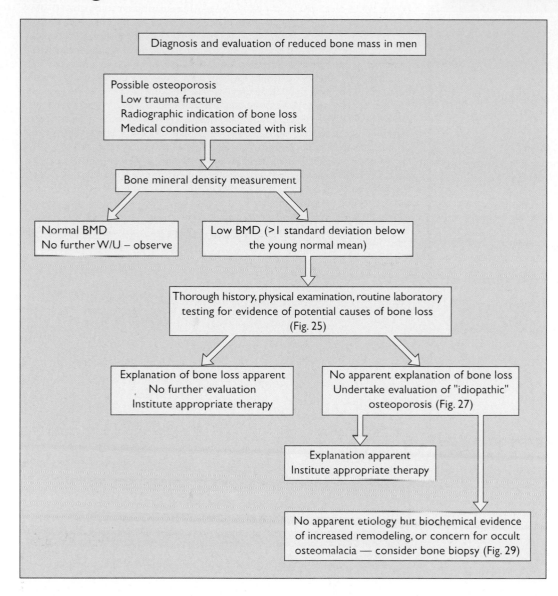

**FIGURE 8-24.** Diagnostic schema for men with suspected osteoporosis. Guidelines for the most efficient cost-effective approach for evaluating patients with low bone mass or suspected of having low bone mass are poorly validated for men and women. Recommendations therefore must be based on existing knowledge of disease epidemiology and clinical characteristics, rather than on models carefully tested in prospective studies. Within these constraints it is possible to formulate an approach to men with osteoporosis. In some men (as in women) the diagnosis of an osteopenic metabolic bone disease can be made with basic clinical information. Most important is a clear history of low trauma fractures in the absence of evidence of a focal pathologic process (malignancy, infection, and Paget disease). Several clinical situations exist in which the presence of osteoporosis cannot be confidently determined but should be considered likely. In these circumstances, further diagnostic steps are appropriate. These situations include the presence of suspicious fractures, radiographic presence of low bone mass, and conditions known to be associated with increased risk of bone loss. BMD—bone mineral density; W/U—work up.

## ASSESSMENT OF A MAN WITH LOW BONE MASS

History
  Environmental factors
    Alcohol consumption
    Exercise
    Fall frequency
    Smoking cigarettes
  Genetic
    Ethnic background
    Family history
  Medical
    Gastrointestinal disease
    Hypogonadism
    Renal disease
  Nutrition
  Transplantation
  Pharmacologic
    Anticonvulsants
    Calcium
    Glucocorticoids
    Heparin
    Malnutrition
    Thyroid hormone
    Vitamin D intake

Physical Examination
  Gait
  Height
  Hip anatomy
  Spine anatomy (degree of dorsal
    kyphosis and lumbar lordosis)
Laboratory Studies
  Complete blood count
  Creatinine, albumin, calcium, phosphorus,
    and alkaline phosphatase
  Liver function tests
  Bioavailable testosterone
  PTH
  Urinary Calcium

**FIGURE 8-25.** The history, physical, and routine biochemical profile can be very helpful in directing a focused evaluation of a man with low bone mass. At this stage of the evaluation, emphasis is placed on determining the specific diagnosis (What is the cause of the low bone mass, osteoporosis or osteomalacia?) and identification of contributing factors in the genesis of the disorder. Risk factors for osteoporosis are explored, including family history, ethnic background, tobacco and alcohol use, lifelong dietary habits, and physical activity. A history of gastrointestinal or renal disease is elicited. Loss of height and fracture histories also are obtained. Medications that cause bone loss are identified. A history of fall frequency is obtained, and factors that increase the propensity to fall are reviewed. The systems review focuses on conditions that cause secondary osteoporosis (eg, endocrinopathies, immobilization, and malabsorption). The physical examination begins with an accurate measurement of height and includes a detailed examination of the spine and hip. The object of the laboratory examination is to find secondary causes of osteopenia. Routine tests, including levels of serum creatinine, albumin, calcium, phosphorus, alkaline phosphatase, and liver function tests, as well as a complete blood count should be carried out. If, on the basis of these tests, there is evidence for medical conditions associated with bone loss (eg, alcoholism, hyperparathyroidism, malignancy, Cushing syndrome, thyrotoxicosis, and malabsorption) a definitive diagnosis should be pursued with appropriate testing.

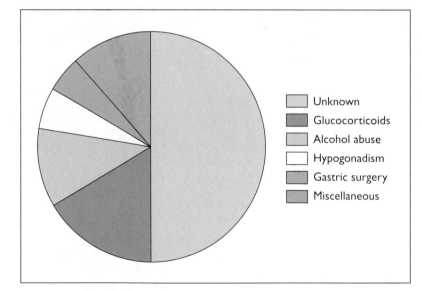

Unknown
Glucocorticoids
Alcohol abuse
Hypogonadism
Gastric surgery
Miscellaneous

**FIGURE 8-26.** Causes of osteoporosis in men with vertebral fracture. A secondary cause of osteoporosis will be identified in approximately half of men with vertebral fracture. Of these, excessive alcohol ingestion, exogenous use of corticosteroids, and hypogonadism will account for more than half [32].

## EVALUATION OF A PATIENT WITH IDIOPATHIC OSTEOPOROSIS

24-hour urine calcium and creatinine (to identify idiopathic hypercalciuria)
24-hour urine cortisol
Serum 25-hydroxyvitamin D
Serum protein electrophoresis (in those >50 y of age to exclude multiple myeloma)
Serum free testosterone
Serum thyroid-stimulating hormone

**FIGURE 8-27.** In men with reduced bone mass in whom no clear pathophysiology is identified by the routine methods listed, it has been considered appropriate to be aggressive diagnostically, primarily because the potential for occult "secondary" causes of osteoporosis is perceived to be high. However, the incidence of occult causes of osteoporosis in men is poorly studied. The diagnostic yield and cost-effectiveness of extensive biochemical studies in men with apparently "idiopathic" osteoporosis is unknown. Nevertheless, lacking this information, a reasonable evaluation of men for whom the cause of osteoporosis is unknown is outlined

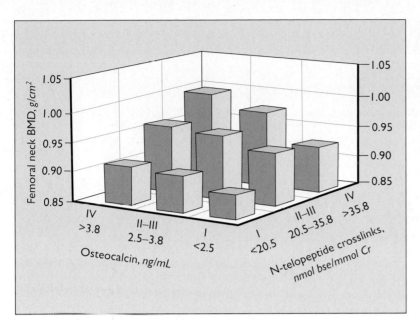

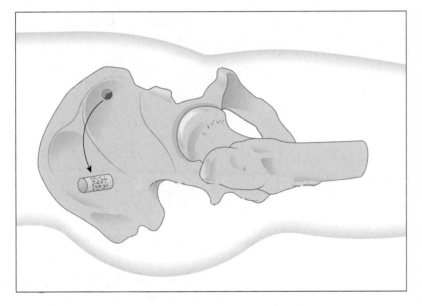

**FIGURE 8-28.** Correlation of bone remodeling markers with bone density. Aging in healthy men is associated with detectable appendicular and substantial axial bone loss. The cause of age-related bone loss in men is unknown but has been speculated to be related to an acceleration in bone turnover. Specific biochemical markers of skeletal metabolism, such as serum levels of osteocalcin and urinary excretion of N-telopeptide cross-links (NTx), correlate well with overall remodeling rates in patients with overt metabolic bone disorders and also may be of use in predicting bone mineral density (BMD) in healthy persons. In a study of 273 healthy men aged 65 to 87 years, Krall and colleagues [33] found both serum osteocalcin and urinary Ntx levels to be inversely related to BMD. The difference between femoral neck BMD between persons in the low-OC low-NTx group and those in the high-OC high-NTx group was 11%. The strength of the relationship between BMD and biochemical markers of turnover is similar to previous findings in women. These observations raise the possibility that biochemical markers of bone turnover could be used as indicators of current bone status in men.

**FIGURE 8-29.** Role of bone biopsy in men with idiopathic osteoporosis. Transiliac bone biopsy is a safe and effective means of assessing skeletal histology and remodeling characteristics. It has been suggested that a transiliac bone biopsy is indicated in those men in whom a thorough biochemical evaluation has failed to reveal a cause for osteoporosis [34]. The rationale for this approach is based on the need to accomplish several objectives: (1) ensure that occult osteomalacia is not present; (2) identify unusual causes of osteoporosis that may be revealed only by histologic analysis, such as mastocytosis; and (3) obtain information concerning the remodeling rate that, in turn, may further direct the differential diagnosis (eg, unsuspected thyrotoxicosis or secondary hyperparathyroidism suggested by the presence of increased turnover) or may be helpful in designing the most appropriate therapeutic approach. However, considerable histologic heterogeneity exists among men with osteoporosis. Whether distinct histologic patterns represent different stages of a single disease entity, separate subtypes of the disease or simply an arbitrary subdivision of a normal distribution of remodeling rates is unknown. Unfortunately, the diagnostic yield or clinical impact of the bone biopsy is unknown. Concern exists that it may be low, thus detracting from its clinical applicability. A reasonable approach to the evaluation of remodeling dynamics in men with idiopathic osteoporosis may be to combine the advantages of the biochemical markers of bone turnover with those of bone biopsy. An initial biochemical assessment of bone turnover should provide an understanding of the remodeling rate. In the presence of an increase in biochemical indices of remodeling, a bone biopsy may be appropriate to identify unusual causes of high-turnover osteoporosis.

# Therapy

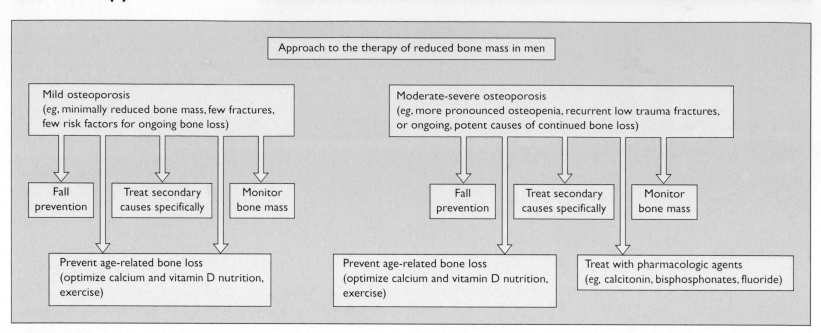

Approach to the therapy of reduced bone mass in men

Mild osteoporosis
(eg, minimally reduced bone mass, few fractures, few risk factors for ongoing bone loss)

Moderate-severe osteoporosis
(eg, more pronounced osteopenia, recurrent low trauma fractures, or ongoing, potent causes of continued bone loss)

Fall prevention

Treat secondary causes specifically

Monitor bone mass

Fall prevention

Treat secondary causes specifically

Monitor bone mass

Prevent age-related bone loss
(optimize calcium and vitamin D nutrition, exercise)

Prevent age-related bone loss
(optimize calcium and vitamin D nutrition, exercise)

Treat with pharmacologic agents
(eg, calcitonin, bisphosphonates, fluoride)

**FIGURE 8-30.** Approach to the therapy of reduced bone mass in men. In any man in whom osteoporosis has developed or is considered a clinically important possibility, efforts should be made to prevent age-related bone loss. Such efforts are the foundation on which a successful treatment plan is based and should always be a part of prevention of and therapy for osteoporosis, regardless of the other causes of bone disease that may also be present. Calcium supplements are safe and may slow bone loss. Based on suggestive but not definitive data a recent National Institutes of Health Consensus Development Conference recommended a calcium intake of 1000 mg/d in young men and 1500 mg/d in men over 65 years of age. Vitamin D deficiency should be suspected in all elderly persons and if present treated with daily vitamin D supplements. Available data strongly suggest a powerful effect of weight and mechanical force on the skeletons of men. In view of the clear decrease in physical activity and muscle strength with aging, senile bone loss in men may partly relate to a diminution of the trophic effects of mechanical force on skeletal tissues. However, a specific exercise prescription is difficult to generate with currently available information. At present, general guidelines include the use of weight-bearing exercise to the extent it can be safely undertaken and avoidance of situations that might materially increase the risk of trauma and fracture. Measures designed merely to prevent further age-related bone loss may be insufficient in men with moderate or severe osteopenia. These men are at high risk for bone loss because of coexisting and unremediable conditions and those in whom sustained bone loss has been demonstrated. In these situations, additional pharmacologic therapies should be considered.

## PREVENTION AND TREATMENT OPTIONS FOR OSTEOPOROSIS IN MEN

Bisphosphonates

Calcitonin

Calcium

Fluoride

Growth hormone

Parathyroid hormone

Testosterone

Thiazide diuretics

Vitamin D

**FIGURE 8-31.** Therapy for osteoporotic disorders in men is virtually unexplored. In the United States, no approved pharmacologic therapies exist for osteoporosis in men. Until results from long-term placebo-controlled trials are reported, androgen replacement therapy should be reserved for men with marked biochemical hypogonadism who can be monitored closely for possible adverse effects. Prolonged exposure to thiazide diuretics is associated with substantial skeletal protection in both men and women; however, the source of the benefit is unclear. Almost no information is available on the use of parathyroid hormone, growth hormone, fluoride, or other anabolic agents in men with osteoporosis. Studies in women with osteoporosis suggest that therapy with drugs such as calcitonin and bisphosphonates appears to be the best options at present. Using drugs in men based on evidence from studies in women, however, is not an appropriate long-term solution. Drug therapy for men must be based on studies of efficacy, safety, and quality of life in men. Very few clinical trials of osteoporosis therapies have been performed specifically in men, although some men with osteoporosis have been included in mixed populations treated with a variety of agents. In general, it is very difficult to ascertain whether the success of these approaches was in any way gender-specific.

# References

1. Donaldson LJ, Cook A, Thomson RG: Incidence of fractures in a geographically defined population. *J Epidemiol Commun Health* 1990, 44:241–245.

2. Karlsson MK, Johnell O, Nilsson BE, et al.: Bone mineral mass in hip fracture patients. *Bone* 1993, 14:161–165.

3. Mallmin H, Ljunghall S, Persson I, et al.: Fracture of the distal forearm as a forecaster of subsequent hip fracture: a population-based cohort study with 24 years of follow-up. *Calcif Tissue Int* 1993, 52:269–272.

4. Melton LJ III, Atkinson EJ, O'Fallon WM, et al.: Long-term fracture risk prediction with bone mineral measurements made at various skeletal sites. *J Bone Miner Res* 1991, 6(suppl 1):S136.

5. Mann T, Oviatt SK, Wilson D, Orwoll ES: Vertebral deformity in men. *J Bone Miner Res* 1992, 7:1259–1265.

6. Diamond TH, Thornley SW, Sekel R, Smerdley P: Hip fracture in elderly men: prognostic factors and outcomes. *Med J Aust* 1997, 167:412–415.

7. Magaziner J, Simonsick EM, Kashner M, et al.: Survival experience of aged hip fracture patients. *Am J Publ Health* 1989, 79:274–278.

8. Cheng S, Suomine H, Sakari-Rantala R, et al.: Bone mineral density predicts fracture occurrence: a five-year follow-up study of elderly people. *J Bone Miner Res* 1997, 12:1075–1082.

9. Nevitt MC: Epidemiology of osteoporosis. *Rheum Dis Clin N Am* 1994, 20:535–559.

10. Gilsanz V, Beochat MI, Roe TF, et al.: Gender differences in vertebral body sizes in children and adolescents. *Radiology* 1994, 190:673–677.

11. Gilsanz V, Beochat MI, Gilsanz R, et al.: Gender differences in vertebral sizes in adults: biomechanical implications. *Radiology* 1994, 190:678–682.

12. Gilsanz V, Kovanlikaya A, Costin G, et al.: Differential effect of gender on the sizes of the bones in the axial and appendicular skeletons. *J Clin Endocrinol Metab* 1997, 82:1603–1607.

13. Beck TJ, Ruff CB, Scott WWJ, et al.: Sex differences in geometry of the femoral neck with aging: a structural analysis of bone mineral data. *Calcif Tissue Int* 1992, 50:24–29.

14. Mosekilde L, Mosekilde L: Sex differences in age-related changes in vertebral body size, density and biomechanical competence in normal individuals. *Bone* 1990, 11:67–73.

15. Soule SG, Conway G, Prelevic GM, et al.: Osteopenia as a feature of the androgen insensitivity syndrome. *Clin Endocrinol* 1995, 43:671–675.

16. Finkelstein JS, Klibanski A, Neer RM, et al.: Osteoporosis in men with idiopathic hypogonadotropic hypogonadism. *Ann Intern Med* 1987, 106:354–361.

17. MacAdams MR, White RH, Chipps BE: Reduction of serum testosterone levels during chronic glucocorticoid therapy. *Ann Intern Med* 1986, 104:648–651.

18. Stepan JJ, Lachman M: Castrated men with bone loss: effect of calcitonin treatment on biochemical indices of bone remodeling. *J Clin Endocrinol Metab* 1989, 69:523–527.

19. Girasole G, Passeri G: Upregulation of osteoclastogenic potential of the marrow is induced by orchidectomy and is reversed by testosterone replacement in the mouse. *J Bone Miner Res* 1992, 7:S96.

20. Vermeulen A: Clinical review 24: androgens in the aging male. *J Clin Endocrinol Metab* 1991, 73:221–223.

21. Katznelson L, Finkelstein JS, Schoenfeld DA, et al.: Increase in bone density and lean body mass during testosterone administration in men with acquired hypogonadism. *J Clin Endocrinol Metab* 1996, 81:4358–4365.

22. Morishima A, Grumbach MM, Simpson ER, et al.: Aromatase deficiency in male and female siblings caused by a novel mutation and the physiological role of estrogens. *J Clin Endocrinol Metab* 1995, 80:3689–3698.

23. Carani C, Qin K, Simoni M, et al.: Effect of testosterone and estradiol in a man with aromatase deficiency. *N Engl J Med* 1997, 337:91–95.

24. Bilezikian JP, Morishima A, Bell J, Grumbach MM: Increased bone mass as a result of estrogen therapy in a man with aromatase deficiency. *N Engl J Med* 1998, 339:599–603.

25. Smith EP, Boyd J, Frank GR, et al.: Estrogen resistance caused by a mutation in the estrogen-receptor in a man. *N Engl J Med* 1995, 331:1056–1061.

26. Slemenda CW, Longcope C, Zhou L, et al.: Sex steroids and bone mass in older men: positive associations with serum estrogens and negative associations with androgens. *J Clin Invest* 1997, 100:1755–1759.

27. Greendale GA, Edelstein ES, Barrett-Connor E: Endogenous sex steroids and bone mineral density in older women and men: the Rancho Bernardo study. *J Bone Miner Res* 1997, 12:1833–1843.

28. Khosla S, Melton LJ III, Atkinson EJ, et al.: Relationship of serum sex steroid levels and bone turnover markers with bone mineral density in men and women: a key role for bioavailable estrogen. *J Clin Endocrinol Metab* 1998, 83:2266–2274.

29. Slemenda CW, Christian JC, Reed T, et al.: Long-term bone loss in men: effects of genetic and environmental factors. *Ann Intern Med* 1992, 117:286–291.

30. Diamond T, Stiel D, Lunzer M, et al.: Ethanol reduces bone formation and may cause osteoporosis. *Am J Med* 1989, 86:282–288.

31. Rico H, Cabranes JA, Cabello J, et al.: Low serum osteocalcin in acute alcohol intoxication: a direct effect of alcohol on osteoblasts. *Bone Min* 1987, 2:221–225.

32. Kanis JA: Assessment of bone mass and osteoporosis. IN *Osteoporosis.* Oxford: Blackwell Science Ltd; 1994:144.

33. Krall EA, Dawson-Hughes B, Hirst K, et al.: Bone mineral density and biochemical markers of bone turnover in healthy elderly men and women. *J Gerontol* 1997, 52A:M61–M67.

34. Klein RF, Gunness M: The transiliac bone biopsy: when to get it and how to interpret it. *Endocrinologist* 1992, 2:158–168.

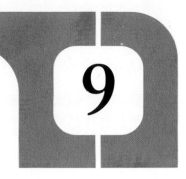

# Osteoporosis Associated with Systemic Illness and Medications

## Paul D. Miller

Osteoporosis is defined as low bone mass, microarchitectural bone deterioration, and susceptibility to fracture. The primary causes of osteoporosis are estrogen deficiency after menopause and advanced age. Ten secondary causes of osteoporosis have been categorized by organ system or systemic disease. Each of these secondary causes is associated with a negative calcium balance or defects in bone formation or resorption at the bone remodeling unit. This chapter focuses on the diagnostic characteristics of these secondary causes.

Osteoporosis may be related to gastrointestinal disorders. In most of these disorders, the bone loss is associated with a rapid gastrointestinal transit time that precludes adequate calcium absorption. Osteoporosis may also be related to chronic liver, kidney, or pancreatic diseases. Chronic liver disease may impair the conversion of cholecalciferol to 25-hydroxycholecalciferol, reduce the production of insulin-like growth factor-I, and cause iron overload in tissues; all of these may be related to bone loss. Renal failure is associated with changes in calcium metabolism, hypogonadism, hyperparathyroidism, inadequate production of 1,25-dihydroxyvitamin D, and chronic metabolic acidosis; these conditions, in turn, cause osteoporosis. Several types of medications have also been associated with osteoporosis. The mechanism of bone loss stems from the type and action of the medication. Low bone mass and fractures may also be related to disorders of bone marrow. Bone resorption and osteoporosis may be associated with immobilization or microgravity environments. Immobilization (affecting the total body, occurring after an accident causing quadriplegia, or required for a single limb) can induce excessive bone resorption and osteoporosis. The same excessive bone resorption is seen in people living in microgravity environments. The accelerated bone resorption seen in these circumstances is associated with increased urinary calcium excretion.

Osteoporosis has also been shown to be related to endocrine disorders. The mechanisms of these disorders are related to endocrine gland malfunction. Osteoporosis has been associated with several genetic disorders of metabolism, including Marfan syndrome, homocystinuria, Ehlers-Danlos syndrome, and hypophosphatasia. These genetic disorders of metabolism may be associated with low bone mass or bone loss. Disorders of connective tissue metabolism may be accompanied by inadequate bone mineralization as well, because the substrate for calcification is defective. Osteoporosis is also often associated with nutritional disorders related to calcium and vitamin D. Finally, osteoporosis may be related to osteomalacia and osteogenesis imperfecta.

This chapter is designed to help physicians understand the characteristics and mechanisms of secondary causes of osteoporosis and to assist with the diagnosis of the many causes of bone loss. It stresses the importance of carefully evaluating each patient with low bone mass before administering therapeutic interventions.

---

### TEN SECONDARY CAUSES OF OSTEOPOROSIS

Gastrointestinal diseases
Liver, kidney, or pancreatic diseases
Medications
Bone marrow disorders
Immobilization and microgravity
Endocrine disorders
Pregnancy
Genetic metabolic disorders
States of nutritional deficiency
Osteomalacia and osteogenesis imperfecta

**FIGURE 9-1.** The 10 secondary causes of osteoporosis listed according to the organ system involved or the system disease associated with bone loss.

# Osteoporosis Related to Gastrointestinal Diseases

## GASTROINTESTINAL DISEASES AND CONDITIONS ASSOCIATED WITH OSTEOPOROSIS

Hemi-gastrectomy or total gastrectomy

Intestinal bypass

Asymptomatic celiac disease

Small intestinal malabsorption conditions (eg, Whipple's disease, scleroderma)

Inflammatory bowel disease

**FIGURE 9-2.** Gastrointestinal diseases and conditions associated with osteoporosis [1]. Patients with hemi-gastrectomy or total gastrectomy may develop osteoporosis or, less frequently, osteomalacia. The osteoporosis is related to a rapid gastrointestinal transit time, which precludes adequate calcium absorption. Osteomalacia, which may develop in selected patients, is due to a lack of bile-salt binding to fat-soluble vitamin D. This causes inadequate vitamin D absorption in the terminal ileum. Surgical intestinal bypass may also cause osteoporosis or osteomalacia by the same pathophysiologic mechanisms. Quantitative bone histology suggests that bone formation is impaired in gastrectomized animal models. Patients with Crohn's disease and asymptomatic nontropical sprue (celiac disease) often have low bone mass.

## DIAGNOSTIC CLUES FOR DETECTION OF ASYMPTOMATIC CELIAC DISEASE

Low bone mass

Normal serum 25-hydroxyvitamin D concentrations

Normal serum bone-specific alkaline phosphatase activity

24-hour urine calcium excretion < 50 mg/d

Elevated levels of serum antigliadin or antiendomysial antibodies (levels may also be normal)

Iron deficiency

Definitive diagnosis on small-bowel biopsy

**FIGURE 9-3.** Diagnostic clues for the detection of asymptomatic celiac disease. Asymptomatic celiac disease (nontropical sprue) is an underdiagnosed bowel condition leading to osteoporosis, not osteomalacia [2]. One of the most important clues is a 24-hour urine calcium excretion less than 50 mg/d. This low value suggests calcium malabsorption or extremely low calcium intake. Low urinary calcium excretion is valid for the determination of calcium malabsorption if the serum calcium level is within the normal range and the glomerular filtration rate exceeds 50 mL/min (determined by creatinine clearance). If hypocalcemia or significant renal failure is present, low urinary calcium excretion may be due to these disorders rather than to calcium malabsorption. High serum antigliadin and antiendomysial antibodies are also associated with celiac disease. However, these antibodies may be undetectable in some patients with this condition. Thus, the absence of these antibodies does not necessarily exclude a diagnosis of celiac disease. Patients with celiac disease often have normal serum 25-hydroxy-vitamin D levels because the disease begins in the proximal small intestine and vitamin D is absorbed in the terminal ileum. Celiac disease causes selective malabsorption of calcium and iron. Therefore, unexplained iron deficiency may also be a clue to the presence of this disease. If a hypocalciuric patient has unexplained low bone mass, bone loss, or fractures, then a small intestinal biopsy is the definitive method for diagnosing celiac disease. Treatment with a gluten-free diet can increase bone mass.

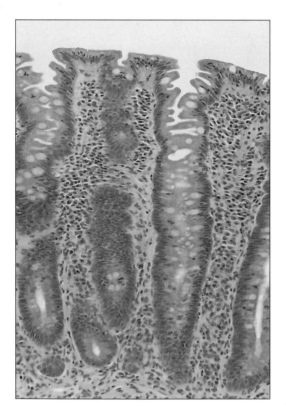

**FIGURE 9-4.** (see Color Plate) Small bowel biopsy specimen from a patient with celiac disease. This condition is diagnosed by histologic features demonstrating the loss of villous architecture and infiltration of the lamina propria with abundant mononuclear cells.

# Osteoprosis Related to Liver, Kidney, or Pancreatic Diseases

## CHRONIC LIVER, KIDNEY, AND PANCREATIC DISEASE RELATED TO OSTEOPOROSIS

Chronic liver disease

Hemochromatosis or iron accumulation over osteoid surfaces

Chronic renal failure

Chronic renal tubular acidosis

Hypercalciuria

Renal phosphate wastage

Chronic pancreatic insufficiency

**FIGURE 9-5.** Chronic liver, kidney, or pancreatic diseases associated with osteoporosis. Chronic liver disease may lead to osteoporosis or osteomalacia [3]. Conversion of cholecalciferol to 25-hydroxycholecalciferol, which normally occurs in the liver, may be impaired by chronic liver disease. This impairment may lead to osteoporosis or osteomalacia. The liver is the primary source of circulating insulin-like growth factor-1 (IGF-1), and some cases of osteoporosis related to liver disease may be due to the inadequate production of this stimulator of bone formation. In this regard, the elevated IGF-1 concentrations observed in patients with chronic hepatitis C may be responsible for the elevated bone mass observed in these patients.

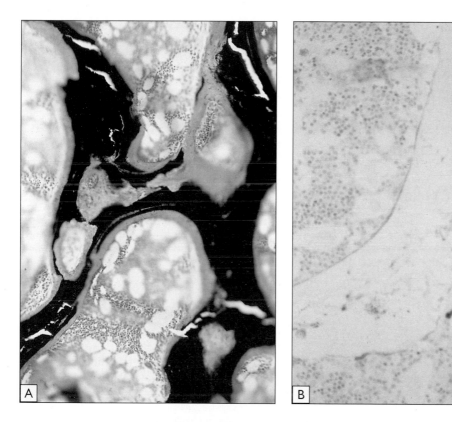

A

B

**FIGURE 9-6.** (see Color Plate) **A**, Bone biopsy specimen from a patient with iron overload and osteomalacia (hemochromatosis). Abundant thick osteoid seams (shown in pink) are the characteristic finding of osteomalacia. **B**, Bone biopsy specimen from a patient with iron overload and osteoporosis. The liver is also responsible for the proper disposal of iron, and iron overload may lead to iron accumulation in other tissues, including bone. Iron deposited in bone (shown in blue) may accumulate on osteoid surfaces and lead to frank osteomalacia or osteoporosis. Although classic hemochromatosis is usually associated with elevated serum iron indices, iron may accumulate in bone in the absence of elevated serum ferritin levels. In cases of unexplained osteoporosis or fracture, iron accumulation can be diagnosed only by bone biopsy.

## CAUSES OF HYPERCALCIURIA

Primary hyperparathyroidism

Absorptive hypercalciuria

Chronic metabolic acidosis

Hypercalcemia

Vitamin D excess

Vitamin A excess

Sarcoidosis and other granulomatosis diseases

Immobilization and microgravity

Glucocorticoid excess (including Cushing disease)

**FIGURE 9-7.** Causes of hypercalciuria. The osteoporosis observed in patients with chronic renal failure may be caused by any of the following: hypogonadism, long-term heparin exposure, secondary hyperparathyroidism, inadequate renal production of 1,25-dihydroxyvitamin D, or chronic metabolic acidosis [4]. Chronic metabolic acidosis, as seen in patients with renal tubular acidosis, may lead to osteoporosis when bone releases calcium to buffer the serum acid load. This process is often associated with hypercalciuria and may also lead to osteomalacia if other renal tubular defects (such as renal phosphate wastage or inadequate proximal tubular production of 1,25-dihydroxyvitamin D) are present. Osteoporosis may be related to hypercalciuria. Hypercalciuria (calcium excretion >250 mg/d in women and >300 mg/d in men) may be due to any of the causes shown in this figure. Osteoporosis may be related to idiopathic hypercalciuria (renal), and normalization of hypercalciuria with thiazides may be associated with increases in bone mass. However, this increase in bone mass may also be due to a direct effect of thiazides on bone. Thiazides may also be used therapeutically to normalize urinary calcium excretion in patients with glucocorticoid-induced hypercalciuria.

# Osteoporosis Related to Medication Administration

### MEDICATIONS ASSOCIATED WITH OSTEOPOROSIS

Short- or long-term glucocorticoid administration

Long-term administration of gonadotropin-releasing hormone agonist

Long-term therapy with antiseizure medication

Long-term heparin treatment

Long-term tetracycline administration

Possible associations: Depo-Provera, cyclosporine, methotrexate, lithium, antidepressant agents, antipsychotic drugs

**FIGURE 9-8.** Medications associated with osteoporosis [5]. Glucocorticoids induce bone loss through many mechanisms [6]. The rate of bone loss is dose dependent. Bone loss occurs even with low dosages (<7.5 mg of prednisone per day or its dose equivalent), suggesting that the effects of glucocorticoids on bone may be cumulative. Use of inhaled steroids over the long term has also been associated with bone loss. Long-term therapy with gonadotropin-releasing hormone (GnRH) agonist, for patients with such disorders as PMS or prostate cancer, induces bone loss. Intermittent therapy with GnRH for infertility may induce temporary bone loss that is reversed after discontinuation of therapy.

Long-term antiseizure therapy may induce bone loss through several mechanisms. Long-term phenytoin sodium or phenobarbital use has been associated with osteomalacia, particularly in institutionalized children with vitamin D deficiency. However, these compounds may cause defects in hepatic activation of 25-hydroxyvitamin D, which is associated with mineralization defects.

Adult patients treated with antiseizure medications generally have high-turnover osteoporosis rather than osteomalacia. Recent data in animals suggest that these medications may directly affect bone turnover, leading to impaired bone formation as well. Long-term heparin or tetracycline administration may induce bone loss and fractures. The bone loss and increased risk for fracture is dose- and duration-dependent, and the mechanism of increased bone resorption is unclear. Depo-Provera has been associated with low bone mass in premenopausal women using it for birth control. The bone loss may not be fully reversed after discontinuation of therapy with the drug. This progestational agent suppresses pituitary secretion of follicle-stimulating hormone and luteinizing hormone sufficiently to result in low concentrations of estradiol, which may explain the bone loss. Prospective studies are under way to determine whether this bone loss is significant. In animal models. administration of cyclosporine or methotrexate has been associated with bone loss. Human studies suggest that this bone loss may not be clinically relevant. Lithium administration may cause hyperparathyroidism and hypercalcemia, which may affect bone. However, this has not been adequately investigated. Certain antidepressant and antipsychotic medications have been associated with elevated prolactin levels and low bone mass in small cross-sectional studies. Elevated prolactin levels may lead to bone resorption; thus, these medications merit further investigation.

# Osteoporosis Related to Bone Marrow Disorders

**FIGURE 9-9.** Bone marrow disorders potentially associated with osteoporosis.

### BONE MARROW DISORDERS ASSOCIATED WITH OSTEOPOROSIS

| | |
|---|---|
| Multiple myeloma | Gaucher disease |
| Mastocytosis | Beta$_2$-macroglobulinemia |
| Thalassemia | Lymphoma |

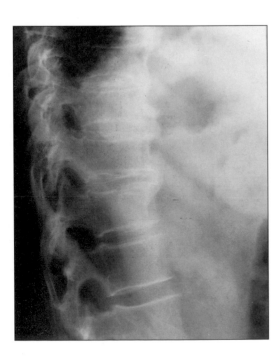

**FIGURE 9-10.** Radiograph of new vertebral compression fracture in a 50-year-old man with multiple myeloma without anemia or elevated erythrocyte sedimentation rate. Multiple myeloma is a common cause of osteoporosis and often presents with vertebral compression fractures [7]. Immunoelectrophoresis should be performed in patients 50 years of age or older who have vertebral fractures.

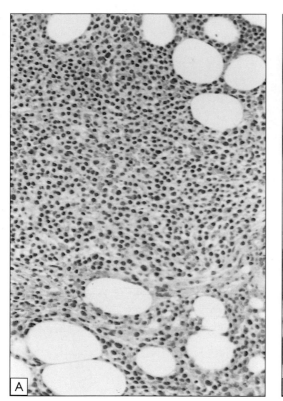

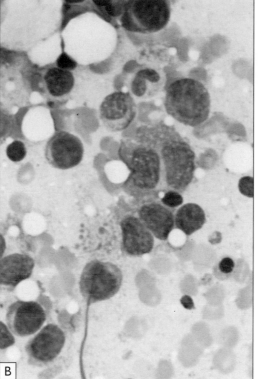

**FIGURE 9-11.** (*see* Color Plate) Bone marrow biopsy specimens from patient shown in Figure 9-10. A monoclonal protein spike should be followed by a bone marrow examination, which will definitively diagnose myeloma. **A**, Diffuse replacement of bone marrow with plasma cells. **B**, Higher magnification shows cells with characteristic halos surrounding the plasma nuclei.

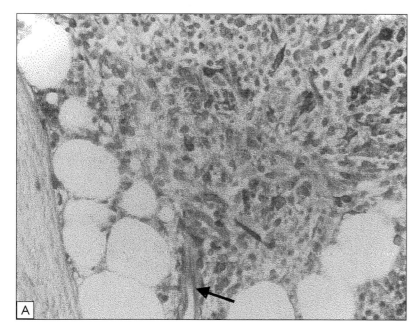

**FIGURE 9-12.** (*see* Color Plate) Histologic findings of bone marrow from a patient with mastocytosis. Mastocytosis is an unusual cause of osteoporosis [8]. Patients with mastocytosis may or may not have skin manifestations (hives or other nonspecific rashes). Unexplained severe low bone mass, bone loss, fractures, or high biochemical markers of bone resorption may be due to mastocytosis. Histologic characteristics of bone marrow may often be diagnostic of mastocytosis. Thalassemia may be associated with osteoporosis and mineralization defects as well. Gaucher disease and its accompanying bone marrow expansion, has been associated with osteoporosis and hip fracture. Beta$_2$-macroglobu-

linemia or amyloid accumulation in bone, sometimes observed in chronic renal failure or amyloidosis, may also be associated with osteoporosis.

**A**, Glycol methacrylate–embedded iliac creat biopsy specimen. A typical mast cell aggregate adjacent to bone is penetrated at one end by a small arteriole (*arrow*). The aggregate consists of large purple elongated spindle-shaped mast cells admixed with small round lymphocytes. (Stain, azure A at a pH of 4.5; original magnification, ×200.) **B**, Section adjacent to that shown in part A. The large mast cells (mc) show only weak cytoplasmic staining and are admixed with smaller eosinophils (e) and lymphocytes (l). (Stain, hematoxylin and eosin; original magnification, ×1000.)

(*Continued on next page*)

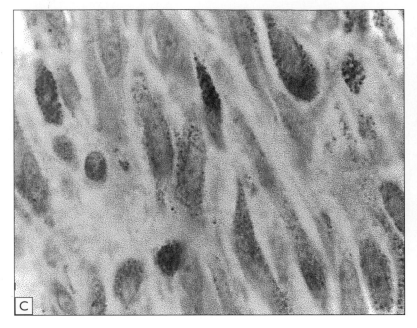

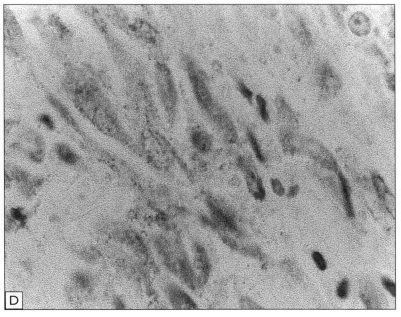

**FIGURE 9-12.** (*Continued*) **C,** Higher-power view of the section shown in part A. Purple staining of mast cells is the result of strong staining of granules with azure. The normal blue absorption peak of azure undergoes a red metachromatic shift induced by the high negative charge density of heparin in the granules. (Original magnification, ×1000.) **D,** Section adjacent to those in parts A and B. The mast cell granules also stain positively for this enzyme. (Stained for tartrate-resistant acid phosphatase; original magnification, ×1000.)

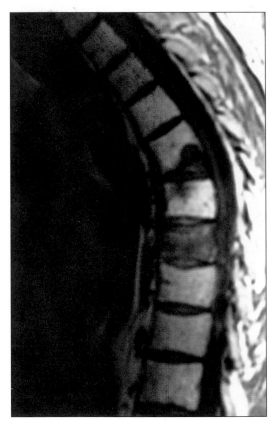

**FIGURE 9-13.** Magnetic resonance imaging scan of a man with an acute vertebral compression fracture. Lymphoma infiltration in the bone marrow may lead to localized osteoporosis and fracture in the involved bone [9]. The lymphoma infiltration is depicted by the "ivory" vertebra. Vertebral biopsy confirmed the diagnosis of lymphoma.

# Osteoporosis Related to Endocrine Disorders

| ENDOCRINE DISORDERS ASSOCIATED WITH OSTEOPOROSIS | |
|---|---|
| Hyperparathyroidism | Hypogonadism (female and male) |
| Cushing syndrome | Male aromatase deficiency |
| Hyperthyroidism | Hypothalamic-pituitary dysfunction |
| Hyperprolactinemia | Acromegaly |

**FIGURE 9-14.** Endocrine disorders associated with osteoporosis.

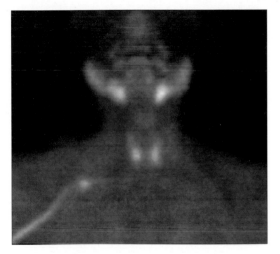

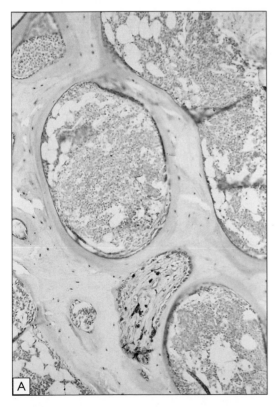

**FIGURE 9-15.** Sestamibi scan showing an enlarged parathyroid gland. Primary hyperparathyroidism may lead to excessive bone resorption and osteoporosis [10]. The cortical bone sites seem to be affected more than the cancellous bone sites, although the latter bone structure may not be spared in subsets of patients. Even if cancellous bone mass is not declining, parathyroidectomy is often followed by increases in bone mass. In some cases, elevated parathyroid hormone and serum calcium levels are sufficient to establish the diagnosis. However, the documentation of enlarged parathyroid glands using newer radioisotope scans (sestamibi) is reassuring and helps guide the parathyroid surgeon.

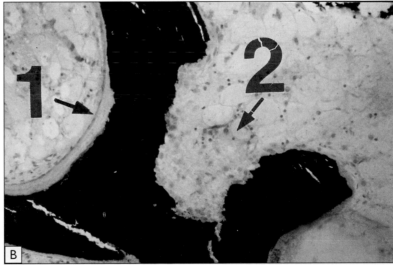

**FIGURE 9-16.** (see Color Plate) Quantitative bone histomorphometry. Increased tetracycline labeling, increased mineralization rates, and increased osteoclast numbers may be useful in cases of hyperparathyroidism, which are difficult to diagnose. **A,** Abundant osteoclast cells in purple. **B,** Two histologic features of hyperparathyroidism: 1) abundant osteoblasts creating bone matrix (pink seam) and 2) osteoclasts inducing bone resorption (scalloped borders).

(Continued on next page)

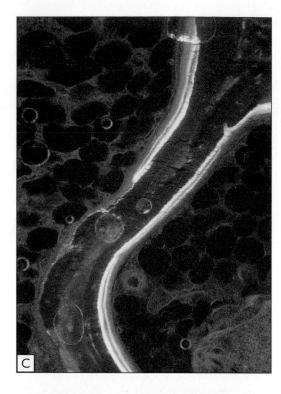

**FIGURE 9-16.** (*Continued*) **C**, Increased mineralization (broad tetracycline bands) related to excess parathyroid activity.

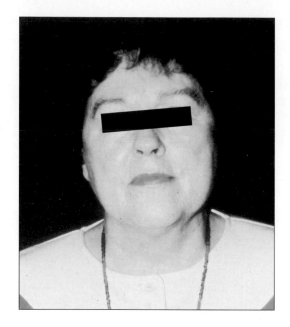

**FIGURE 9-17.** Facial characteristics of a patient with Cushing disease.

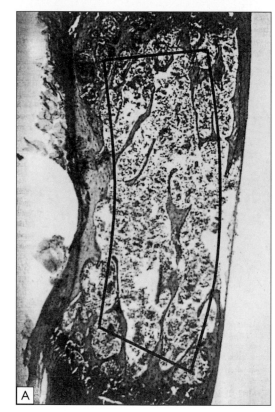

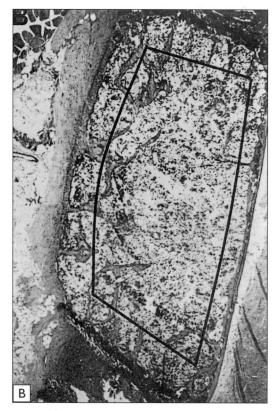

**FIGURE 9-18.** Photomicrographs of the effects of placebo (**A**) and prednisolone (**B**) on murine vertebral cancellous bone. Cushing syndrome is characterized by excess glucocorticoid production from an adrenal tumor, adrenal hyperplasia due to pituitary adrenocorticotropic (ACTH) excess, or ectopic ACTH excess, all of which lead to increased bone resorption and osteoporosis [11]. Bone histologic characteristics in patients with glucocorticoid excess are distinct from those in patients with osteoporosis due to estrogen deficiency. Trabecular connectivity is preserved with glucocorticoid excess, and trabecular bone is often perforated with patients with osteoporosis due to estrogen deficiency. Bone histology in chronic glucocorticoid exposure exhibits reduced cancellous bone area and decreased trabecular width. Trabecular profiles can be entirely resorbed. Finally, glucocorticoid exposure decreases long-bone area and is associated with a reduction in the rate of bone formation. Bone density often increases after the glucocorticoid excess is corrected, even in patients with long-standing Cushing syndrome.

Hyperthyroidism may also lead to increased bone resorption and osteoporosis. The mechanism may be a direct effect of thyroid hormone on osteoclast activity. Excessive exogenous thyroid hormone replacement may also be associated with bone loss. However, the clinical significance of this relationship, as well as its association with fracture, is unclear. (*From* Weinstein *et al.* [12]; with permission.)

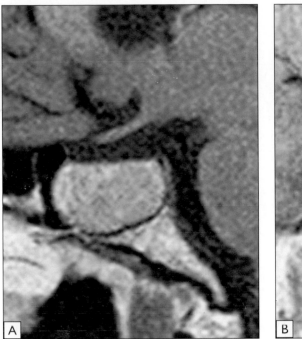

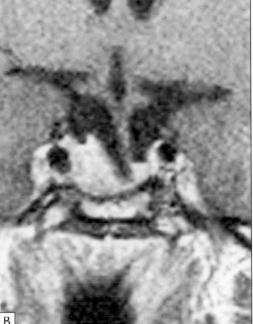

**FIGURE 9-19.** Magnetic resonance images (**A** and **B**) of an enlarged pituitary gland that is producing excess prolactin. Excess prolactin secretion, which is typical of prolactinomas, may be associated with increased bone resorption. This effect may be independent of the hypogonadism that often accompanies prolactinomas. In patients with low bone mass, bone loss, or unexplained fractures, magnetic resonance imaging of the pituitary may be diagnostic if elevated prolactin levels are detected.

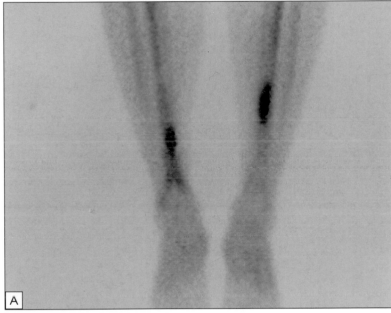

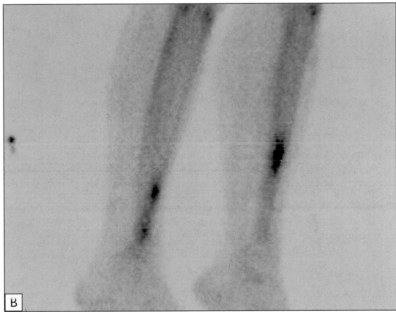

**FIGURE 9-20.** Radionuclide bone scan obtained from a young woman with hypomenorrhea, stress fractures, and painful shins but normal routine radiographs of the legs. **A,** Anterior view. **B,** Right lateral and left medial views. In both men and women, hypogonadism may lead to osteoporosis at any age. Postmenopausal osteoporosis is the most prevalent form of osteoporosis in women. Low testosterone concentrations in men may also be an etiologic factor for osteoporosis. Recently, osteoporosis in men has also been linked to deficiency of aromatase (the enzyme responsible for converting testosterone to estrogen). In men with unexplained low bone mass, elevations in circulating levels of follicle-stimulating hormone and luteinizing hormone, low concentrations of free or bioavailable testosterone, low plasma estradiol-estrone concentrations, or low insulin-like growth factor-1 levels suggest this enzymatic disorder.

Androgen replacement does not correct the defect in these patients, and estrogen replacement may be required to prevent further bone loss.

Osteoporosis may also occur in young women and men with hypothalamic-pituitary dysfunction related to excessive exercise or eating disorders. In affected young women, amenorrhea or hypomenorrhea results from inadequate production of follicle-stimulating hormone and luteinizing hormone and bone mass is lost. Such patients often present with painful feet or tibial pain. Routine radiographs are often normal, but a bone scan confirms the diagnosis of stress fractures. It is important to emphasize that these women are losing bone systemically. Some of these women have a hip fracture as their first fracture. Bone density may not be extremely low in these cases, and bone fragility may be related to the high rate of bone turnover associated with gonadal deficiency and nutritional inadequacies.

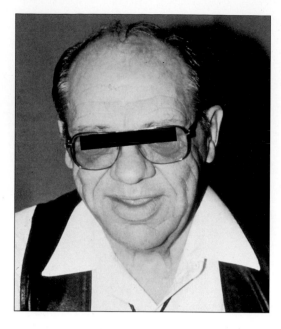

**FIGURE 9-21.** Patient with acromegaly and vertebral fractures. Osteoporosis may be seen in patients with acromegaly, a body habitus that would not be expected to be associated with low bone mass. This association is probably related to the hypogonadism that occurs in patients with these pituitary tumors. Despite elevated growth hormone levels, gonadal insufficiency dominates the metabolic milieu of these patients.

## Osteoporosis Related to Pregnancy

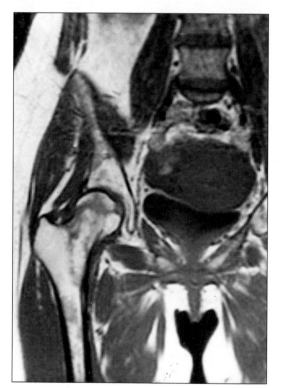

**FIGURE 9-22.** Magnetic resonance image of a pregnant woman's hip. Osteoporosis of the hip is a specific condition associated with pregnancy and lactation. The mottled decreased signal on a T1-weighted image of the femoral head distinguishes this condition from aseptic necrosis of the femur. Osteoporosis of pregnancy is painful, even without a fracture. It heals spontaneously after delivery or cessation of lactation [13].

# Osteoporosis Related to Nutritional Deficiency

## STATES OF NUTRITIONAL DEFICIENCY ASSOCIATED WITH OSTEOPOROSIS

Poor calcium consumption

Vitamin D deficiency

Anorexia nervosa or bulimia

Deficiencies in vitamin K or vitamin C

**FIGURE 9-23.** States of nutritional deficiency associated with osteoporosis [14]. Osteoporosis, which is not accompanied by osteomalacia, has been described in populations with chronic low intake of dietary calcium. In fact, calcium replacement alone in late postmenopausal women may retard bone loss and reduce fractures. Although vitamin D deficiency is often associated with osteomalacia, patients with low vitamin D levels may also lose bone density and sustain fractures in the absence of osteomalacia. Vitamin D replacement may also reduce fractures in subsets of postmenopausal women. These effects are mediated by a combination of mechanisms, including positive calcium balance, reduction in bone turnover, and improvement of muscle tone and balance. Recent data indicate that vitamin K and vitamin C also have important roles in bone metabolism.

# Osteoporosis Related to Osteomalacia and Osteogenesis Imperfecta

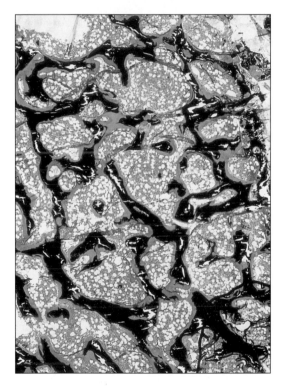

**FIGURE 9-24.** (see Color Plate) Histologic findings on bone biopsy specimen from a patient with osteomalacia. Low bone mass may also be associated with very different types of metabolic bone diseases, including osteomalacia and osteogenesis imperfecta. Osteomalacia is the accumulation of excess osteoid (nonmineralizing bone) caused by impaired mineralization of osteoid (thick pink outer layer on black calcified bone surface). This impairment can result from several clinical and pathophysiologic conditions. The strict quantitative histomorphometric criteria used to diagnose osteomalacia are 1) osteoid surface greater than 80%, 2) osteoid thickness greater than 14 microns, and 3) mineralization lag time of 100 days or more. In addition, there are subclassifications of "preosteomalacia" and "focal" osteomalacia with separate criteria; these conditions may be less severe and are related to lesser degrees of vitamin D deficiency. These alternative classifications of osteomalacia may simply represent different developmental stages of the disorder.

## CLINICAL CONDITIONS ASSOCIATED WITH OSTEOMALACIA

Malabsorption

Chronic liver disease

Hemigastrectomy

Chronic hypophosphatemia

Chronic hypophosphatemia or phosphaturia with inadequate 1,25-dihydroxyvitamin D levels (oncogenic osteomalacia or proximal renal tubular defects)

Severe reduction in 25-hydroxyvitamin D levels

Chronic metabolic acidosis

Medications such as phenytoin sodium, phenobarbital, continuous high-dose etidronate therapy, excess fluoride

Chronic renal failure

**FIGURE 9-25.** Clinical entities associated with osteomalacia. Low 25-hydroxy-vitamin D concentrations are often seen in patients without osteomalacia. A spectrum of calcium metabolism disorders may be related to both the duration and severity of vitamin D deficiency. Osteomalacia occurs more often in patients whose 25-hydroxyvitamin D values are less than 6 ng/mL. This level of reduction often leads to decreases in 1,25-dihydroxyvitamin D levels and osteoporosis. Levels of 25-hydroxyvitamin D greater than 12 ng/mL may still be associated with elevated circulating parathyroid hormone levels, which may aggravate bone loss. Osteomalacia can be present with normal vitamin D levels and normal bone alkaline phosphatase activity. The condition cannot be diagnosed by assuming that it is present in patients with elevated bone alkaline phosphatase activity and clinical entities that may be associated with osteomalacia [15].

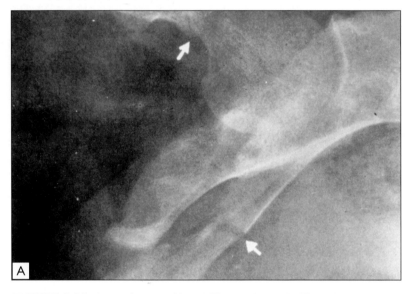
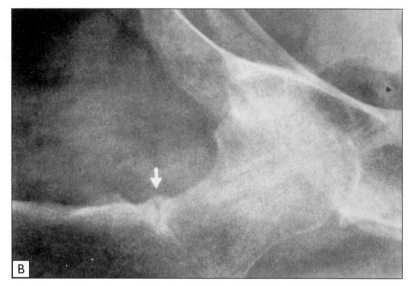

**FIGURE 9-26.** Looser's zones (**A** and **B**) on radiography. These lines occur only in advanced cases of osteomalacia. The diagnosis can be made only by quantitative bone histomorphometry.

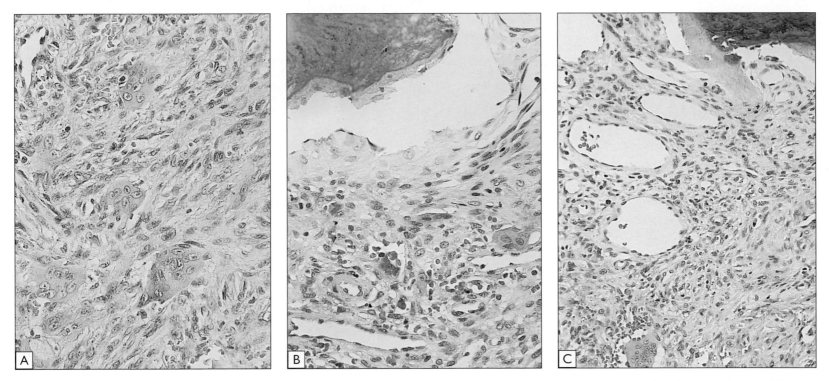

**FIGURE 9-27.** (*see* Color Plate)  Histologic characteristics of a tumor associated with oncogenic osteomalacia. Bone biopsy should be considered in clinical situations related to osteomalacia, particularly in patients with fractures or chemical abnormalities that are associated with oncogenic osteomalacia [16]. Establishing the correct diagnosis in these cases is important because pharmacologic treatment (phosphorus and 1,25-dihydroxyvitamin D replacement) must be tailored to the condition. Clinicians should continue to search for the mesenchymal cell line tumor that will appear months to years after diagnosis. **A**, multinucleated giant cells admixed with spindle-shaped mesenchymal cells. There are vascular spaces filled with blood and yellow-brown pigment most compatible with hemosiderin. **B**, Giant cells and mesenchymal cells with a focus of ossification. **C**, A lower magnification of *panel B*, which also shows prominent dilated vascular spaces.

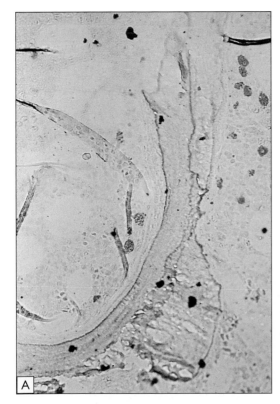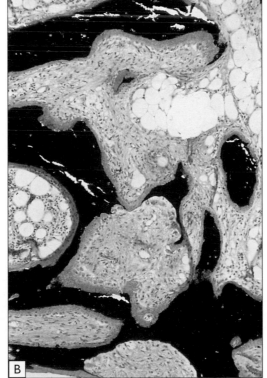

**FIGURE 9-28.** (*see* Color Plate)  Bone biopsy specimens in patient with chronic renal failure. Bone biopsy may be the only method to determine whether the observed hypercalcemia or elevated alkaline phosphatase level is related to osteomalacia, aluminum accumulation, or hyperparathyroidism. This determination is particularly important if desferrioxamine therapy, long-term 1,25 dihydroxyvitamin D treatment, or surgical parathyroidectomy is being considered. In some patients, serum parathyroid hormone levels and alkaline phosphatase activity may help distinguish between hyperparathyroid and aluminum bone disease. However, sufficient overlap exists in individual patients that bone histologic characteristics become the definitive way to make a specific diagnosis. **A**, Aluminum, shown in red, covering osteoid surfaces. **B**, Features of osteitis fibrosa cystica: fibrosis of the bone marrow, excess bone resorption shown by scalloping, and abundant osteoid shown by the thick pink layer.

The patient shown in this figure was receiving long-term dialysis and had hypercalcemia and intact parathyroid hormone concentrations that were eight times the upper limit of normal. Aluminum covered 100% of this patient's osteoid surfaces [17]. Proceeding with parathyroidectomy just on the basis of the chemical aberrations, before aluminum chelation, would have been a serious error because of the high likelihood of postoperative aluminum-related adynamic bone disease, a crippling disorder.

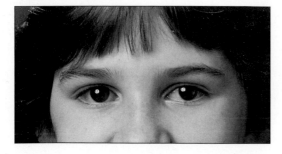

**FIGURE 9-29.** *(see Color Plate)* Blue sclera in a child with osteogenesis imperfecta. Low bone mass and fractures are seen in patients with osteogenesis imperfecta. In children with this disorder, it is often difficult to discriminate osteogenesis imperfecta from idiopathic juvenile osteoporosis [18]. If the patient has blue sclera, the diagnosis of osteogenesis imperfecta is clear. Tissue culture of skin biopsy specimens may also be helpful in diagnosing osteogenesis imperfecta.

# References

1.  Rao SD, Kleerekoper M, Rogers M, *et al.*: Is gastrectomy a risk factor for osteoporosis? In: *Osteoporosis*. Edited by Christiansen C, Arnaud CD, Nordin BEC, *et al.* Glostrop, Denmark: Aalborg Stiftsbogtrykkeri; 1984:775–777.

2.  Trier JS: Celiac sprue. *N Engl J Med* 1991, 325:1709–1719.

3.  Long RG, Meinhard E, Skinner RK, *et al.*: Clinical, biochemical and histological studies of osteomalacia, osteoporosis and parathyroid function in chronic liver disease. *Gut* 1978, 19:85–90.

4.  Malluche HH, Langub MC, Monier-Faugere MC: Pathogenesis and histology of renal osteodystrophy. *Osteoporosis Int* 1997, 7:S184–S187.

5.  Bonnick SL: *Bone Densitometry in Clinical Practice.* Totowa, NJ: Humana Press; 1998:152–166.

6.  Chiodini I, Carnevale V, Torlantano M, *et al.*: Alterations on bone turnover and bone mass at different skeletal sites due to pure glucocoroticoid excess: a study in eumenorrheic patients with Cushing's syndrome. *J Clin Endocrinol Metab* 1998, 83:1863–1867.

7.  Riggs BL: Osteoporosis. In: *Textbook of Endocrinology*. Edited by DeGroot LJ. Orlando, FL: Grune and Stratton; 1987.

8.  Chines A, Pacifici R, Avioli LA, *et al.*: Systemic mastocytosis and osteoporosis. *Osteoporosis Int* 1993, S1:S147–S149.

9.  Gebhardt MC, Mankin HJ: The diagnosis and management of bone tumors. In: *Metabolic Bone Disease and Clinically Related Disorders*. Edited by Avioli LV, Krane SM. Philadelphia: WB Saunders; 1990:777–780.

10.  Silverberg SJ, Shane E, de la Cruz L, *et al.*: Skeletal disease in primary hyperparathyroidism. *J Bone Miner Metab* 1989, 4:283–291.

11.  Seeman E, Wahner HW, Offord KP, *et al.*: Differential effects of endocrine dysfunction on the axial and the appendicular skeleton. *J Clin Invest* 1982, 69:1302–1309.

12.  Weinstein RS, *et al.*: *J Clin Invest* 1998, 102:274–282.

13.  Pitkin RM: Calcium metabolism in pregnancy. A review. *Am J Obstet Gynecol* 1975, 12:724–737.

14.  Heaney RP: Nutritional factors in osteoporosis. *Ann Rev Nutr* 1993, 13:287–316.

15.  Parfitt AM: Osteomalacia and related disorders. In: *Metabolic Bone Disease and Clinically Related Disorders*. Edited by Avioli LV, Krane SM. Philadelphia: WB Saunders; 1990:329–396.

16.  Hirano T, Tanizawa T, Endo N, *et al.*: Oncogenic osteomalacia: pre- and postoperative histomorphometric studies. *J Bone Miner Metab* 1997, 15:227–231.

17.  Coburn JW, Norris KC, Nebeker HG: Osteomalacia and bone disease arising from aluminum. *Semin Nephrol* 1986, 6:68–89.

18.  Glorieux FH, Bishop NJ, Plotkin H, *et al.*: Cyclic administration of pamidronate in children with severe osteogenesis imperfecta. *N Engl J Med* 1998, 339:947–952.

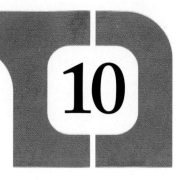

# GLUCOCORTICOID-INDUCED OSTEOPOROSIS

## Lorraine A. Fitzpatrick

Skeletal decalcification was recognized as a feature of Cushing disease as early as 1932. With the isolation of cortisol, the anti-inflammatory, antineoplastic, and immunosuppressive properties of glucocorticoids have been useful for treating many diseases. Patients exposed to long-term glucocorticoid therapy have distinct clinical features associated with the suppression of the hypothalamic-pituitary-adrenal axis [1]. Glucocorticoid-induced osteoporosis is probably the most common cause of secondary osteoporosis. Although the true incidence of osteoporosis in this population remains unknown, patients receiving high-dose glucocorticoid therapy experience rapid bone loss and vertebral compression fractures that can occur within weeks to months of initiation of therapy [2]. Overall, 30% to 35% of patients receiving glucocorticoid therapy sustain vertebral crush fractures and have a 50% increased risk for hip fracture [3].

The bone loss caused by excess glucocorticoids is diffuse and affects both the cortical and axial skeleton. Glucocorticoids damage trabecular bone to a greater extent than cortical bone, perhaps because of the greater surface area of trabecular bone. The osteopenia is caused by several mechanisms: suppression of osteoblast function, inhibition of intestinal calcium absorption leading to secondary hyperparathyroidism, and increased osteoclast-mediated bone resorption. Bone resorption is promoted by the direct stimulation of renal excretion of calcium by glucocorticoids and hypogonadism associated with the suppressive effects of glucocorticoids.

The minimum glucocorticoid dose associated with rapid bone loss is not well established. Patients with juvenile chronic arthritis ingesting a cumulative prednisone dose of 5 g sustain vertebral fractures. The authors recommend no more than 5 mg of prednisone per day [4]. Studies that evaluate mineral density of trabecular bone indicate that loss of this type of bone is significantly greater than loss of cortical bone, probably because of the differential effect of glucocorticoid therapy on trabecular versus cortical bone. Traditional risk factors associated with osteoporosis also influence glucocorticoid-induced osteoporosis. Retrospective analysis also suggests that certain factors are associated with increased risk for glucocorticoid-induced bone loss. Osteoporosis is more severe in patients younger than 15 years or older than 50 years of age and in postmenopausal women [4,5]. In older, immobilized, or postmenopausal patients, a pre-existing low level of bone mass may lead to rapid development of clinically significant osteopenia. In the younger patient, a higher rate of bone turnover results in more rapid bone loss. The improved longevity in transplant recipients has also raised issues about glucocorticoid-associated bone loss. The additional immuno-suppressive agents that these patients are prescribed makes the relative contribution of each agent to bone loss difficult to assess. The incidence of fracture rates range from 8% to 65% during the first year after transplantation, and rates of fracture and bone loss are greatest in the first 6 to 12 months after transplantation [6]. Other risk factors include low body mass index [7]; disorders associated with interleukin-1 production, such as rheumatoid arthritis; and the general osteoporosis risk factors.

# Epidemiology and Risk Factors

### EPIDEMIOLOGY OF GLUCOCORTICOID-INDUCED OSTEOPOROSIS

Incidence estimated at 30% to 50% [18,19]

Studies limited because of confounding variables (eg, additional immunosuppressive therapy, altered drug clearance rates, autoimmune disease, or changing doses of glucocorticoids)

Bone loss is greatest in first 6 to 12 months of therapy [20–22]

Bone loss is related to duration and total cumulative dose [7,23]

**FIGURE 10-1.** Epidemiology of glucocorticoid-induced osteoporosis.

### RISK FACTORS FOR GLUCOCORTICOID-INDUCED OSTEOPOROSIS

Age < 15 years or > 50 years of age associated with risk for severe osteoporosis [4,5]

Postmenopausal women are at higher risk

High total cumulative dose of glucocosteroids

Low body mass index [7]

Secondary risk factors

  Duration of therapy

  Disorders associated with interleukin-1 production, such as rheumatoid arthritis

  General osteoporosis risk factors (age, race, sex, body habitus, immobilization, genetics)

Relative risk of each factor remains unknown, although certain factors are associated with an acceleration of glucocorticoid-induced bone loss

**FIGURE 10-2.** Risk factors for glucocorticoid-induced osteoporosis.

## Pathophysiology

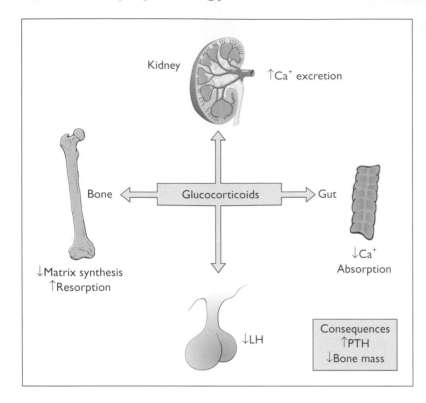

FIGURE 10-3. Pathophysiology of glucocorticoid-induced bone loss. Several interrelated factors affect mineral metabolism in patients with an excess of endogenous or exogenous glucocorticoids. Glucocorticoids directly affect the bone, alter calcium absorption from the intestine, change the ability of the kidney to reabsorb calcium, and inhibit gonadal hormone secretion. Secondary hyperparathyroidism has been documented in patients receiving glucocorticoid therapy.

Intestinal absorption of calcium determines the amount of substrate available to meet the needs of bone remodeling. Glucocorticoids decrease net intestinal calcium absorption by an unknown mechanism [8]. Glucocorticoids may alter vitamin D metabolism; this would also inhibit calcium absorption. Bone constantly undergoes remodeling and can be greatly affected by administration of glucocorticoids [9]. Suppression of bone formation is the major impairment in bone physiology caused by glucocorticoids [10]. Glucocorticoids directly inhibit differentiation of preosteoblasts and alter the oncoproteins that regulate the genes for alkaline phosphatase, osteocalcin, and other growth factors [11,12]. Calcium kinetic studies support the hypothesis that glucocorticoids enhance bone resorption [13]. At the level of the kidney, glucocorticoids enhance calcium excretion.

Glucocorticoids can alter levels of gonadal hormones in both men and women. Glucocorticoids reduce testosterone levels in men [14,15] and interfere with normal ovulation in women [16]. Serum follicle-stimulating hormone and luteinizing hormone are suppressed by exogenous glucocorticoid administration. The cause of secondary hyperparathyroidism is attributable to the decrease in calcium absorption, and direct action of glucocorticoids on the parathyroid gland has been documented [17].

## Bone Histomorphometry

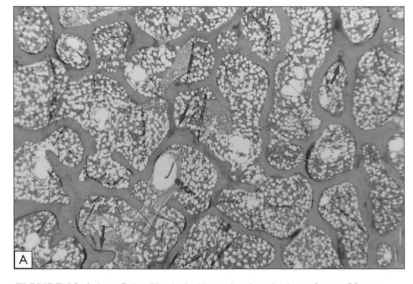

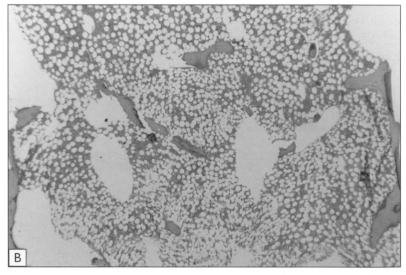

FIGURE 10-4. (see Color Plate) A, Normal trabecular bone from a 30-year-old patient. Note the thick, serpiginous trabecular plates with excellent connectivity. Arrows indicate areas of osteoid, consistent with bone formation. B, Severe osteoporosis in a 30-year-old patient receiving long-term glucocorticoid therapy. Multiple isolated bone islands are present, and little evidence of bone formation is noted. Histomorphometrically, dynamic measures of bone formation are profoundly reduced, indicating that remodeling has been uncoupled. The larger surface of trabecular bone suggests that it is more affected by glucocorticoids than is cortical bone; however, reduction in cortical bone volume can be seen. It is estimated that 30% loss of bone occurs during each remodeling cycle in patients receiving glucocorticoid therapy.

## Physical Findings

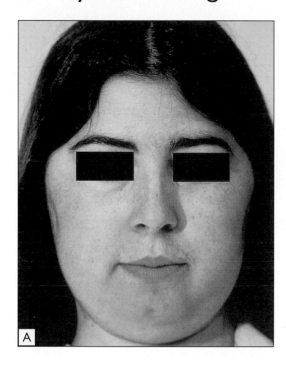

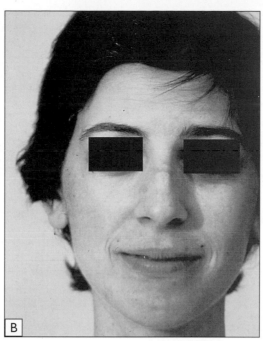

A

B

**FIGURE 10-5.** Symptoms and physical findings that can identify patients with excessive glucocorticoids. Increased deposition of fat is one of the earliest signs to occur in almost all patients (**A**). Fat distribution is increased in the peritoneal cavity, mediastinum, and, as shown here, subcutaneous sites on the face and neck. The "moon facies" with increased fat in the supraclavicular or temporal fossae and dorso-cervical area ("buffalo hump") are rarely seen in normal individuals. Filling of the temporal fossae may prevent eyeglass frames from fitting properly. Rarely, long-term exogenous steroid use results in fat accumulation in the epidural space and can cause neurologic deficits. Alterations in fat distribution resolve when glucocorticoid therapy is stopped (**B**).

## Radiographic Diagnosis

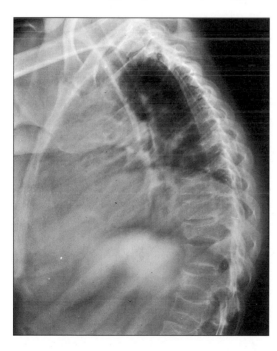

**FIGURE 10-6.** Osteopenia on spine radiography. High circulating levels of glucocorticoids, either endogenous or exogenous, cause marked loss of bone mineral density. Both cortical and cancellous bone is lost, and vertebral collapse, as shown in this figure, is not uncommon.

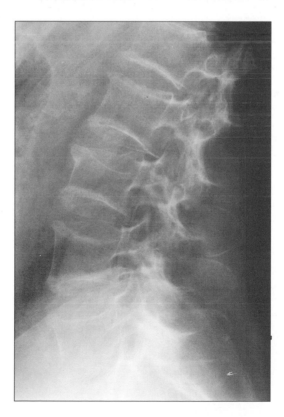

**FIGURE 10-7.** Radiograph of a 50-year-old woman who has been receiving daily steroid therapy for systemic lupus erythematosus for 2 years. Osteoporosis with ballooning of the thoracic and lumbar interspaces is present. Sclerosis of the vertebral endplates is also noted. The patient also had avascular necrosis of the right femoral head.

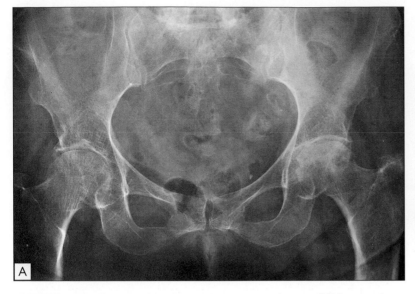

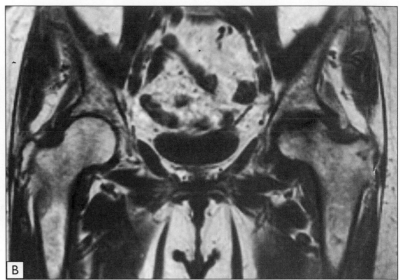

**FIGURE 10-8.** Radiograph and magnetic resonance imaging (MRI) scan of the hip. The left hip film (**A**) shows irregularity and sclerosis of the left femoral head with collapse of the articular cortex. The T1-weighted coronal MRI of the hips (**B**) shows a region of decreased signal in the superior portion of the left femoral head. The plain film and MRI finding are characteristic of avascular necrosis of the left hip. By using MRI technique, the death of marrow fat cells can be detected as early as 12 to 48 hours after its onset. Plain film findings may appear months after the onset of clinical symptoms.

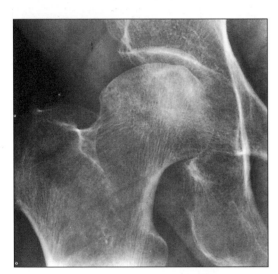

**FIGURE 10-9.** Osteonecrosis of the right femoral head. Sclerosis of the right femoral head with irregularity of the superior articular surface is consistent with avascular necrosis in this 71-year-old woman receiving steroids. Complications of avascular necrosis include secondary degenerative arthritis, intra-articular osteochondral loose bodies, and cystic degeneration.

## DIFFERENTIAL DIAGNOSIS OF AVASCULAR NECROSIS OF THE FEMORAL HEAD

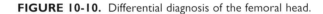

| | |
|---|---|
| Trauma | Dysbaric conditions (Caisson disease) |
| Hemoglobinopathies | Collagen vascular diseases |
| Exogenous or endogenous steroid use | Gaucher disease |
| Renal transplantation | Gout |
| Alcoholism | Irradiation |
| Pancreatitis | Synovitis |

**FIGURE 10-10.** Differential diagnosis of the femoral head.

**FIGURE 10-11.** Bone scan of a 53-year-old woman with a history of systemic lupus erythematosus and hip pain who had been receiving steroids for many years. The bone scan shows focal areas of increased uptake in the proximal right humerus and both femoral heads. The areas of increased uptake in the femoral heads surround photopenic defects. The appearance of uptake is classic for avascular necrosis.

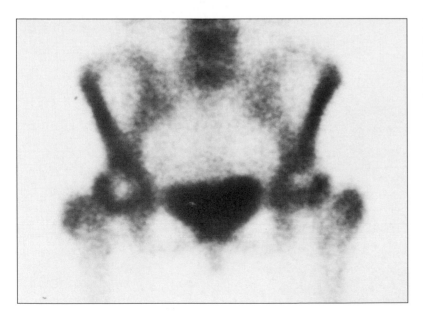

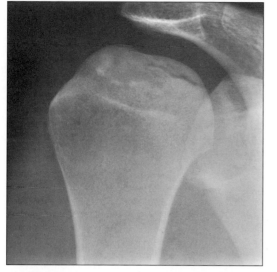

**FIGURE 10-12.** Radiograph of a 26-year-old man with right shoulder pain who had been receiving long-term glucocorticoid therapy for systemic lupus erythematosus. The film shows avascular necrosis of the right humeral head with collapse, subchondral fracture, and sclerosis.

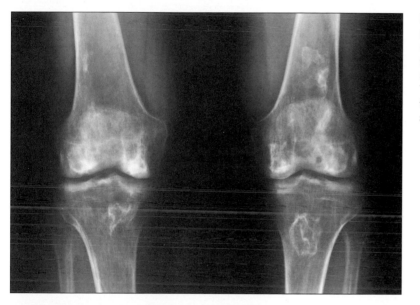

**FIGURE 10-13.** Radiograph of a 42-year-old man with a history of high-dose steroid therapy given for hepatitis. Regular but discrete areas of increased density can been seen in the medullary region of both distal femurs and proximal tibials; these areas are most pronounced at the periphery of the lesions. This finding is consistent with multiple bone infarctions secondary to exogenous steroid use. The pathogenesis of steroid-induced infarction is not known, but attention has focused on the presence of microscopic fat emboli in the end arteries of bone and other organ systems.

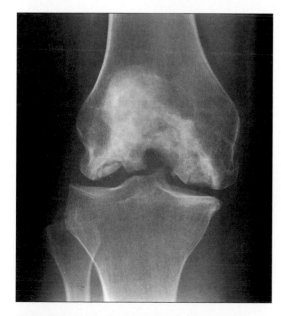

**FIGURE 10-14.** Radiograph of a 30-year-old woman with Crohn's disease who has been receiving prednisone for 15 years. Extensive avascular necrosis involving the femoral condyle is present. The femoral head, humeral head, distal femur, and proximal tibia are common sites of steroid-induced avascular necrosis.

### STAGING OF ISCHEMIC NECROSIS OF THE FEMORAL HEAD

| Stage | Findings |
|-------|----------|
| 0 | Suspected necrosis but no clinical findings; normal radiographs and bone scan |
| I | Clinical findings, normal radiographs, and abnormal bone scan |
| II | Osteopenia, cystic area, and bone sclerosis on radiographs |
| III | Crescent sign and subchondral collapse without flattening of the femoral head on radiographs |
| IV | Flattening of the femoral head and normal joint space on radiographs |
| V | Joint space narrowing and acetabular abnormalities on radiographs |

**FIGURE 10-15.** Staging of avascular necrosis of the femoral head.

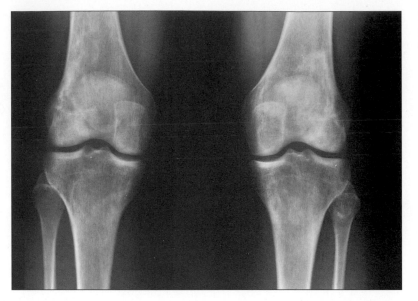

**FIGURE 10-16.** Knee radiographs of a 26-year-old woman with systemic lupus erythematosus receiving prednisone therapy. The film shows symmetric infarctions around both knees with mottled appearance and serpentine sclerosis.

## Bone Scans

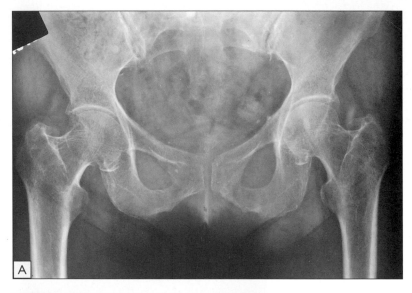

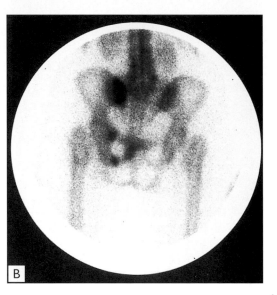

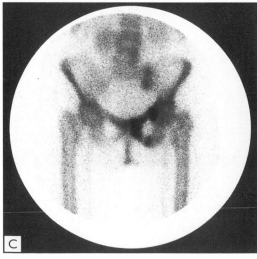

**FIGURE 10-17.** Bone scan and radiograph of the pelvis in a 73-year-old woman receiving glucocorticoids who experienced bilateral hip pain. The initial radiograph of the pelvis (**A**) showed slight sclerosis at the site of the fractures. This was confirmed on bone scan, which revealed foci of increase uptake in the superior and inferior left pubic rami, left pubic bone, and the left sacroiliac region (**B** and **C**).

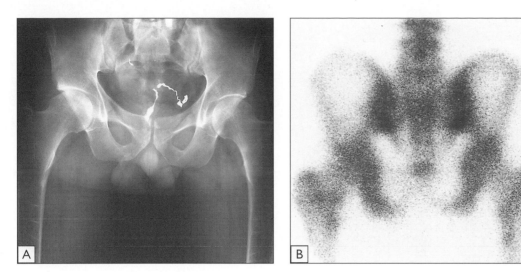

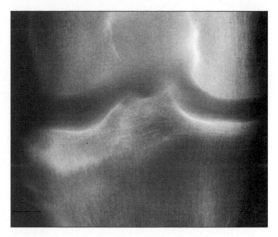

**FIGURE 10-18.** Radiograph (**A**) and bone scan (**B**) of a 34-year-old man with a history of Crohn's disease and long-term steroid use. The patient's short bowel syndrome also contributes to decreased calcium absorption. Both radiograph and bone scan showed bilateral stress fractures in the region of the lesser trochanter. The bone scan was positive before the plain film revealed the stress fractures. Stress fractures of the hip are particularly dangerous because they can become displaced fractures.

**FIGURE 10-19.** Knee radiograph indicating osteopenia and faint linear band sclerosis at the right lateral proximal tibia. This is consistent with a compression or stress fracture in the right lateral tibial plateau.

# References

1. Fitzpatrick LA: Glucocorticoid-induced osteoporosis. In: *Osteoporosis*. Edited by Marcus R. Boston: Blackwell Scientific; 1994:202–226.

2. Baylink DJ: Glucocorticoid-induced osteoporosis. *N Engl J Med* 1983, 309:306–308.

3. Bressot C, Meunier PJ, Chapuy MC, *et al.*: Histomorphometric profile, pathophysiology and reversibility of corticosteroid-induced osteoporosis. *Metab Bone Dis Rel Res* 1979, 1:303–319.

4. Varanos S, Ansell BM, Reeve J: Vertebral collapse in juvenile chronic arthritis: its relationship with glucocorticoid therapy. *Calcif Tissue Int* 1987, 41:75–78

5. Als OS, Gotfredsen A, Christiansen C: The effect of glucocorticoids on bone mass in rheumatoid arthritis patients: influence of menopausal state. *Arthritis Rheum* 1985, 28:369–375.

6. Rodino MA, Shane E: Osteoporosis after organ transplantation. *Am J Med* 1998, 104:459–469.

7. Thompson JM, Modin GW, Arnaud CD, *et al.*: Not all postmenopausal women on chronic steroid and estrogen treatment are osteoporotic: predictors of bone mineral density. *Calcif Tissue Int* 1997, 61:377–381.

8. Klein RG, Arnaud SB, Gallagher JC, *et al.*: Intestinal calcium absorption in exogenous hypercortisonism. Role of 25-hydroxyvitamin D and cortico-steroid dose. *J Clin Invest* 1977, 60:253–259.

9. Wong GL: Basal activities and hormone responsiveness of osteoclast-like and osteoblast-like bone cells are regulated by glucocorticoids. *J Biol Chem* 1979, 254:6337–6340.

10. Weinstein RS, Jilka RL, Parfitt AM, *et al.*: Inhibition of osteoblastogenesis and promotion of apoptosis of osteoblasts and osteocytes by gluco-corticoids: potential mechanisms of their deleterious effects on bone. *J Clin Invest* 1998, 102:274–282.

11. Canalis E: Effect of glucocorticoids on type I collagen synthesis, alkaline phosphatase activity and deoxyribonucleic acid content in cultured rat calvariae. *Endocrinology* 1983, 112:931–939.

12. Subramaniam M, Colvard D, Keeting P, *et al.*: Glucocorticoid regulation of alkaline phosphatase, osteocalcin and proto-oncogenes in normal human osteoblast-like cells. *J Cell Biochem* 1992, 50:411–424.

13. Lund B, Storm TL: Bone mineral loss, bone histomorphometry and vitamin D metabolism in patients with rheumatoid arthritis on long-term glucocorticoid treatment. *Clin Rheumatol* 1985, 4:143–149.

14. Doerr P, Pirke KM: Cortisol-induced suppression of plasma testosterone in normal adult males. *J Clin Endocrinol Metab* 1976, 43:622–628.

15. MacAdams MR, White RH, Chipps BE: Reduction of serum testosterone levels during chronic glucocorticoid therapy. *Ann Intern Med* 1986, 104:648–651.

16. Crilly RG, Cawood M, Marshall DH, *et al.*: Hormonal status in normal, osteoporotic and corticosteroid-treated postmenopausal women. *J R Soc Med* 1978, 71:733–736.

17. Lukert BP, Adams JS: Calcium and phosphorus homeostasis in man: effect of corticosteroids. *Arch Intern Med* 1976, 136:1249–1253.

18. Cryer PE, Kissane JM: Vertebral compression fractures with accelerated bone turnover in a patient with Cushing's disease (clinicopathologic conference). *Am J Med* 1980, 68:932–940.

19. Greenberger PA, Hendrix RW, Patterson R: Bone studies in patients on prolonged systemic corticosteroid therapy for asthma. *Clin Allergy* 1982, 12:363–368.

20. Sambrook PN, Birmingham J, Kempler S: Corticosteroid effects on proximal femur bone loss. *J Bone Miner Res* 1990, 5:1211–1216.

21. Gennari C, Civitelli R: Glucocorticoid-induced osteoporosis. *Clin Rheum Dis* 1986, 12:637–654.

22. LoCascio V, Bonucci E, Imbimbo B: Bone loss in response to long-term glucocorticoid therapy. *Bone Miner* 1990, 8:39–51.

23. Reed IR, Heap SW: Determinants of vertebral mineral density in patients receiving long-term glucocorticoid therapy. *Arch Intern Med* 1990, 150:2545–2548.

# IMMOBILIZATION OSTEOPOROSIS

**11**

## B. Jenny Kiratli

Bone loss occurs with inactivity and immobilization. Just as bone mass increases during growth and development and with exercise attributable to increases in mechanical loading, bone mass decreases along with reduced mechanical use. This response has been recognized for more than 50 years and has been evaluated in many clinical conditions. However, much remains unknown about underlying mechanisms and prevention or treatment. Clinical immobilization includes a variety of situations, and site-specific bone loss seems to be relative to the magnitude of immobilization. Although osteopenia has been reported in various diseases and conditions that cause temporary or partial immobilization, few detailed studies have been devoted to most of these. A larger body of literature concerns bone loss with complete paralysis due to spinal cord injury [1]. The concepts discussed here for bone response to paralysis are expected to apply to other immobilizing conditions, but perhaps with reduced severity.

Spinal cord injury is the most extreme case of clinical immobilization: Complete paralysis of particular body parts is frequently the outcome, and the observed osteopenia may be considered a worst-case scenario of skeletal response to reduced mechanical loading. Paralysis caused by spinal cord injury reflects the location and extent of neurologic damage. Injuries in the cervical region of the spinal cord result in quadriplegia because they affect both upper- and lower-extremity function. Injuries below this area cause paraplegia because the brachial plexus is preserved and only lower-extremity function is affected. This simple distinction does not address the multitude of other organ and regulatory functions that are affected by the level of the injury; however, because most of this chapter explores bone atrophy with regard to motor function, body and limb mobility are the primary focus of this discussion. The spinal level of injury also determines the amount of motor and sensory function that is preserved or absent, such that quadriplegia does not mean total loss of upper-extremity function unless the injury occurs above C4. Furthermore, injury to the spinal cord may also include partial interruption of neural transmission: Some but not all neurons in the injured part of the cord are damaged. This results in "incomplete" paralysis and preservation of motor function relative to intact neurons. Thus, even spinal cord injury does not always lead to complete cessation of mechanical loading.

Acute immobilization is characterized by hypercalciuria and heterotopic ossification (the incidence rate was previously 25% but has recently been decreasing). Hypercalcemia is infrequent, except in younger patients. Most bone loss seems to occur in the first year after injury, and bone turnover stabilizes within 4 years after injury.

As with other instances of bone loss, osteopenia is not in itself a problem until it contributes to elevated risk for fracture. Both the patterns and treatment of fracture are unique in patients with spinal cord injury. The underlying risk factors and risk profiles may also differ from those of patients with other forms of osteoporosis.

This chapter covers some basic concepts regarding bone biomechanics and the manner in which bone responds to alterations in its mechanical environment; clinical evidence of osteopenia resulting from disuse and immobilization, with primary focus on spinal cord injury; relevant information about fractures in patients with spinal cord injury, and a theoretical framework for understanding bone loss and fracture risk with decreased mechanical loading, specifically in patients with spinal cord injury.

# Bone Biomechanics

## TYPES OF MECHANICAL LOADING

| External Loads on the Body | Internal Loads on Bone |
|---|---|
| Ground Reaction Forces/Gravity | Compression |
| Body Weight | Tension |
| Body Segmental Mass | Torsion |
| Muscle Activity | Shear |
| Impact | |

**FIGURE 11-1.** Types of mechanical loading. During normal movement, the human skeleton is constantly subjected to external and internal loads, and these loads so strongly influence bone tissue that the tissue adapts structurally. Bone becomes deformed from bending, compression, and torsion loads. External loads might include ground reaction forces generated during walking, running, climbing steps; compression and torsion imposed by the mass of body segments at rest and during movement; forces generated by muscular contractions, and impact loading (such as hitting a tennis ball). Internal compressive, tensile, torsional, and shear strain (deformation) are generated within the bone tissue as a result of these external loads. Strain direction, strain distribution, strain rate and frequency, and stimulus duration are all components of the mechanical control of bone response.

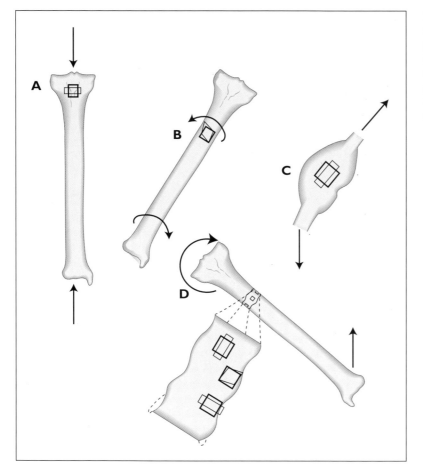

**FIGURE 11-2.** Bone deformation in response to loading. Bone deformation initiates the bone remodeling response. These diagrams show the internal strains generated within the bone by mechanical loading. The thick lines are the undistorted shapes, and the thin lines are the distorted ones. The deformations, much exaggerated, are: compression (**A**); torsion, producing shear (**B**); tension, as in the patella (**C**); and bending (**D**). In *D*, the deformations are shown on a piece of bone unwrapped from the whole bone. The lower part shows tension; the middle, shear; and the top, compression. (*Adapted from* Currey [2]; with permission.)

## EXAMPLES OF BONE ADAPTATION TO MECHANICAL LOADING

| Influence | Effect |
| --- | --- |
| Growth and development | Increased bone mass |
| Exercise and increased physical activity | Increased bone mass |
| Disuse or immobilization | Decreased bone mass |

**FIGURE 11-3.** Examples of bone adaptation to mechanical loading. Much clinical and experimental evidence indicates that bone tissue adapts to alterations in mechanical use. Bone accretion occurs during adolescence as a result of normal growth and development. Evidence that body mass predicts bone mass increment during growth supports the expectation that mechanical loading is an important factor [3]. In other words, the loads imposed on the developing child by his or her body weight influence skeletal regulation. Physical activity, especially resistance exercise, leads to increased bone formation in the young adult and reduction in bone loss in the older adult; increase in bone mass has been demonstrated in older adults with impact loading [4]. Decreased loading in experimental or therapeutic recumbency or in diseases and condition of immobilization causes decreased bone mass.

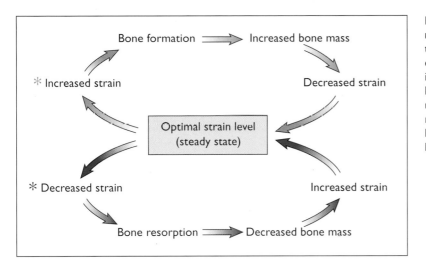

**FIGURE 11-4.** Regulation of bone mass. Bone accommodates to a customary mechanical loading environment. Increased external loading leads to increased tissue-level strain, and bone formation is initiated to regain the customary strain environment. Increasing bone mass reduces the strain level, and a feedback loop is established until a new equilibrium is achieved. Bone responds to dynamic loading rather than static loading, and only a short duration of loading, if the magnitude is sufficient, is necessary to initiate bone adaptation [5]. Conversely, reduction in external loads causes initiation of bone resorption and decreased bone mass in order to maintain customary strain level. Several theories have been proposed regarding the regulatory mechanisms of this adaptive effect [6].

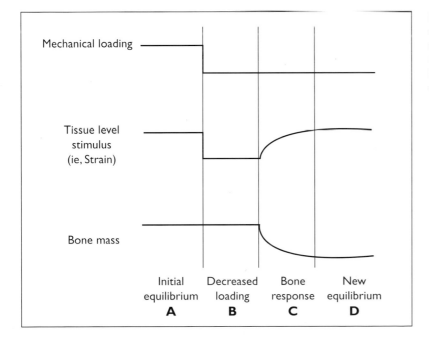

**FIGURE 11-5.** Adaptation of bone mass to immobilization. **A,** An equilibrium exists within bone in relation to its mechanical environment. **B,** If habitual mechanical use declines, tissue-level strain declines. **C,** Bone tissue responds by reducing mass; this allows the strain level to return to normal or to an optimal level. **D,** A new equilibrium is established in relation to the now habitual condition of decreased loading.

## EFFECTS OF MECHANICAL USAGE ON MODELING AND REMODELING

| Effects on Skeletal Envelopes | Modeling | Remodeling |
|---|---|---|
| *Increased Strain* | *Activated* | *Inhibited* |
| Periosteal | Expansion | Expansion ?? |
| Endosteal | Loss retarded | Loss retarded |
| Trabecular | Loss retarded | Loss retarded |
| Intracortical | No effect | Activation retarded; increased mass |
| *Decreased Strain* | *Inhibited* | *Activated* |
| Periosteal | Apposition retarded ?? | Apposition retarded ?? |
| Endosteal | Loss accelerated | Loss accelerated |
| Trabecular | Loss accelerated | Loss accelerated |
| Intracortical | No effect | Activation stimulated; loss of bone mass |

**FIGURE 11-6.** Differential response by bone tissue. Bone adapts by different mechanisms in the bone envelopes in response to alteration in the local mechanical environment. Mechanical loading includes a complex set of stimuli that are not uniform throughout the bone. This table summarizes expected responses in periosteal, endosteal, trabecular, and intracortical bone envelopes caused by elevated and decreased loading, in circumstances of both modeling (accretion of new bone) and remodeling (reorganization of existing bone). (*Adapted from* Martin and Burr [6]; with permission.)

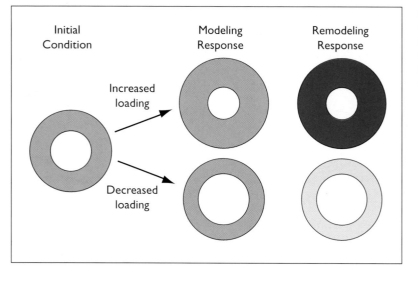

**FIGURE 11-7.** Modeling and remodeling responses to the increased and decreased mechanical loading described in Fig. 11-6. Periosteal expansion and increased cortical thickness occur with increased loading, and intracortical density may increase (indicated by darker color) with remodeling. Cortical thinning is found with decreased mechanical loading, and intracortical density may be reduced with remodeling.

# Clinical Evidence

## MODELS OF IMMOBILIZATION

Animal Models
  Tendon resection: rabbit
  Hindlimb suspension: rat
  Intact, isolated wing: turkey
  Spinal cord transection: cats
  Limb casting: dogs
  Body cast immobilized: monkey
Spaceflight
  Astronauts
Bedrest
  Healthy volunteers

**FIGURE 11-8.** Models of immobilization. Evidence of bone atrophy in circumstances of immobilization or disuse is available from animal studies and studies of hypogravity and voluntary bedrest. Various techniques have been used to simulate disuse and immobilization in animal studies. This figure presents the more frequently used animal models, including examples of both irreversible and reversible immobilization. Data are available on histologic responses and mechanical properties of atrophied bone, as well as quantification of muscle atrophy and its correlation with bone response. Many of these studies have also yielded specific information about the amount and type of loading stimulus necessary to maintain normal bone homeostasis. In the 1970s, NASA began to investigate the effects of weightlessness on the skeleton and studied astronauts participating in space flight and earthbound volunteers put to extended bedrest. The findings are applicable to understanding clinical conditions of immobilization. These studies have also included attempts at counter-measures to prevent bone loss, including pharmacologic therapy (bisphosphonates) and physical means (eg, recumbent cycling and impact or compressive loads applied to the feet). Currently, astronauts engage in treadmill exercise during space flight, in part to prevent bone atrophy. In animal and human models, much of the bone loss appears to be reversible with return to normal mechanical loading.

## CLINICAL EXAMPLES OF IMMOBILIZATION

Temporary immobilization
  Therapeutic bedrest (eg, prolapsed disc)
  Injury
Paretic disorders
  Poliomyelitis
  Cerebral Palsy
  Multiple Sclerosis
  Stroke
Paralysis
  Spinal Cord Injury
Other conditions
  Amputation
  Total joint replacement
  Regional disorder (eg, frozen shoulder)

**FIGURE 11-9.** Clinical examples of immobilization. Physical activity may be temporarily reduced in cases of injury or therapeutic bedrest, and long-standing reduction in physical activity is concomitant with aging or general health decline in many individuals. Overall or specific weakness (paresis) and even paralysis are found with disorders that may occur primarily in childhood, such as cerebral palsy and poliomyelitis; some degenerative diseases in adulthood, such as multiple sclerosis; and with stroke. Complete or partial paralysis is associated with traumatic spinal cord injury. Normal mechanical loading is also decreased in conditions: for example, limb amputation, where muscle attachments are severed and muscles proximal to the amputation are immobilized; total joint replacement, in which stress-shielding occurs as the normal loads are essentially diverted from the bone to the prosthesis; and localized joint immobility. In all of these conditions, localized bone loss has occurred concurrently with reduction in mechanical use. In hemiparetic conditions, such as stroke, compensatory increase in use (and bone mass) may occur on the unaffected side.

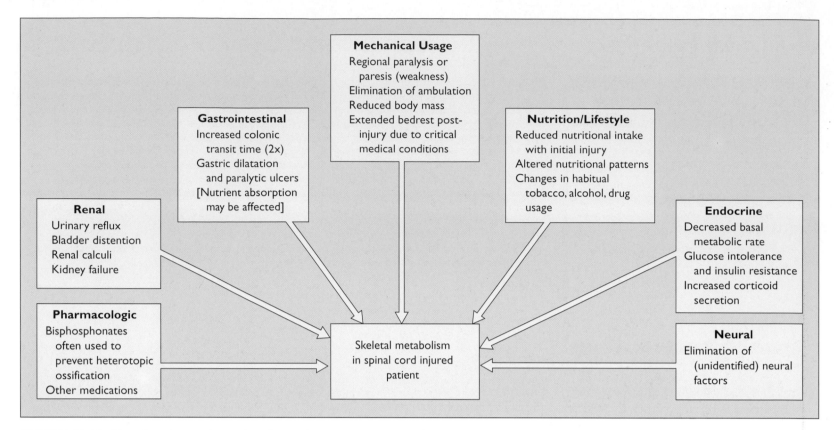

**FIGURE 11-10.** Physiologic factors that might influence bone response in spinal cord injury. Myriad medical and lifestyle changes occur with spinal cord injury, and several of these factors might contribute to bone response. Although it is commonly thought that motor paralysis is the predominant factor underlying bone loss after paralysis (hence the common term "disuse osteoporosis"), other, unidentified neural factors may also contribute (an alternate term is "neurogenic bone loss," which is more open-ended). In addition to the regional paralysis and resultant loss of ambulation ability, there may be additional medical conditions, such as traumatic bone fractures, head injury, or other critical injuries that necessitate extended bedrest. As these medical conditions resolve, the patient will be encouraged to sit and move as much as he or she is able, and wheelchair mobility will be initiated. Muscle mass is rapidly lost with acute spinal cord injury because of reduced use and denervation. The reduction in muscle mass and activity removes a primary factor of bone maintenance (mechanical loading). Patients also frequently experience great weight loss in the acute stage after a spinal cord injury. Nonmechanical factors that may influence bone response include endocrine, gastrointestinal, renal, and nutritional changes and changes in substance use (ie, tobacco, alcohol, drugs) and prescribed medications. No specific data on these latter effects are available, but they should not be forgotten as potential factors.

## MARKERS OF BONE TURNOVER IN ACUTE AND CHRONIC SPINAL CORD INJURY

| Bone Metabolism | Acute Response | Chronic Response |
|---|---|---|
| Formation markers: | | |
| Osteocalcin | elevated | normal |
| C terminus peptide, type I procollagen | elevated | ? |
| Resorption markers | | |
| Hydroxyproline/creatinine ratio (urinary) | elevated | normal |
| Pyridinolines | elevated | ? |
| C-terminus telopeptide, type I procollagen | elevated | ? |
| Turnover markers | | |
| Serum ionized calcium | normal | normal |
| Calcium/creatinine ratio (urinary) | elevated | normal |
| Calcitonin | elevated | elevated/normal |
| Parathyroid hormone | decreased | decreased |
| 25-hydroxycholecalciferol (Vitamin D) | decreased | decreased |

**FIGURE 11-11.** Markers of bone turnover in acute and chronic spinal cord injury. Much of the early literature on bone loss with immobilization (before the advent of densitometry) described effects of paralysis, specifically from poliomyelitis and spinal cord injury, on markers of bone metabolism, such as alkaline phosphatase and hydroxyproline. Recent work with more specific markers has borne out the findings of these early researchers [7–10]. Immediately after injury, markers of bone formation and bone resorption increase, with greater and more sustained increases in resorption markers. Thus, the initial bone remodeling response appears to represent an uncoupling of the osteoblast–osteoclast cellular actions that normally maintain a balance of bone formation and resorption. Hormone and metabolite levels of resorption markers remain elevated for up to 8 months and then return to normal levels. By 12 months after injury, most markers are within the normal range and there is little evidence of abnormal bone metabolism in patients with chronic spinal cord injury. However, several recent studies indicate persistent vitamin D deficiency and parathyroid hormone depression [11–13]. Relatively few studies on this topic have been done, and results of existing studies are inconsistent. Furthermore, not all patients conform to group findings; some disparate results may be attributable to underlying disease or other conditions. Finally, data are not yet available for some of the newer markers for patients with long-standing spinal cord injury (these are indicated by "?" in the table).

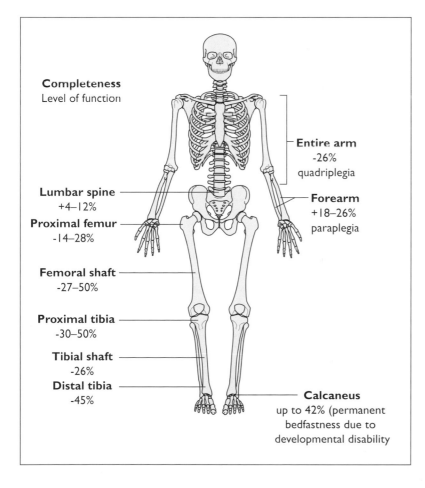

**Completeness**
Level of function

**Entire arm**
-26%
quadriplegia

**Lumbar spine**
+4–12%

**Forearm**
+18–26%
paraplegia

**Proximal femur**
-14–28%

**Femoral shaft**
-27–50%

**Proximal tibia**
-30–50%

**Tibial shaft**
-26%

**Distal tibia**
-45%

**Calcaneus**
up to 42% (permanent
bedfastness due to
developmental disability)

**FIGURE 11-12.** Regional bone loss after spinal cord injury. Local osteopenia is observed in relation to changes of mechanical loading. Thus, bone loss occurs only in skeletal regions below the level of the lesion where motor function is reduced. Data are available from many studies; these results are summarized in the figure [14–25]. Although the results vary, the findings are mostly consistent. While the level of the neurologic lesion determines which body parts are affected (ie, regions distal to the injury), the severity of the injury or "completeness" also contributes to the magnitude of the effect; this might explain some of the variability in studies that have not controlled for completeness. Voluntary motor function may be preserved to varying degrees below the level of the lesion with an incomplete injury. Thus, some amount of mechanical loading is preserved, and the bone response is less. Total leg bone mass is reduced by approximately 50%, with regional changes as shown in the figure. Equivalent bone decrement occurs in the lower limbs of both paraplegic and quadriplegic individuals; this is not surprising because the mechanical environment (eg, paralysis and absence of standing) of the lower extremity is essentially the same for both patient populations. Upper-extremity bone loss occurs with quadriplegia, but bone mass is increased with paraplegia; these findings correspond with decreases and increases in upper-extremity function in quadriplegia and paraplegia, respectively. In both paraplegic and quadriplegic patients, lumbar spine bone mass increases. No evidence suggests an independent age effect on bone response, and there is little evidence of increasing bone loss with greater duration of injury (although some reports indicate such an effect).

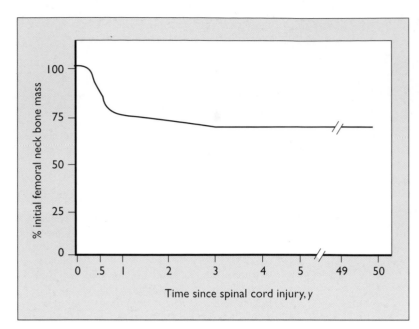

**FIGURE 11-13.** Femoral neck bone response with acute and chronic spinal cord injury. Few data are available on bone mass for the first few days after spinal cord injury because of logistic problems with making these measurements. In fact, even though the metabolic changes have begun, little observable change would be expected immediately in bone mass because of the time delay of bone remodeling (ie, 4 to 6 weeks for bone mass change). This schematic, based on available data, shows bone response in the femoral neck. Individual responses vary greatly, and measurement intervals are often variable for individual patients and across studies. Reduction in femoral neck bone mineral density is greater in the early months after acute immobilization (approximately 2% per month for the first 5 to 7 months) than in the later months (less than 1% per month for the remainder of the year). The average loss over the first year is approximately 20%. Few data are available for the loss rate within the next few years after injury, but some continuing loss seems to occur as the average total loss up to 30%. Bone mass appears to stabilize by the fourth year, with little evidence of later loss even after many decades of paralysis. Bone response in the leg does not differ between quadriplegic and paraplegic patients.

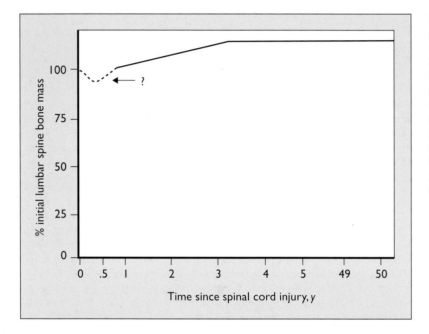

**FIGURE 11-14.** Lumbar spine bone response with acute and chronic spinal cord injury. Bone response at the lumbar spine shows a different pattern. Essentially no reduction attributable to paralysis occurs in this region. However, an initial but reversible decline may occur in patients subjected to extreme recumbency because of additional medical complications. In fact, some evidence suggests a slight increase in bone mineral density of the lumbar spine in chronic paralysis (up to 12% above normative values). As with bone mineral density of the femoral neck, duration of injury has no effect, and there is no difference between quadriplegic and paraplegic patients. The commonly accepted explanation for maintenance of lumbar spine bone mass is that patients with spinal cord injury carry their body weight during daily activities via a sitting position; thus, normal loading patterns may not be substantially disrupted and may be similar to those of ambulatory individuals.

## THERAPIES TO PREVENT BONE LOSS IN SPINAL CORD INJURED PATIENTS

| Therapy | Effect on Bone Mass |
| --- | --- |
| Upright loading | No evidence |
| Electrical stimulation exercise | Some evidence of reduction in bone loss |
| Pharmacologic | Suggestive evidence (yet unpublished) of reduction in bone loss |

**FIGURE 11-15.** Therapies to prevent bone loss in patients with spinal cord injury. For many decades, clinicians and researchers have sought effective countermeasures for the bone loss associated with disuse and immobilization. Few reports in the literature describe successful treatments, however. Much attention has focused on physical countermeasures based on the expectation that the primary cause of atrophy is elimination of mechanical loading; thus, replacement or simulation of mechanical loading should reverse bone loss. Upright standing in a standing frame or with braces has not been shown to reduce osteopenia.

However, standing protocols have involved relatively brief frequency of stimulus (1 hour per day, 3 times per week) and include static loading only; dynamic loading, which causes bone deformation, is required to elicit a bone response. Electrical stimulation of leg musculature during cycling exercise has recently been shown to positively affect bone mass [26], although many prior studies have not shown such an effect. Pharmacologic treatments (including calcitonin, etidronate, clodronate, and toludronate) have also been attempted, with mostly negative results; some evidence indicates a positive effect on bone turnover assessed by biopsy and with metabolic markers [27–30], but no data on bone mass change have been published. Bisphosphonate treatment (primarily etidronate) has been found to be successful in preventing heterotopic ossification [31].

# Long Bone Fractures after Spinal Cord Injury

## SYMPTOMS AND INDICATIONS OF FRACTURE IN THE SPINAL CORD INJURED PATIENT

Swelling and erythema

Increased autonomic dysreflexia

Increased spasticity

Patient experienced a sound ("pop" or "crack") that indicated fracture

Limb deformity

**FIGURE 11-16.** Symptoms of fracture in patients with spinal cord injury. Fractures frequently occur in such patients without evidence of trauma and often go undiagnosed acutely because of absent sensation and lack of a traumatic event. In some instances, the patient is aware of a sound (loud crack or pop) when the limb fractures (eg, while performing a leg-stretching exercise or during dressing). Common symptoms include local swelling and redness, increased spasticity or autonomic dysreflexia, and, occasionally, deformity. Essentially, the untransmitted pain of the fracture acts as an internal noxious stimulus that heightens the nervous system responses (spasticity and potentially life-threatening autonomic dysreflexia). In the absence of obvious causes of autonomic dysreflexia, the examining physician should evaluate the possibility of a pathologic or unnoticed bone fracture in these patients.

## LOCATION AND FREQUENCY OF LONG BONE FRACTURES IN SPINAL CORD INJURED PATIENTS

| Skeletal Region | Prevalence (Published Data) | Prevalence (Current Study) |
|---|---|---|
| Femoral neck | 12.5% | 13% - all proximal |
| Inter/Subtrochanteric | 4.9% | |
| Femoral shaft | 12.8% | 19% |
| Supracondylar (femoral) | 29.6% | 22% |
| Tibial plateau | 2.3% | 19% - all proximal |
| Tibial proximal shaft | 6.6% | |
| Tibial midshaft | 8.6% | 13% |
| Tibia distal shaft | 13.2% | 13% |
| Other leg (not specified) | 10.5% | |

**FIGURE 11-17.** Location and frequency of long bone fractures. Most long bone fractures that occur after spinal cord injury are in the lower extremity. This is consistent with the expectation of specific bone loss with regional paralysis or paresis. The morphologic types and locations of these fractures are distinct from those seen in other osteoporotic populations. The predominant fracture types and sites are spiral fracture of the femoral shaft; displaced, bending fractures of the femoral (distal) condylar region; and simple fractures of the proximal tibia. Estimates of the proportion of fracture types are provided from the literature [32–36] and a recent study [Kiratli BJ: Unpublished data]. The prevalence of long bone fractures is estimated at approximately 6%, but this may be an under-representation because of data collection methods. The current rate may be much closer to 20%.

## CHARACTERISTICS OF SPINAL CORD INJURED PATIENTS WHO SUSTAIN LONG-BONE FRACTURES

More common in paraplegia

More common with flaccid paralysis

More common with complete paralysis

Average duration of spinal cord injury: 14 y

High frequency of multiple fractures

**FIGURE 11-18.** Characteristics of patients with spinal cord injury who sustain long bone fractures. The proportion of fractures is higher in paraplegic than in quadriplegic patients; flaccidity and complete injury are also more common patient characteristics. Although these fractures can occur at any time after spinal cord injury, the median time after injury is 14 years. Multiple fractures are common, although this does not include refracture of previous fracture sites.

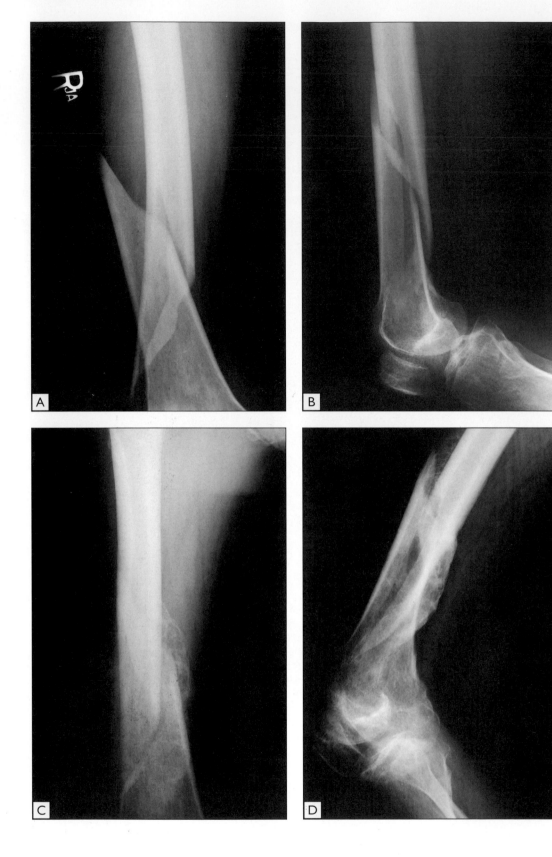

**FIGURE 11-19.** Spiral fracture of the femoral shaft. One of the most common and spectacular fractures in patients with spinal cord injury is the spiral fracture of the femoral shaft. This figure shows the antero-posterior and lateral views of an initial (**A** and **B**) and healed (**C** and **D**) femoral fracture in a 47-year-old, complete quadriplegic man whose spinal cord (C7) injury occurred 12 years before the fracture. Although neither internal not external fixation was performed, these fractures tend to heal solidly, albeit sometimes in malalignment.

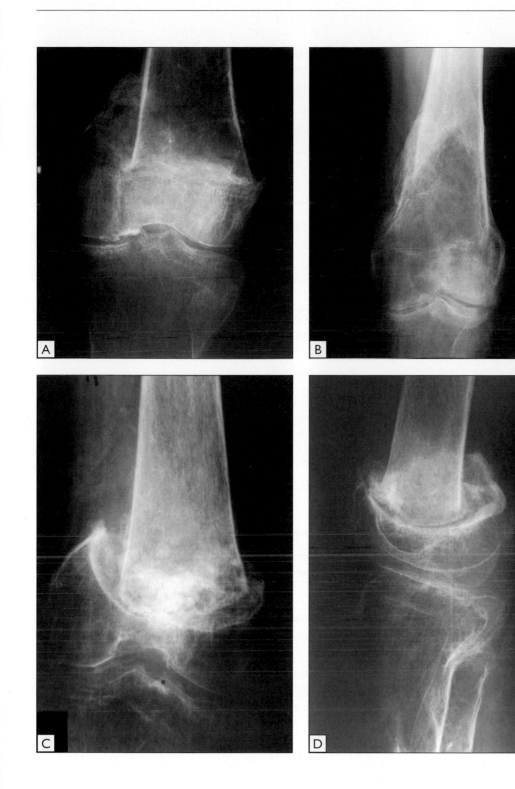

**FIGURE 11-20.** Displaced fracture of the distal femur. Another common fracture occurs in the highly cancellous region of the distal femur. Treatment is conservative, and orthopedic fixation is not usually offered. This type of fracture is more likely to result in nonunion or pseudoarthrosis, or it may involve excessive bone formation within the distal joint. Several healing responses after this type of fracture are shown. Successful healing is shown for (**A**) an 80-year-old complete paraplegic man whose spinal cord injury (T12) occurred 54 years before the fracture and (**B**) a 37-year-old complete quadriplegic man whose spinal cord injury (C6) occurred 11 years before the fracture. A nonunion is shown in anteroposterior (**C**) and lateral (**D**) views in a 76-year-old complete paraplegic man whose spinal cord injury (T4 and T5) occurred 19 years before the fracture. The more distal fractures seem to have worse healing outcomes. In some cases, joint fusion occurs as a sequela of extensive heterotopic bone formation that extends into the femorotibial joint space. Resection may be offered to patients with this condition to regain joint mobility, but excessive bone formation may recur after resection surgery. Furthermore, bone resection in this area may be difficult because of the potential for damage to the neurovascular bundle encased in bony tissue. The clinical decision should include consideration of the effect of the immobile joint on activities of daily living, such as sitting, transferring, and wheelchair mobility.

## TREATMENT REGIMEN FOR LONG-BONE FRACTURES IN SPINAL CORD INJURED PATIENTS

| Treatment Approach | Indication | Reason |
| --- | --- | --- |
| Conservative treatment soft (pillow) splint and external brace | Commonly used | Safe, effective to promote healing in most cases |
| Cast fixation | Contraindicated; less risk with bivalve cast | Skin fragility - risk of skin breakdown. Bivalve cast allows skin checks |
| Surgical fixation: prosthesis, plates, and rods | Contraindicated | Risk of infection, poor bone stock, skin fragility |

**FIGURE 11-21.** Treatment regimen. Although no consensus papers in the orthopedic literature concern optimal fracture management in patients with spinal cord injury, conservative, nonoperative treatments (such as pillow splinting or external bracing) are generally recommended; casts are used only if they are well-padded and can be frequently removed for skin inspection. Surgical interventions (open reduction internal fixation) are generally contraindicated because of preexisting osteopenia, skin fragility, and heightened risk for further complications, including infection, continuous drainage, edema, hematoma, secondary hemorrhage, and refracture. Prolonged immobilization has associated risks, such as joint contractures, postural deformities, general loss of cardiovascular fitness, and possible increase in bone turnover leading to accentuated osteopenia. The patient's prefracture functional abilities should be assessed, and treatment should be directed to maximize return to equivalent function. Treatment regimens vary, however, and are based mostly on the experience of the treating physicians in the absence of consensus protocols.

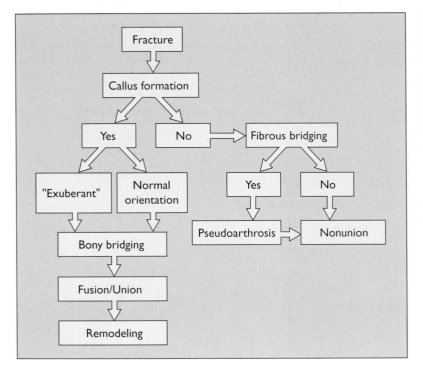

**FIGURE 11-22.** Healing response. Healing responses also vary. Adequate healing (bony union) occurs in many patients, although complications may occur; some patients, in contrast, do not form callus and tend not to heal (malunion or nonunion). Acute complications of fractures include hemorrhage and autonomic dysreflexia, and secondary complications such as infection and heterotopic bone formation often follow. Without proper management, outcomes can include spontaneous arthrodesis and loss of joint motion; malalignment resulting in functional deformity; and nonunion, which may develop into a pseudoarthrosis. Unfused fractures can produce pain in patients with intact sensation and can interfere in activities of daily living because of abnormal limb mobility or stability. Nonetheless, healing is often reported as rapid, and nonunion is relatively rare. Little is known about the reasons for these different healing responses, nor about how often fractures might heal spontaneously in satisfactory positions without intervention. Orthopedic treatment decisions are influenced by fracture location and structure, as well as the medical and physical status of the patient.

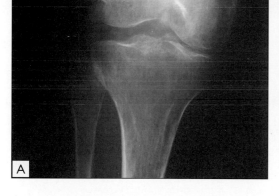

**FIGURE 11-23.** Exuberant callus formation. One of the distinctive features of long bone fracture healing with spinal cord injury is the formation of "exuberant" callus. This type of callus has a cloudy, disorganized appearance with no alignment along stress lines. Although typical in spinal cord injury, it is not characteristic of all fractures, and callus formation often appears normal in these patients. The formation of exuberant callus does not seem to interfere with the healing process. The patient shown here is a 32-year-old complete paraplegic man whose spinal cord injury (T12) occurred 8 years before the fracture. Anteroposterior (**A**) and lateral (**B**) views are shown.

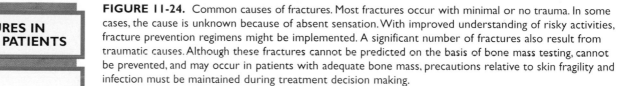

## CAUSES OF FRACTURES IN SPINAL CORD INJURED PATIENTS

Nontraumatic
    Fall from wheelchair
    During transfer activity
    Activity of daily living
    Range of motion exercise
    Unknown
Traumatic
    Fall, other than from wheelchair
    Motor vehicle accident
    Other accident

**FIGURE 11-24.** Common causes of fractures. Most fractures occur with minimal or no trauma. In some cases, the cause is unknown because of absent sensation. With improved understanding of risky activities, fracture prevention regimens might be implemented. A significant number of fractures also result from traumatic causes. Although these fractures cannot be predicted on the basis of bone mass testing, cannot be prevented, and may occur in patients with adequate bone mass, precautions relative to skin fragility and infection must be maintained during treatment decision making.

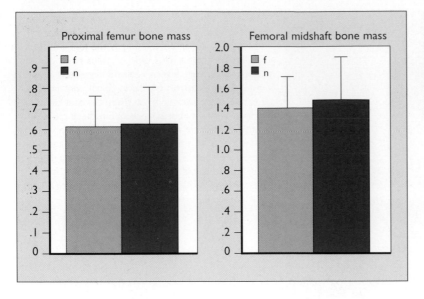

**FIGURE 11-25.** Bone mass and fracture history in patients with spinal cord injury. Mean bone mass of the proximal femur and femoral midshaft are slightly, but not significantly, lower in patients with spinal cord injury who have a history of fracture (*light blue*) than in those with no history of fracture (*dark blue*). The bone values in these cohorts overlap, and no clear threshold of elevated fracture risk is available to discriminate between the cohorts [Kiratli BJ: Unpublished data]. This may indicate that most patients with spinal cord injury are at greatly increased risk but have not yet sustained a fracture-causing event.

# Theoretical Framework for Fracture Risk Prediction

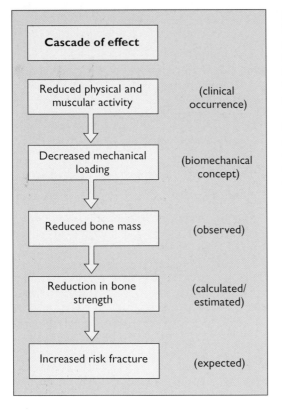

**FIGURE 11-26.** Cascade of effect summarizing the course of immobilization osteopenia. The result of an immobilizing disease or condition is regional paralysis and/or paresis or reduced physical activity and movement, relative to the extent of the immobilization. By definition, decreased activity means decreased habitual mechanical loading. The observed effect is regional bone loss, although other neurogenic or endocrine factors may also influence skeletal response. Although bone mineral density is only moderately correlated with breaking strength, bone mass is commonly used to represent bone strength. However, geometric and architectural factors should not be ignored. Reduced bone mass and bone strength imply elevated fracture risk. Although this cascade is mostly accurate, other components need additional consideration. First, we have little information about the structural and geometric bone responses to immobilization and whether compensatory mechanisms preserve bone strength. Second, we know little about the risk factors underlying fractures in patients with paralytic or immobilizing conditions. Specifically, these patients are not subjected to the same habitual loading patterns as ambulatory persons (eg, repetitive loading 1 to 1.5 times body weight during ambulation); thus, the interpretation of fracture risk based on bone mass may be inadequate in these populations.

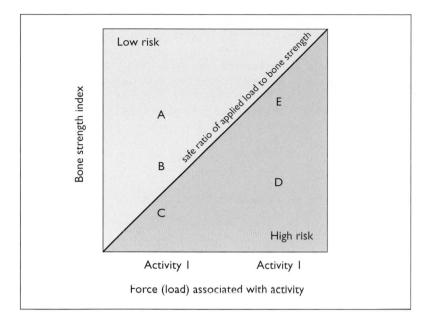

**FIGURE 11-27.** Risk profile comparing bone strength with fracture event. Does low bone mass indicate high fracture risk? For a fracture to occur, the applied load must be greater than the bone can withstand, and the type and location of fracture depend on characteristics of the loads applied to the skeleton as well as the strength of the bone. Essential data that influence the mechanical failure (fracture) of bone are the type, direction, and velocity of applied loads. Therefore, an event that would cause fracture in one individual might not produce the same effect in someone with stronger bones. Furthermore, the forces applied to the bone during various activities differ according to individual variables such as weight, height, body segmental lengths and mass, and velocity during the activity.

This graph describes an approach for estimation of individualized fracture risk. Whether a given activity imparts a fracture risk depends on the force of the activity relative to the strength of the bone. For example, activity 1 may represent falling out of a wheelchair. This imposes no risk to person A (ambulatory person) or person B (person with spinal cord injury) because both have bones that are strong enough to withstand the force of the fall. Person C (person with spinal cord injury), however, is expected to sustain a fracture during the fall because his bone strength is below the safe level (ie, the applied load exceeds the bone failure strength). Thus, the clinician must be aware of the heightened fracture risk that might be associated with activities that would pose no risk for ambulatory individuals, such as stretching a leg or lower-extremity dressing. Precautions can be suggested to reduce the applied loads (eg, "don't pull your leg so hard during stretching exercise") and reduce fracture risk. Conversely, some activities involve high loads, and the bone would be expected to fracture regardless of bone strength. Activity 2 may represent a motor vehicle accident in which the applied loads exceed bone strength in both person D (person with spinal cord injury) and person E (ambulatory person). Risk prediction based on bone mass would be pointless in this case.

In summary, bone fracture occurs when the applied load exceeds the bone strength, and bone does not fracture when bone strength is greater than the applied load. Although calculation of individualized risk profiles is not readily available, a general awareness of this approach should be useful in clinical interactions with patients to guide prevention.

# References

1. Kiratli BJ: Immobilization osteopenia. In: Osteoporosis. Edited by Marcus R, Feldman D, Kelsey J. San Diego: Academic Press; 1996:833–854.

2. Currey. *The Mechanical Adaptations of Bone.* Princeton: Princeton University Press; 1984.

3. van der Meulen MCH, Ashford MW, Kiratli BJ, Bachrach LK, et al.: Determinants of femoral geometry and structure during adolescent growth. *J Ortho Res* 1996, 14:22–29.

4. Snow CM, Matkin CC, Shaw JM: Physical activity and risk for osteoporosis. In: Osteoporosis. Edited by Marcus R, Feldman D, Kelsey J. San Diego: Academic Press; 1996:511–528.

5. Turner CH: Three rules for bone adaptation to mechanical stimuli. *Bone* 1998, 23:399–407.

6. Martin RB, Burr DB: *Structure, Function, and Adaptation of Compact Bone.* New York: Raven Press; 1989.

7. Hangartner TN: Osteoporosis due to disuse. *Phys Med Rehab Clin North Am* 1995, 6:579:594.

8. Roberts D, Lee W, Cuneo RC, et al.: Longitudinal study of bone turnover after acute spinal cord injury. *J Clin Endocrinol Metab* 1998, 83:415–422.

9. Szollar SM, Martin EM, Sartoris DJ, et al.: Bone mineral density and indexes of bone metabolism in spinal cord injury. *Arch Phys Med Rehab* 1998, 77:28–35.

10. Uebelhart D, Hartmann D, Vuagnat H, et al.: Early modifications of biochemical markers of bone metabolism in spinal cord injury patients. A preliminary study. *Scand J Rehab Med* 1994, 26:197–202.

11. Bauman WA, Zhong YG, Schwartz E: Vitamin D deficiency in veterans with chronic spinal cord injury. *Metabolism* 1995, 44:1612–1616.

12. Mechanick JI, Pomerantz F, Flanagan S, et al.: Parathyroid hormone suppression in spinal cord injury patients is associated with the degree of neurologic impairment and not the level of injury. *Arch Phys Med Rehab* 1997, 78:692–696.

13. Vaziri ND, Pandian MR, Segal JL, et al.: Vitamin D, parathyroid, and calcitonin profiles in persons with long-standing spinal cord injury. *Arch Phys Med Rehab* 1994, 75:766–769.

14. Biering-Sørensen F, Bohr H, et al.: Longitudinal study of bone mineral content in the lumbar spine, the forearm and the lower extremities after spinal cord injury. *Eur J Clin Invest* 1990, 20:330–335.

15. Biering-Sørensen R, Bohr H: Bone mineral content of the lumbar spine and lower extremities years after spinal cord lesion. *Paraplegia* 1988, 26.293–301.

16. Demirel G, Yilmaz H, Paker N, et al.: Osteoporosis after spinal cord injury. *Spinal Cord* 1998, 36:822–825.

17. Finsen V, Indredavik B, Fougner K: Bone mineral and hormone status in paraplegics. *Paraplegia* 1992, 30:343–347.

18. Garland D, Stewart C, Adkins R, et al.: Osteoporosis after spinal cord injury. *J Ortho Res* 1992, 10:371–378.

19. Hancock DA, Reed GW, Atkinson PJ, et al.: Bone and soft tissue changes in paraplegic patients. *Paraplegia* 1980, 17:267–271.

20. Hangartner T, Rodgers M, Glaser R, et al.: Tibial bone density loss in spinal cord injured patients: effects of FES exercise. *J Rehab Res Develop* 1994, 31:50–61.

21. Kiratli BJ: Skeletal adaptation to disuse: longitudinal and cross-sectional study of the response of the femur and spine to immobilization (paralysis). PhD Thesis. Madison: University of Wisconsin-Madison; 1989.

22. Leslie W, Nance P: Dissociated hip and spine demineralization: a specific finding in spinal cord injury. *Arch Phys Med Rehab* 1993, 74:960–964.

23. Lussier L, Knight J, Bell G, et al.: Body composition comparison in two elite female wheelchair athletes. *Paraplegia* 1983, 21:16–22.

24. Saltzstein R, Hardin S, Hastings J: Osteoporosis in spinal cord injury: using an index of mobility and its relationship to bone density. *J Am Paraplegia Soc* 1992, 15:232–234.

25. Vose G, Keele, D: Hypokinesia of bedfastness and its relationship to x-ray determined skeletal density. *Texas Report of Biology and Medicine* 1970, 28:123–130.

26. Bloomfield SA, Mysiw WJ, Jackson RD: Bone mass and endocrine adaptations to training in spinal cord injured individuals. *Bone* 1996, 19:61–68.

27. Chappard D, Minaire P, Privat C, et al.: Effects of tiludronate on bone loss in paraplegic patients. *J Bone Mineral Res* 1995, 10:112–118.

28. Meythaler JM, Tuel SM, Cross LL: Successful treatment of immobilization hypercalcemia using calcitonin and etidronate. *Arch Phys Med Rehab* 1993, 74:316–319.

29. Minaire P, Depassio J, Berard E, et al.: Effects of clodronate on immobilization bone loss. *Bone* 1987, 8:S63–S68.

30. Pearson EG, Nance PW, Leslie WD, et al.: Cyclical etidronate: its effect on bone density in patients with acute spinal cord injury. *ArchPhys Med Rehab* 1997, 78:269–272.

31. Banovac K, Gonzalez F: Evaluation and management of heterotopic ossification in patients with spinal cord injury. *Spinal Cord* 1997, 35:158–162.

32. Comarr AE, Hutchinson RH: Extremity fractures of patients with spinal cord injuries. *Am J Surg* 1962, 103:732–739.

33. Freehafer A, Mast W: Lower extremity fractures in patients with spinal cord injury. *J Bone Joint Surg* 1965, 47A:683–694.

34. Freehafer A, Coletta M, Becker C: Lower extremity fractures in patients with spinal cord injury. *Paraplegia* 1981, 19:367–372.

35. Ingram R, Suman R, Freeman P: Lower limb fractures in the chronic spinal cord injured patient. *Paraplegia* 1989, 27:133–139.

36. Ragnarsson K, Sell G: Lower extremity fractures after spinal cord injury: a retrospective study. *Arch Phys Med Rehab* 1981, 62:418–423.

# 12

# ETIOLOGY AND BIOMECHANICS OF HIP AND VERTEBRAL FRACTURES

## Mary L. Bouxsein

Fractures are one of the most dramatic and devastating sequelae of the aging of the human skeleton. In the United States alone, more than 1.5 million age-related fractures occur annually, including 280,000 hip and 500,000 vertebral fractures. Associated medical expenditures are nearly $14 billion. Moreover, on the basis of current demographic trends predicting a dramatic increase in the number of individuals older than 70 years of age, the number of fractures is projected to double or triple in the next 50 years. Clearly, interventions to reduce the incidence of fracture are needed. To be most effective, these interventions must be based on a sound understanding of the cause of fractures. In the past, the predominant view was that age-related fractures were strictly a consequence of bone loss. This view was based on studies showing a dramatic increase in fracture incidence with age and a greater fracture rate in women than in men (*see* chapter 1). However, recent evidence indicates that factors related not only to skeletal fragility but also to skeletal loading influence risk for fracture.

This chapter reviews the cause of age-related fractures of the hip and spine, introduces a standard engineering concept used to evaluate structural failures, and applies this concept to skeletal fractures. The inter-related roles of skeletal fragility and skeletal loading are also discussed.

## Determinants of Fracture Risk and Introduction of the Factor of Risk

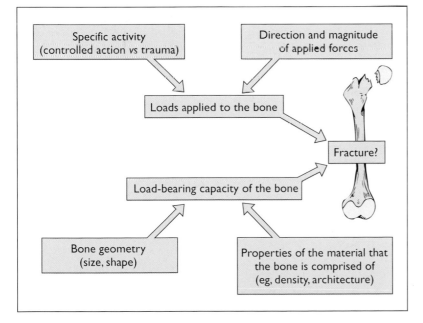

**FIGURE 12-1.** Cause of fractures. From a mechanical viewpoint, a hip or vertebral fracture represents a structural failure of the bone whereby the forces applied to the bone exceed its load-bearing capacity (or failure load). The load-bearing capacity of a bone depends on the properties of the materials that the bone is made of and on how this material is arranged to give the bone its particular size and shape. The magnitude and direction of the loads applied to the bone are associated with a specific loading event, whether it be a controlled activity, such as bending or lifting, or traumatic loading, such as that associated with a fall.

## Factor of risk (φ)

φ = **Applied load/structural capacity**

φ >> 1, fracture unlikely

φ <<, fracture unlikely

**FIGURE 12-2.** Factor of risk. To express the related roles of skeletal loading and skeletal fragility, Hayes [1] introduced the concept of the factor of risk. The numerator of the factor of risk is the forced applied to a bone during a given activity of interest, and the denominator is the structural capacity (or failure load) of the bone during that same activity. When this ratio is greater than one (ie, the force applied to the bone is much higher than the structural capacity of the bone), then a fracture is predicted to occur. A high factor of risk may result from a low bone mineral density and therefore very weak bones, or it may occur because of an activity wherein high forces are applied to the skeleton, such as during a motor vehicle accident or a fall. For example, to implement the factor of risk concept for hip fractures, it is essential to 1) identify activities associated with a hip fracture, 2) determine the loads applied to the proximal femur during those activities, and 3) estimate the failure load of the proximal femur during those activities.

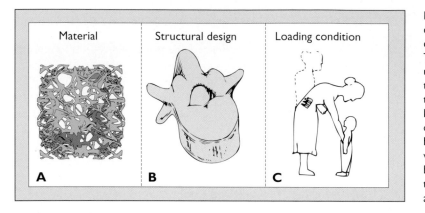

| Material | Structural design | Loading condition |
| A | B | C |

**FIGURE 12-3.** Factors that determine the amount of force a skeletal structure can withstand. In this figure, the vertebral body is used to demonstrate the characteristics of the spine that determine its capacity to resist mechanical loads. The ability of a structure to carry loads is determined by the matter that makes up the structure, the corresponding mechanical behavior of that matter, the way that the matter is arranged to form a skeletal structure, and the loading conditions to which the structure is subjected. In the spine, the vertebral bodies carry a large proportion of the compressive loading. The vertebral body primarily consists of trabecular bone (**A**). The structural design of the vertebral body is determined by the organization of this trabecular bone and by the size and shape of the vertebral body itself (**B**). Finally, the behavior of the structure is also determined by the loading conditions that arise from activities of daily living (**C**) or from traumatic loading situations (eg, falls or motor vehicle accidents). (From Myers and Wilson [2]; with permission.)

# Basic Bone Properties and Age-Related Changes

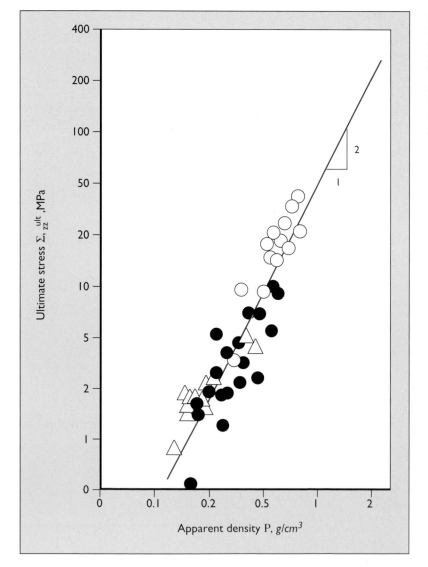

**FIGURE 12-4.** The strong relationship between density and the mechanical behavior of trabecular bone. The relationship between these two variables is linear on a log-log scale and therefore can be described by a power law of the form $y = ax^b$. Several studies have shown that the exponent $b$ is approximately 2. Therefore, small changes in density can result in dramatic changes in compressive strength. For example, a 25% decrease in apparent density, approximately equivalent to 20 to 25 years of age-related bone loss, would be predicted to cause an approximately 45% decrease in the compressive strength of trabecular bone. (Adapted from Carter and Hayes [3]; with permission.)

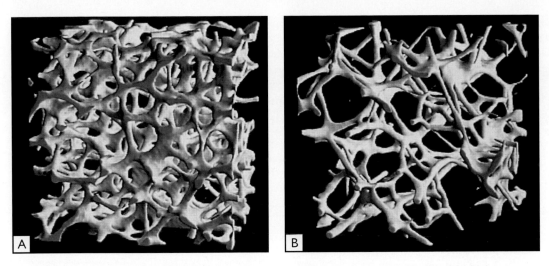

**FIGURE 12-5.** Dramatic age-related change in bone mass and architecture of vertebral trabecular bone. Trabecular bone strength depends not only on its density (Fig. 12-4) but also on the arrangement and structure of the trabecular elements themselves. This trabecular architecture can be described by the number, orientation, spacing, thickness, and connectivity of trabeculae. This figure clearly shows that the changes in the architecture of trabecular bone accompany the age-related changes in bone density

(42-year-old man [L2 level] [**A**] compared with 84-year-old woman [L2 level] [**B**]). The thickness and number of trabecular elements decrease, and the spacing between trabeculae increases with decreases in density. In addition, there may be an accentuated loss of trabeculae that are oriented horizontally. It may be useful to picture the vertical trabeculae as columns that support compressive loads and to view the horizontal trabeculae as cross-struts that brace the columns. In this scenario, the thinning or loss of horizontal trabeculae would reduce the stability of the vertical trabecular "columns" and may lead to failure of the vertical trabeculae by buckling. The contribution of trabecular bone to overall bone strength varies with skeletal site. For example, the proportion of trabecular bone is approximately 60% to 90% at the vertebral body, 50% at the intertrochanteric region of the hip, 25% at the femoral neck, and less than 5% at the femoral and radial diaphyses [4]. (*Courtesy of* Dr. Ralph Müller, Orthopedic Biomechanics Laboratory, Beth Israel Deaconess Medical Center and Harvard Medical School, Boston, Massachusetts.)

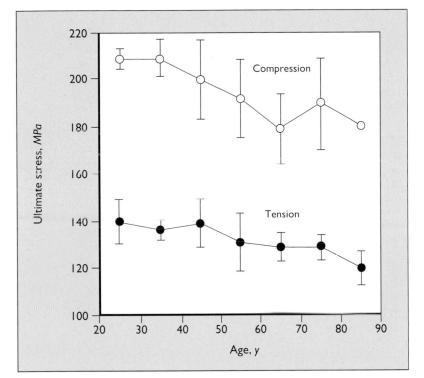

**FIGURE 12-6.** Age-related changes in the ultimate stress of human femoral cortical bone in tension and compression (error bars represent 1 standard deviation). These data indicate that the intrinsic mechanical properties of cortical bone decrease with age and that cortical bone therefore weakens. The mean change is −2.1% per decade for tensile strength and −2.5% per decade for compressive strength. Thus, in normal individuals, the strength of cortical bone decreases by approximately 15% to 20% from 20 to 80 years of age [5].

## AGE-RELATED CHANGES IN VERTICAL TRABECULAR BONE SPECIMENS THAT WERE COMPRESSED IN THE VERTICAL OR HORIZONTAL DIRECTION

| Variable | Specimens Compressed in Supero-Inferior (Vertical) Direction | | Specimens Compressed in Horizontal Direction | |
|---|---|---|---|---|
| | Change per Decade, % | Correlation with Age | Change per Decade, % | Correlation with Age ($r$) |
| Ash density | -9 | -0.85* | -9 | Not reported |
| Ultimate stress | -12.8 | -0.79† | -15.5 | -0.87† |
| Elastic modulus | -13.5 | -0.83† | -15.9 | -0.83† |
| Energy to failure | -14 | -0.75† | -15.2 | -0.88† |

*P<0.01,
†P<0.001.
0.05<P<0.06.

**FIGURE 12-7.** Age-related changes in the mechanical properties human vertebral trabecular bone specimens. To study age-related changes in vertebral trabecular bone, Mosekilde et al. [6] collected cadaveric vertebrae from 42 persons aged 15 to 87 years. Trabecular bone specimens, oriented either parallel or perpendicular to the superior-inferior axis, were removed from the vertebral bodies and tested in compression. A strong relationship was seen between age and density, ultimate strength, elastic modulus, and the energy absorbed before failure. The density decreased approximately 9% per decade, whereas the mechanical properties decreased 12% to 15% per decade [6]. (Data from Mosekilde et al. [6]; with permission.)

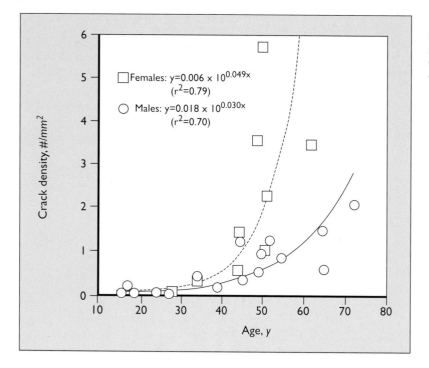

**FIGURE 12-8.** Dramatic age-related increase in microdamage, as measured by the concentration of microcracks in the femoral cortex of human cadaveric specimens. This damage accumulation seems to occur about twice as rapidly in women as in men and may contribute to the higher fracture incidence in women than in men [7].

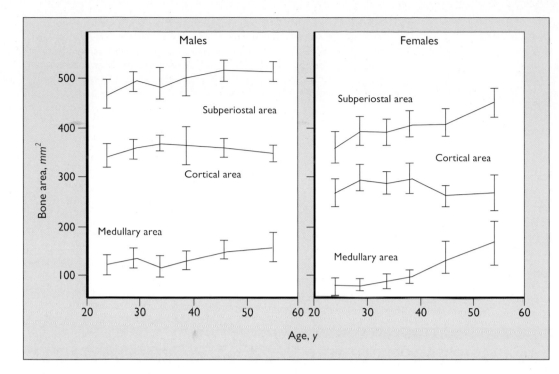

**FIGURE 12-9.** Age-related changes in the cross-sectional geometry of the femoral diaphysis. These data indicate that women undergo more endosteal resorption than men, leading to a reduced cortical area. Both men and women, however, appear to undergo a slight periosteal expansion with age. This geometric adaptation increases the cross-sectional moment of inertia of the specimen and leads to an increased resistance to bending and torsional loads. This geometric change probably helps to offset the detrimental effects of an age-related increase in intra-cortical porosity, which tends to weaken the bone [8].

# Biomechanics of Hip Fractures

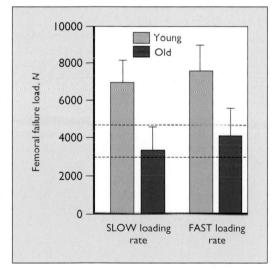

**FIGURE 12-10.** Mean failure loads for cadaveric proximal femurs from young (light blue bars) and elderly (dark blue bars) donors. The femurs were mechanically tested to failure at slow (2 mm/sec) and fast (100 mm/sec) loading rates in a configuration designed to simulate a sideways fall with impact to the greater trochanter. For both the slow and fast loading rates, femurs from the young donor group were 80% to 100% stronger than femurs from elderly individuals. Femurs from both the young and elderly group were approximately 20% to 30% stronger, and absorbed 20% to 30% more energy when tested at the fast loading rate than when tested at the slow loading rate. The two dashed horizontal lines represent the 95% confidence interval for the load that is predicted to be applied to the femur during a sideways fall from standing height. Thus, this cadaveric study indicates that most elderly individuals would be at high risk for hip fracture during a fall from standing height because the load applied to the femur is close to or exceeds the load required to break it. (Adapted from Courtney, et al., [9,12].)

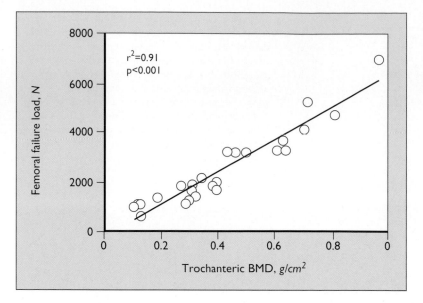

**FIGURE 12-11.** Trochanteric bone mineral density (BMD) versus femoral failure load of cadaveric proximal femurs. There is a strong linear relationship between femoral BMD and the failure load of elderly cadaveric femurs tested in a configuration designed to simulate a fall to the side with impact to the greater trochanter. The load required to fracture the proximal femur ranges from approximately 800 N to 7000 N (or about 200 to 1700 pounds).

## MULTIPLE LOGISTIC REGRESSION ANALYSIS OF FACTORS ASSOCIATED WITH HIP FRACTURE IN COMMUNITY-DWELLING MEN AND WOMEN WHO FELL

| Factor | Adjusted Odds Ratio | (95% Confidence Interval) | P Value |
|---|---|---|---|
| Fall to the side | 5.7 | (2.3–14) | <0.001 |
| Femoral neck bone mineral density* | 2.7 | (1.6–4.6) | <0.001 |
| Potential energy of fall† | 2.8 | (1.5–5.2) | <0.001 |
| Body mass index* | 2.2 | (1.2–3.8) | 0.003 |

*Calculated for a decrease of 1 standard deviation.
†Calculated for an increase of 1 standard deviation.

**FIGURE 12-12.** Risk factors associated with hip fracture in community-dwelling men and women who fell. This case-control study demonstrates that fall severity and bone mineral density are independent risk factors for hip fracture. In a case-control study of 149 community-dwelling men and women, 72 persons fell and sustained a hip fracture (case-patients) and 77 persons fell and did not sustain a hip fracture (controls). Multiple logistic regression analysis of the data showed that in the case-patients, characteristics related to fall severity, femoral bone mineral density (BMD), and body habitus were strong and independent risk factors for hip fracture. For example, persons who fell to the side were six times more likely to sustain a hip fracture than were persons who fell in any other direction. The risk for hip fracture increased nearly three times for every one–standard deviation decrease in femoral BMD compared with the mean BMD, and approximately doubled for each standard deviation decrease in body mass index [11].

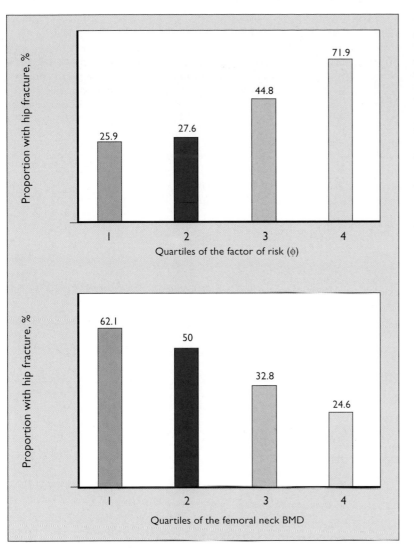

**FIGURE 12-13.** Association between the factor of risk and the presence or absence of hip fracture in persons who have fallen. In this case-control study [12], 98 of 231 persons older than 65 years who had sustained a fall had suffered a hip fracture (case-patients); 133 of these persons had not (controls). The height, weight, and circumstances of the fall for each person was recorded. Femoral bone mineral density (BMD) was assessed by using dual-energy x-ray absorptiometry. The factor of risk was calculated as the ratio of estimated applied load to the hip divided by the estimated maximum failure load of the proximal femur. The applied load was estimated from previous pelvis-release experiments [13]. The maximum failure load of the femur was based on a linear relationship between femoral neck BMD and ultimate load measured in a sideways fall configuration [14]. The factor of risk averaged 2.0 in fracture cases and 1.5 in controls, and there was a strong association between the factor of risk and hip fracture. The odds of hip fracture increased by 9.5 for every unit increase in factor of risk. Bone mineral density by itself was also significantly associated with hip fracture, with an odds ratio of 3.6 for a change in BMD of two standard deviations [12].

# Biomechanics of Vertebral Fractures

### RESULTS OF SURVEY OF PATIENTS WITH VERTEBRAL FRACTURE

| Activity | Patients, % |
|---|---|
| Controlled (eg, Lifting) | 25 |
| Fall | 55 |
| Slow onset/unknown | 19 |

**FIGURE 12-14.** Circumstances surrounding vertebral fracture. It has always been understood that only a small fraction of vertebral fractures are acutely symptomatic and cause the patient to seek medical assistance. However, only recently have large-scale clinical trials estimated the relative incidence of symptomatic and asymptomatic fractures. Results from the Fracture Intervention Trial (FIT), representing the experience of 2000 elderly women who had already sustained at least one vertebral fracture, now address this question [15]. Among approximately 1000 women assigned to receive placebo, new vertebral fractures occurred at an annual rate of 18%, as determined by periodic follow-up spine radiographs. By contrast, the annual incidence of clinically evident fractures was only 6%. Thus, patients are not aware of 2 of every 3 vertebral compression fractures at the time the fracture occurs. Consequently, understanding of the antecedent events that contribute to fracture must remain incomplete.

In one study of consecutive patients reporting to an emergency department with vertebral fracture, patients underwent a structured interview within 1 week of the event to ascertain activities associated with fracture [16]. The prevalence of falls in these patients is surprisingly high. Thus, efforts aimed at preventing falls should be undertaken to prevent both hip and vertebral fracture.

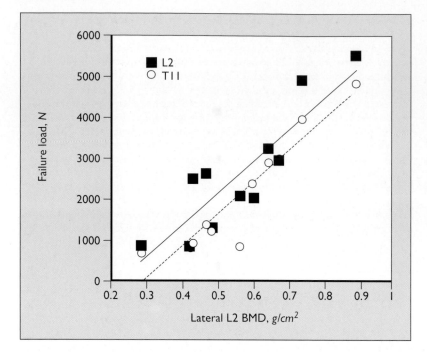

**FIGURE 12-15.** Linear relationship between lumbar spine bone mineral density (BMD) and compressive failure loads of the 11th thoracic (T11) and second lumbar (L2) vertebral bodies. Cadaveric spines from elderly donors (mean age, 72 years; range, 48–87) were subjected to compressive forces to determine their load-bearing capacity and to determine the relationship between lumbar BMD and the failure loads of both lumbar and thoracic vertebral bodies. The correlation coefficients between lumbar BMD and failure loads of T11 and L2 were $r = 0.94$ $(P < 0.001)$ and $r = 0.89$ $(P < 0.001)$, respectively. These findings indicate that, in general, lumbar spine BMD is a reasonably good predictor of the load-bearing capacity of both thoracic and lumbar vertebral bodies. However, the standard error of the estimate (ie, the error that could be expected when trying to predict the failure load of an individual vertebral body from a single BMD value) was substantial. (*Adapted from* Moro *et al.* [17].)

**FIGURE 12-16.** Predicted compressive loads on the second lumbar (L2) and 11th thoracic (T11) vertebrae during various activities. The loads were computed for a woman who weighs 58 kg and is 162 cm tall [18]. N—newtons.

## PREDICTED COMPRESSIVE LOADS ON THE L2 AND T11 VERTEBRAE DURING VARIOUS ACTIVITIES

| Activity | Predicted Load on T11 | | Predicted Load on L2 | |
|---|---|---|---|---|
| | N | Body Weight, % | N | Body Weight, % |
| Relaxed standing | 240 | 41 | 290 | 51 |
| Rising from a chair, without use of hands | 340 | 60 | 980 | 173 |
| Standing, holding 8 kg of weight close to body | 320 | 57 | 420 | 74 |
| Standing, holding 8 kg of weight with arms extended | 660 | 117 | 1302 | 230 |
| Standing, trunk flexed 30°, arms extended | 370 | 65 | 830 | 146 |
| Standing, trunk flexed 30°, holding 8 kg of weight with arms extended | 760 | 135 | 1830 | 323 |
| Lift 15 kg of weight from floor, knees bent, arms straight down | 593 | 104 | 1810 | 319 |

## FACTOR OF RISK FOR VERTEBRAL FRACTURE ASSOCIATED WITH COMMON ACTIVITIES

| Activity | Bone Mineral Density (g/cm$^3$) | | | | | | |
|---|---|---|---|---|---|---|---|
| | 0.3 | 0.4 | 0.5 | 0.6 | 0.7 | 0.8 | 0.9 |
| Get up from sitting | 1.5 | 0.6 | 0.4 | 0.3 | 0.2 | 0.2 | 0.2 |
| Lift 15 kg of weight with knees straight | 2.6 | 1.1 | 0.7 | 0.5 | 0.4 | 0.3 | 0.3 |
| Lift 30 kg of weight with knees straight | 2.1 | 0.9 | 0.6 | 0.4 | 0.3 | 0.3 | 0.2 |
| Lift 30 kg of weight with deep knee bend | 3.7 | 1.5 | 1.0 | 0.7 | 0.6 | 0.5 | 0.4 |
| Open window with 50 N of force | 3.0 | 1.3 | 0.8 | 0.6 | 0.5 | 0.4 | 0.3 |
| Open window with 100 N of force | 1.1 | 0.5 | 0.3 | 0.2 | 0.2 | 0.1 | 0.1 |
| Tie shoes while sitting down | 1.4 | 0.6 | 0.4 | 0.3 | 0.2 | 0.2 | 0.2 |
| | 1.4 | 0.6 | 0.4 | 0.3 | 0.2 | 0.2 | 0.2 |

**FIGURE 12-17.** Factor of risk for vertebral fracture associated with selected common activities, as a function of lumbar bone mineral density. The numerator of the factor of risk was determined from models of spine loading at L2 for an elderly woman of average height and weight. The denominator was determined from regression analysis between lateral lumbar bone mineral density (BMD) and the load-bearing capacity of the L2 vertebrae.

The values for lateral BMD cover a wide range of densities, in particular very osteopenic. The t-score (number of standard deviations from the mean value for BMD in young women) is approximately +1 for a BMD of 0.9 g/cm$^2$ and is −5 for a BMD of 0.4 g/cm$^2$. The factor of risk is predicted to be greater than or close to one for low BMD values *(shaded area). (From* Myers and Wilson [2]; with permission.)

## VERTEBRAL FRACTURES: SUMMARY

Spine forces generated during controlled activities: 200 to 2500 N

Structural capacity of vertebrae from elderly cadavers: 800 to 6000 N

Therefore, common activities can result in spine forces that exceed the structural capacity of the vertebrae

**FIGURE 12-18.** Summary of risk for vertebral fracture. Vertebral bodies were obtained from the T10–T12 and L1–L3 regions of 25 elderly cadaveric spines (15 women, 10 men; 64 to 95 years of age). Bone mineral density was measured in each specimens by dual-energy x-ray absorptiometry. Specimens were also taken to failure in a forward-bending configuration to determine the failure load. Spine BMD was highly correlated to failure load of the L2 vertebral body ($r^2 = 0.79$). These results, taken together with those of the Fig. 12-17, indicate that common activities of daily living, such as shoe tying or rising from a chair, can place persons in the lowest BMD categories in jeopardy of fracture.

## FRACTURE PREVENTION STRATEGIES

Maintain or increase bone strength

Exercise

Diet

Pharmacologic interventions

Antiresorptive (estrogen, SERMs, calcitonin, and bisphosphonates) and potential anabolic agents (fluoride, parathyroid hormone)

Reduce the loads applied to bone mineral density

Decrease fall frequency

Decrease fall severity

Avoid lifting/bending activities

Proper lifting techniques

**FIGURE 12-19.** Fracture prevention. Two strategies should be used to reduce the risk for fracture: 1) improve the quantity and quality of bone and 2) reduce the risk for falls. The first approach requires adequate attention to standard hygienic interventions; dietary adequacy; supplemental calcium and vitamin D use; regular, frequent physical exercise; and various pharmacologic interventions. The second goal requires interventions aimed at reducing loads applied to bone via decreasing the risk for falling, decreasing the severity of falls that do occur, and minimizing damage caused by routine activities. Because leg muscle weakness is an independent risk factor for falls and hip fracture, a cautious program of progressive resistance strength training is an attractive option. Although such a program does not consistently provide important gains in bone mineral density, it does lead to striking gains in muscle strength that are accompanied by improved performance of tasks, such as rising from a chair and walking. SERMs—selective estrogen receptor modulators.

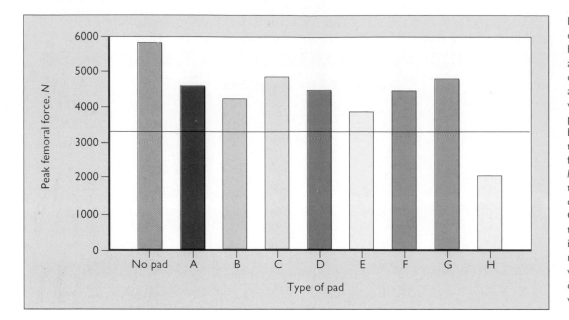

**FIGURE 12-20.** Effect of hip pads on the force delivered to the femur during a sideways fall. Wearing hip padding directly over the greater trochanter is an interesting strategy aimed at minimizing the force of a fall that is transmitted to the bone. To be effective, a padding system must attenuate forces under real-world impact conditions, must be worn by vulnerable patients, and must be able to reduce impact force below the level at which a fracture would be predicted to occur. This figure shows the reduction in impact force provided by various padding systems. The *solid horizontal line* represents the average force required to fracture an elderly femur in a sideways fall configuration (m=50, mean age=81, range=53–99). Only system H substantially reduced the peak force to a clinically useful degree. In one study conducted in a nursing home, patients wearing hip pads experienced far fewer fractures than those who were not wearing pads [19]. Indeed, the only fractures that occurred in the active intervention group occurred when the pad was not being used.

# References

1. Hayes WC: Biomechanics of cortical and trabecular bone: implications for assessment of fracture risk. In: *Basic Orthopaedic Biomechanics*. Edited by Mow VC, Hayes WC. New York: Raven Press; 1991:93–142.

2. Myers E, Wilson S: Biomechanics of osteoporosis and vertebral fractures. *Spine* 1997, 22:25S–31S.

3. Carter DR, Hayes WC: The compressive behavior of bone as a two-phase porous structure. *J Bone Joint Surg* 1977, 59-A:954–962.

4. Einhorn TA: Bone strength: the bottom line. *Calcified Tissue Int* 1992, 51:333–339.

5. Burstein A, Reilly D, Martens M: Aging of bone tissue: mechanical properties. *J Bone Joint Surg* 1976, 58-A:82–86.

6. Mosekilde L, Mosekilde L, Danielson CC: Biomechanical competence of vertebral trabecular bone in relation to ash density and age in normal individuals. *Bone* 1987, 8:79–85.

7. Burr D, Forwood M, Fyhrie D, *et al.:* Bone microdamage and skeletal fragility in osteoporotic and stress fractures. *J Bone Min Res* 1997, 12:6–15.

8. Ruff C, Hayes W: Subperiosteal expansion and cortical remodeling of the human femur and tibia with aging. *Science* 1982, 217:945–947.

9. Courtney A, Wachtel EF, Myers ER, *et al.:* Age-related reductions in the strength of the femur tested in a fall loading configuration. *J Bone Joint Surg* 1995, 77:387–395.

10. Robinovitch SN, Hayes WC, McMahon TA: Prediction of femoral impact forces in falls on the hip. *J Biomech Eng* 1991, 113:366–374.

11. Bouxsein ML, Courtney AC, Hayes WC. Ultrasound and densitometry of the calcaneus correlate with the failure loads of cadaveric femurs. *Calcif Tissue Int* 1995, 56:99–103.

12. Courtney A, Wachtel EF, Myers ER, *et al.:* Effects of loading rate on the strength of the proximal femur. *Calcif Tissue Int* 1994, 55:53–58.

13. Greenspan SL, Myers ER, Maitland LA, *et al.:* Fall severity and bone mineral density as risk factors for hip fracture in ambulatory elderly. *JAMA* 1994, 217:128–133.

14. Myers ER, Robinovitch SN, Greenspan SL, *et al.:* Factor of risk is associated with frequency of hip fracture in a case-control study. *Trans ORS* 1994, 526.

15. Cooper C, Atkinson E, O'Fallon W, *et al.:* Incidence of clinically diagnosed vertebral fractures: a population-based study in Rochester, Minnesota, 1985-1989. *J Bone Min Res* 1992, 7:221–227.

16. Myers E, Wilson S, Greenspan S: Vertebral fractures in the elderly occur with falling and bending. *J Bone Min Res* 1996, 11:S355.

17. Moro M, Hecker AT, Bouxsein ML, *et al.:* Failure load of thoracic vertebrae correlates with lumbar bone mineral density measured by DXA. *Calcif Tissue Int* 1995, 56:206–209.

18. Wilson SE: Development of a Model to Predict the Compressive Forces on the Spine Associated with Age-Related Vertebral Fractures. Master's Thesis. Cambridge: Massachusetts Institute of Technology; 1994.

19. Lauritzen JB, Peterson MM, Lund B: Effect of external hip protectors on hip fractures. *Lancet* 1993, 341:11–13.

# ROLE OF NONPHARMACOLOGIC APPROACH TO FRACTURE AND OSTEOPOROSIS

## Richard L. Prince

In view of the extremely high rates of osteoporotic fracture occurring in all developed and many developing countries, a population-based nonpharmacologic approach to the treatment and prevention of fracture and osteoporosis has many attractions. The major reason for the increasing importance of a public health approach to osteoporotic fracture is the increasing longevity of both men and women. Average life expectancy in most developed countries is about 85 years for women and 78 years for men. The incidence rates for all fractures show a peak in adolescence and a rising age-specific incidence from approximately 50 years on in both men and women. Thus, nonpharmacologic public health prevention should be directed specifically to these two times of life.

In childhood, and especially in adolescence, while the skeleton is developing, lifestyle influences have been shown to increase bone mass in the short term. Some of these gains may be reflected in a higher peak bone mass. It is also important to realize that part of the reason for the peak in fractures in adolescence relates to skeletal insufficiency as well as excessive force applied as a result of accidents. Thus, improving skeletal integrity in childhood may contribute to fracture prevention in adolescence.

Although optimization of peak bone mass theoretically is important in prevention of fracture in old age, fracture rates are in fact lowest in middle age. A more logical, cost-effective approach may be to prevent the loss of bone occurring in old age, thereby reducing fractures. There are two general approaches to be considered. The first is to detect patients at high risk of fracture using historical demographic factors and bone densitometry and treat these subjects with a pharmacologic agent such as a bisphosphonate or estrogen. The other approach discussed here is to apply public health approaches to the whole population with the aim of decreasing common risk factors. It is likely that dietary intervention with calcium, vitamin D, or both can reduce fracture rates by approximately 30%. The figures in this chapter elaborate on the mechanisms and likely effects of these interventions, which concentrate principally on diet and exercise.

## Overview of Bone Acquisition and Maintenance

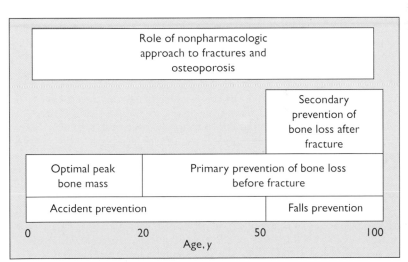

**FIGURE 13-1.** Role of nonpharmacologic approach to fractures and osteoporosis. Different interventions are needed at different times of life. A broadly based public health approach would include programs to reduce accidents in the earlier part of life and falls in the later part of life. Programs aimed at developing optimal peak bone mass and preventing bone loss before and after the first fracture also are integral to this overall approach.

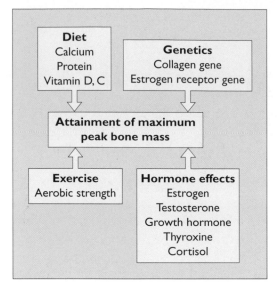

**FIGURE 13-2.** Attainment of maximum bone mass. Peak bone mass is attained at different ages at different sites of the skeleton. In the axial skeleton, it usually is attained at around the age of 18 years. Periosteal bone formation continues in the appendicular skeleton until approximately the age of 25 years. Thus, factors affecting the development of peak bone mass must be considered until this age.

Environmental factors such as diet and exercise act only within the genetic limitations imposed upon the individual. The genetic determinants of peak bone mass currently are an active area of research. It is clear that genetic abnormalities of the estrogen and vitamin D receptors are associated with some cases of impairment of peak bone mass [1,2]. In addition, deficiencies of various hormones resulting from specific endocrine disorders can induce osteoporosis. Examples of these are deficiencies of estrogen, testosterone, and growth hormone. Similarly, excess production of hormones (eg, thyroxine and cortisol) also can impair skeletal integrity. Much more common than the hormonal deficiencies, however, are nutritional deficiencies and the effects of suboptimal exercise.

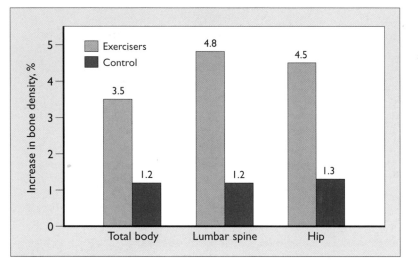

**FIGURE 13-3.** Effects of exercise in childhood. Data on exercise in childhood suggest that significant short-term increases in bone mass can be achieved by increasing forces on the skeleton within achievable limits. Regular physical activity for at least 1 hour three times per week should be considered as part of an exercise prescription for children [3].

**FIGURE 13-4.** Effects of calcium supplementation in adolescent girls. The nutrient most fully investigated in relation to the growing skeleton is calcium. There is no agreement on the minimum calcium intake required, in part because there is no agreement as to the best determinant of clinically meaningful outcome. Much emphasis has been placed on short-term calcium balance studies. In these, the data point to small beneficial effects of increasing calcium intake from 800 to 1300 mg per day. These data have been criticized because the dependent variable—calcium balance—includes the independent variable—calcium intake—as a dominant factor in the calculation of balance. Furthermore, all of the studies have been short-term and may merely reflect delayed adaptation to low calcium intake. The delay may relate not only to delay in increasing gut calcium absorption and renal calcium excretion but also to delay in calcification of preformed osteoid.

Bone density has been used as an end point. Several studies have shown short-term gains in bone density that have not persisted when the calcium supplement is stopped. Thus, the clinical benefit is not clear. If such supplementation could reduce the incidence of childhood fractures, it might be a worthwhile intervention. If, however, the aim is to increase peak adult bone mass, the definitive answer to the question of optimal dietary calcium intake in childhood requires a long-term supplementation study. The only 5-year study showed no treatment benefit from increasing calcium intake from 980 to 1135 mg per day [4]. It seems reasonable to recommend an intake of at least 800 mg per day, because there is evidence for small, short-term increases in bone density when calcium intake is increased from 908 to 1612 mg per day [5].

Childhood deficiency of vitamin D results in osteomalacia. Although exposure to sunlight is the major source of vitamin D, it can be restricted in northern climates. It is therefore recommended that 200 to 400 IU (5 to 10 μg) of vitamin D be consumed each day. The role of protein deficiency in skeletal growth also must be considered.

## PREVENTION OF CHILDHOOD FRACTURE BY PREVENTION OF TRAUMA

Provision of a safe environment
   Home
   Playground
   Roads
Education
   Road safety awareness

FIGURE 13-5. Prevention of childhood fracture by prevention of trauma. A broadly based public health approach should be taken to increasing safety of children's environments in the home, playground, and on the road. In addition, children should receive specific education on avoidance of road trauma.

## NONPHARMACOLOGIC FRACTURE PREVENTION IN ADULTS

| | |
|---|---|
| Adequate diet | Adequate exercise |
| High calcium | Maintenance of bone mass |
| Vitamin D | Avoidance of toxins |
| Low salt | Smoking |
| Phytoestrogens | Excess alcohol |

FIGURE 13-6. Nonpharmacologic fracture prevention in adults. Maintenance of peak bone mass can be considered under three headings: diet, exercise and skeletal toxins. The effects of smoking on the skeleton have been assessed in observational studies. Smoking 20 cigarettes a day for 20 years reduced bone density at the spine by 9%, at the femoral neck by 6%, and at the femoral shaft by 6% [6]. The deleterious effects of alcohol are apparent only at high intakes, where other effects from poor nutrition and falls may be more important.

# Dietary Intervention for Bone Maintenance

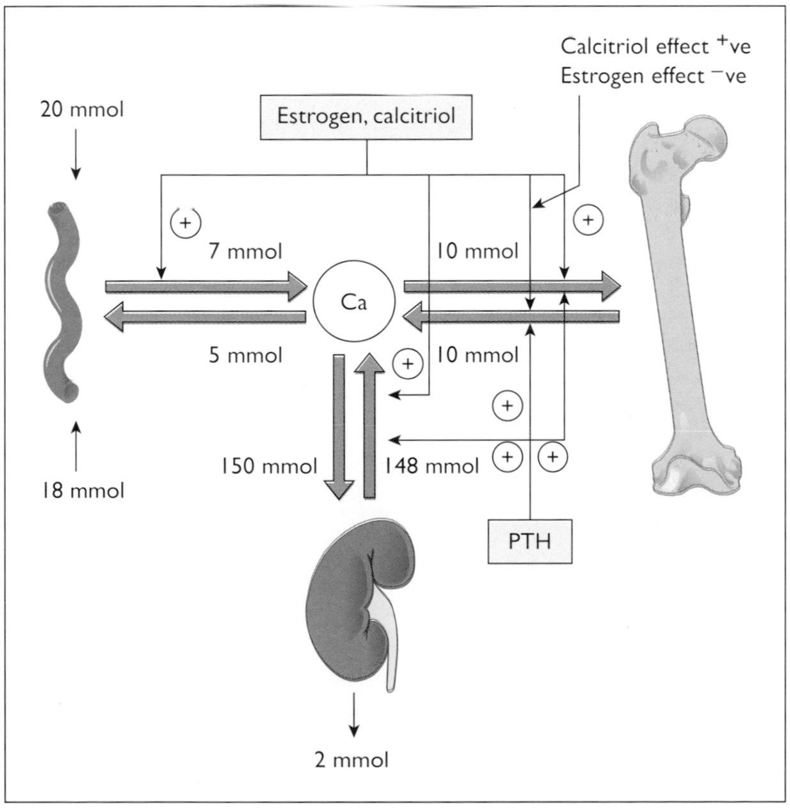

FIGURE 13-7. Regulation of organs involved in calcium transport. Dietary calcium supplementation can be considered in the context of calcium transport around the body. Calcium enters the bowel by ingestion of food and also by intestinal secretion of calcium. Net absorption into the extracellular space is from 2 to 4 mmol per day. This absorption is regulated by calcitriol and estrogen, both of which act to increase the absorbed fraction. Most of this absorbed calcium is excreted in the urine, although calcium also is lost in sweat. When the subject is in calcium balance, the amount of calcium entering the bone and leaving the bone is identical. In periods of dietary calcium deficiency, however, parathyroid hormone (PTH) rises. The rise in PTH induces an increase in bone resorption, an increase in calcium resorption from the urine, and an increase in calcitriol, which increase gut calcium absorption. If dietary calcium intake is low, more calcium leaves the bone than enters the bone to maintain extracellular calcium concentrations, resulting in osteoporosis. PTH stimulates new osteoid formation ready for calcification at the time of an increase in dietary calcium.

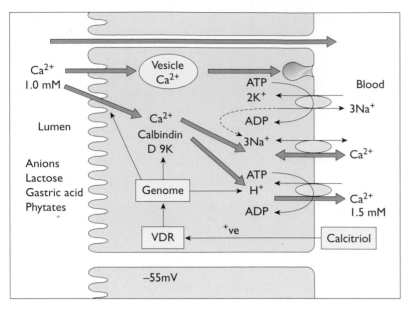

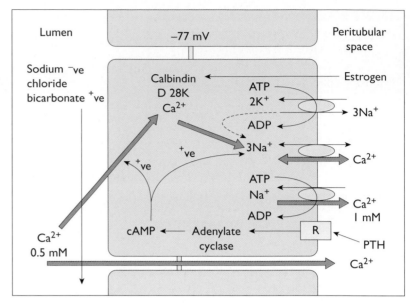

**FIGURE 13-8.** Factors associated with calcium transport across the bowel wall. The molecular biology of calcium absorption in the bowel is complex. In addition to paracellular absorption, which, although largely unregulated, is the major source of calcium absorption at high calcium loads, transcellular calcium absorption is strongly regulated. Vitamin D, in the form of its active metabolite, calcitriol, is the main regulator of gut calcium absorption, although there is some evidence that high concentrations of 25-hydroxy vitamin D may have an effect on calcium absorption. It is believed that genomic effects of calcitriol act to stimulate calcium absorption as well as calcium transport across the cell and calcium efflux at the basal lateral membrane. This latter effect occurs by stimulation of both calcium ATPase and the sodium-calcium cotransporter [7]. Luminal factors affecting the physiochemical state of the calcium can influence absorption, especially the lack of gastric acid in the case of calcium carbonate [8,9]. Associated anions, such as citrate, appear to stimulate absorption. Dietary factors such as phytates [10] impair absorption, whereas lactose, in the presence of lactase, stimulates absorption [11]. The molecular basis of these effects is uncertain but may be associated with paracellular absorption. ADP—adenosine diphosphate; ATP—adenosine triphosphate; VDR—vitamin D receptor.

**FIGURE 13-9.** Factors regulating calcium transport via the distal tubule. Renal calcium transport also is vigorously regulated throughout the distal tubule. In the distal tubule there is evidence that both parathyroid hormone (PTH) and estrogen stimulate calcium reabsorption via effects on the sodium-calcium exchanger and calcium ATPase [12,13]. The luminal concentration of other ions, including sodium chloride [14] and bicarbonate [15], also can affect calcium absorption, which occurs principally by the transcellular route. ADP—adenosine diphosphate; ATP—adenosine triphosphate; cAMP—cyclic adenosine monophosphate; PTH—parathyroid hormone.

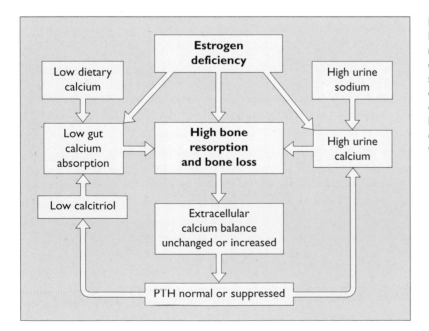

**FIGURE 13-10.** Role of dietary factors in early postmenopausal bone loss. Dietary calcium plays a small role in the bone loss that occurs close to the menopause. The principal cause of bone loss at this time relates to estrogen deficiency, which actually increases extracellular calcium concentrations, thereby suppressing renal calcium reabsorption and gut calcium absorption via effects on parathyroid hormone and calcitriol. Thus, the principal cause of the low gut calcium absorption and high renal calcium excretion at that time is the bone loss itself. In specific circumstances, a low dietary calcium or high urine sodium can exacerbate these losses and induce further bone loss [16]. PTH—parathyroid hormone.

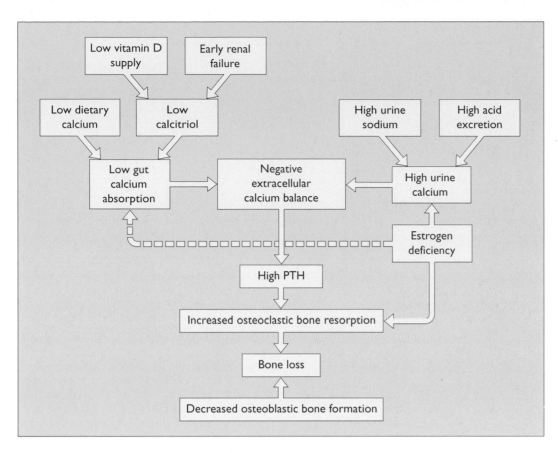

**FIGURE 13-11.** Dietary factors contributing to age-related bone loss. Age-related bone loss is dependent on a negative extracellular calcium balance inducing a high parathyroid hormone. The negative extracellular balance is derived in approximately equal parts by a high urine calcium and relatively low gut calcium. The high urine calcium is driven by estrogen deficiency and excessive ingestion of salt and high-acid foods.

Dietary calcium deficiency is exacerbated by impaired gut calcium absorption resulting from relatively low circulating levels of calcitriol and 25-hydroxy vitamin D. These levels are low because of early renal failure, preventing the formation of calcitriol, and lack of vitamin D supply because of lack of exposure to sunlight. Estrogen deficiency also may play a role in the intrinsic defect in gut calcium absorption that occurs with aging.

The negative extracellular calcium balance induces a high parathyroid hormone level, which increases osteoclastic bone resorption. Because of the age-related osteoblastic defect, increased bone turnover is associated with bone loss. PTH—parathyroid hormone.

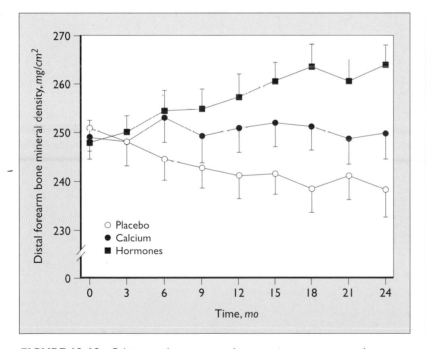

**FIGURE 13-12.** Calcium and estrogen replacement in postmenopausal women. In women less than 10 years past the menopause, calcium supplementation prevented forearm bone loss, but estrogen replacement increased bone mass slightly and was more effective than calcium alone [17]. This demonstrates that calcium is effective and that estrogen deficiency is associated in part with direct effects on calcium balance. (*From* Prince, *et al.* [17]; with permission.)

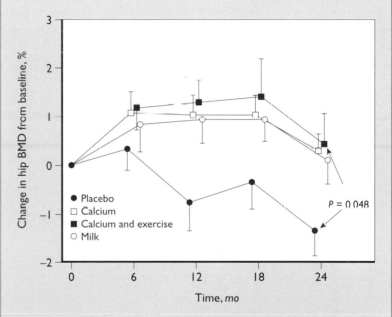

**FIGURE 13-13.** Effects of calcium supplementation and exercise on bone density at the hip. In women 15 years past the menopause, calcium supplementation of 1000 mg per day, either as a tablet or as milk powder, completely prevented hip bone loss over 2 years. Exercise offered little extra benefit [18]. BMD—bone mineral density. (*From* Prince, *et al.* [18]; with permission.)

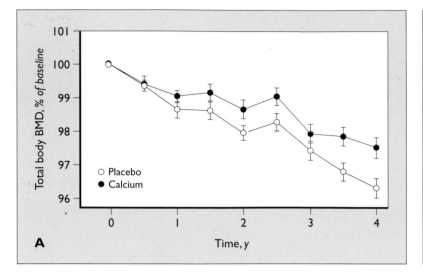

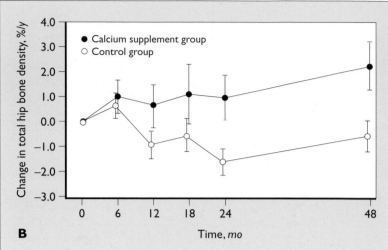

**FIGURE 13-14.** Effects of calcium supplementation on bone loss. Four years of calcium supplementation did not completely prevent total body bone density loss in women 10 years past the menopause (**A**). However, at the hip site calcium supplementation was completely effective in stopping bone loss in women 15 years past the menopause (**B**) [19,20]. BMD—bone mineral density. (Part A *from* Reid, *et al.* [19]; with permission; Part B *from* Devine, *et al.* [20]; with permission.)

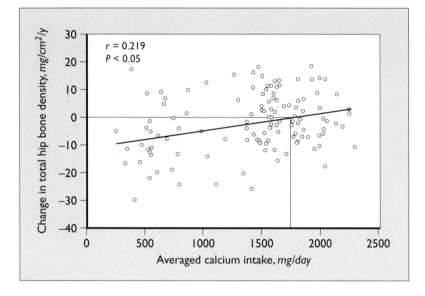

**FIGURE 13-15.** Effect of increasing calcium intake on bone loss in postmenopausal women. The dose of calcium required to prevent bone loss in postmenopausal women is uncertain. Data from 120 women followed prospectively over 2 years suggest that calcium intake to prevent bone loss at the hip should be more than 1500 mg per day. These values match the calcium requirement calculated from balance studies, in which the threshold is approximately 1200 mg per day [20]. (*From* Devine, *et al.* [20]; with permission.)

## CONTROLLED TRIALS OF CALCIUM: EFFECTS ON FRACTURE RATES

| Study | Baseline Characteristics | Baseline Calcium Intake (mg/day) | Intervention | Fracture Outcome in Control Group | Fracture Outcome in Treatment Group | Relative Risk | Absolute Risk Reduction (fractures per 100 patient years, 95% CI) | Number Needed to Treat |
|---|---|---|---|---|---|---|---|---|
| Chevalley et al. [21] | 11 males; 82 females; mean age, 73 y; 44% prevalent vertebral fractures | 650 | $CaCO_3$ or osseino complex 800 mg/day for 15 y | New vertebral fractures— 10.7% | New vertebral fractures—7.4% | 0.69 | 33 (range, -7.8 to 14.3) | 30 |
| Reid et al. [19] | 135 women baseline; 78 women completed; Mean age, 56 y; nonprevalent fractures | 700 | Calcium lactate gluconate1000 mg/d for 4 y | New fractures— 18% | New fractures—5% | 0.3 | 31 (range, -0.4 to 6.5) | 32 |
| Recker et al. [22] | 92 women; mean age, 75 y; prevalent vertebral fractures | 450 | $CaCO_3$ 1200 mg/day for 43 y | New vertebral fractures—51% | New vertebral fractures—28% | 0.55 | 53 (range, 0.7 to 9.8) | 19 |
| Recker et al. [22] | 99 women; mean age, 73 y; nonprevalent vertebral fractures | 414 | $CaCO_3$ 1200 mg/day for 43 y | New vertebral fractures—21% | New vertebral fractures—28% | 1.33 | — | |

**FIGURE 13-16.** Effects of calcium supplementation on fracture rates. Three small randomized controlled trials of calcium supplementation have been undertaken. These show an absolute risk reduction of three to five fractures per hundred patient years, or an absolute risk reduction ranging between 31% and 70% [19,21,22]. The Recker study showed no benefit in elderly women with nonprevalent vertebral fractures. The confidence intervals for these effects are large, and further studies are needed.

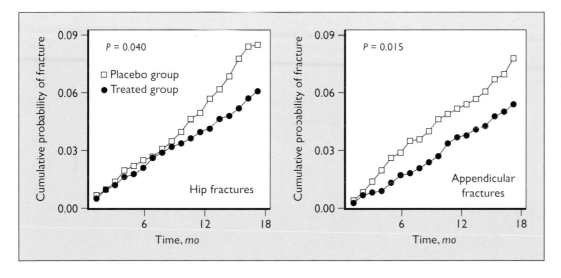

**FIGURE 13-17.** Effects of calcium plus vitamin D on fractures in elderly women. In women in institutional care (mean age, 84 years), calcium plus vitamin D not only prevented bone loss but also reduced hip fractures by 43% and non-vertebral fractures by 32% [23]. )*From* Chapuy, *et al.* [23]; with permission.)

## CONTROLLED TRIALS OF CALCIUM AND VITAMIN D: EFFECTS ON FRACTURE RATES

| Study | Baseline Characteristics | Baseline Calcium Intake (mg/day) | Intervention (per day) | Fracture Outcome in Control Group | Fracture Outcome in Treatment Group | Relative Risk (range) | Absolute Risk Reduction (fractures per 100 patient years, 95% CI) | Number Needed to Treat |
|---|---|---|---|---|---|---|---|---|
| Chapuy et al. [23] | 2303 women Mean age, 84 y | 511 | Ca₃(PO₄)₂ 1200 mg Vitamin D 800 IU for 3 y | Appendicular fractures— 27.3% | Appendicular fractures— 21.6% | 0.72 (0.6–0.84) | 1.9 (0.7–3.1) | 52 |
| Chapuy et al. [23] | 2303 women Mean age, 84 y | 511 | Ca₃(PO₄)₂ 1200 mg Vitamin D 800 IU for 3 y | Hip fractures— 15.8% | Hip fractures— 11.6% | 0.73 (0.62–0.84) | 1.4 (0.4–2.3) | 71 |
| Dawson-Hughes et al. [24] | 176 men 213 women Mean age, 72 y | 700 | Calcium citrate malate 500 mg Vitamin D 700 IU for 3 y | Appendicular fractures— 12.8% | Appendicular fractures— 5.9% | 0.5 (0.2–0.9) | 2.3 (0.4–4.2) | 43 |
| Dawson-Hughes et al. [24] | 213 women Mean age, 73 y | 700 | Calcium citrate malate 500 mg Vitamin D 700 IU for 3 y | Appendicular fractures— 19.6% | Appendicular fractures— 11.6% | 0.6 (0.2–0.8) | 4.6 (0.8–8.4) | 22 |

**FIGURE 13-18.** Effects of calcium and vitamin D on fracture rates. Two larger intervention studies examining calcium plus vitamin D have been undertaken. The Chapuy study showed an absolute reduction of 1.4 hip fractures per hundred patients treated and 1.9 appendicular fractures per hundred patients treated [23]. A smaller study in Boston studied both men and women. That study showed a 2.3% reduction in appendicular fractures [24,25]. Analysis of the data for the women alone showed a 4.6% reduction in fractures. These rates indicate that it is necessary to treat only between 20 and 50 individuals to prevent any appendicular fracture and 70 individuals to prevent hip fracture in 1 year.

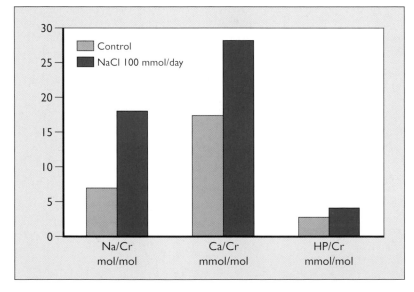

**FIGURE 13-19.** Effects of sodium loading on renal excretion. Increasing salt intake increases sodium excretion and calcium excretion in the kidney. It is also associated with an increase in bone resorption as measured by the hydroxy-proline creatinine ration [26]. Cr—creatinine; HP—hydroxyprolene. (*Adapted from* Goulding [26]; with permission.)

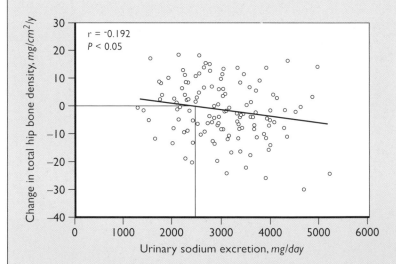

**FIGURE 13-20.** Effects of increasing sodium intake on bone loss at the hip in postmenopausal women. In postmenopausal women, the higher the sodium excretion over 2 years the greater the bone lost at the hip [27]. (*From* Devine, et al. [27]; with permission.)

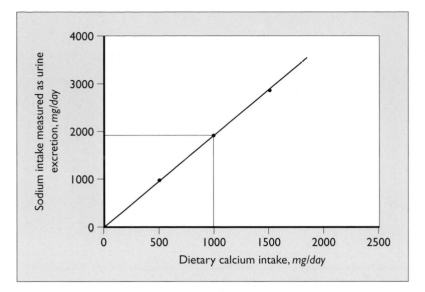

**FIGURE 13-21.** Determinants of hip bone density. Two determinants of hip bone density are dietary calcium intake and salt intake, as measured by sodium excretion. The higher the dietary calcium intake, the lower the bone loss. The higher the salt intake, the higher the bone loss. It is, therefore, possible to balance intakes of these two nutrients. The data show that with a dietary calcium intake of 1000 mg per day, providing sodium intake is less than 2000 mg, no bone loss of the hip will occur [27]. *(From* Devine, *et al.* [27]; with permission.)

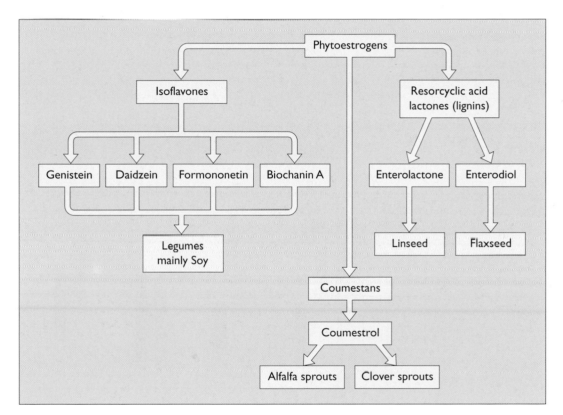

**FIGURE 13-22.** Types and sources of phyto-estrogens. There are three major groups of phyto-estrogens: isoflavones, coumestans, and resorcyclic acid lactones. In terms of human disease, soy has been most extensively studied, containing mostly isoflavones although it also contains a small amount of coumestrol. The coumestans are more potent ligands for the estrogen receptor, however.

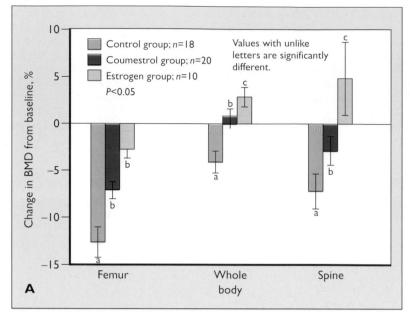

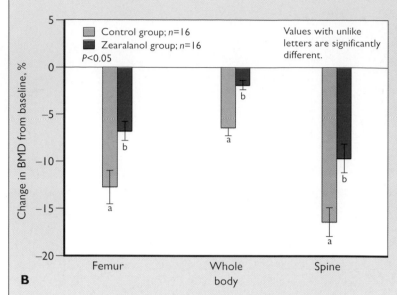

**FIGURE 13-23.** Effects of phytoestrogens on bone density in aging rats. Studies in the aged rat model of postmenopausal osteoporosis indicate that coumestrol significantly reduces bone loss at the spine and hip and completely prevents bone loss in the whole body (**A**). Another phytoestrogen, zearalanol, also demonstrates efficacy in reducing bone loss after oophorectomy (**B**). Dose calculations suggest that consumption of 350 g of alfalfa sprouts per week may provide enough coumestrol to provide beneficial effects on bone in humans [28]. *(From* Draper, *et al.* [28]; with permission.)

# Role of Activity and Exercise

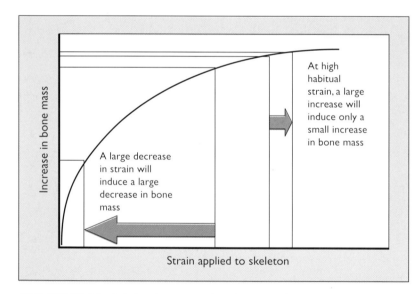

**FIGURE 13-24.** Relation between induced strain and osteogenic response. Strain relationships applied to the skeleton show very significant effects on periosteal bone formation in animal models of stress-strain relationship. Studies in healthy adults show small effects of increasing stress-strain relationships to increase bone density at the site in which the strain has been applied. Similarly, immobilization studies as a result of hemiplegia or stroke show dramatic reductions in bone density. Studies that show a significant increase in bone density with exercise in patients previously immobilized have not yet been performed.

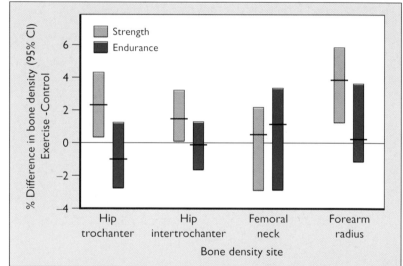

**FIGURE 13-25.** Effects of exercise on bone density. The effects of exercise on bone density depend on the site of maximum change in stress-strain relationship. Adjacent sites in the hip can show significant effects or no effects. The figure shows that the strength regimen, which included weight training, significantly increased the bone density at the trochanter and intertrochanter site, but had no effect at the femoral neck site. The endurance regimen, which did not increase stress-strain relationships as much as did the weight lifting regimen, showed no overall effect on bone density [29]. *(Adapted from* Kerr, *et al.* [29].)

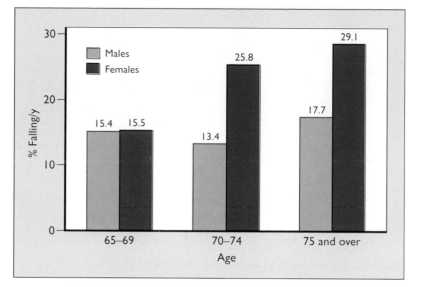

**FIGURE 13-26.** Incidence of falls in elderly men and women. Prevention of falls is a potentially important public health approach to the prevention of osteoporotic fractures. The incidence of falls is highly age dependent, especially in women [30]. *(From* Australian Bureau of Statistics [30].)

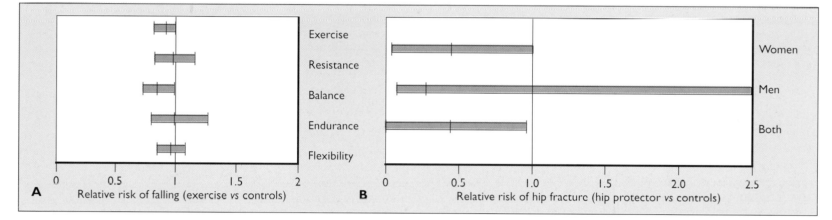

**FIGURE 13-27.** Prevention of trauma resulting from falls. Preliminary studies of exercise regimens show that some interventions can significantly reduce falls, although this has not yet been shown to prevent fractures. **A,** The effects of various types of exercise regimens on the relative time to first fall. Regimens involving balance and exercise appear to be better than those involving resistance

weight training and flexibility [31]. Another approach to fracture prevention is to apply hip protectors over the greater trochanter to cushion the fall. **B,** The relative risk of hip fracture in subjects randomized to wear hip protectors or not. In this small study a significant reduction in hip fractures in subjects wearing hip protectors is shown [32]. (Part A *From* Province, *et al.* [31]; with permission.)

# References

1. Smith EP, Boyd J, Frank GR, *et al.*: Estrogen resistance caused by a mutation in the estrogen-receptor gene in a man. *N Engl J Med* 1994, 331:1056–1061.

2. Sainz J, Van Tornout JM, Loro L, *et al.*: Vitamin D-receptor gene polymorphism and bone density in prepubertal American girls of Mexican descent. *N Engl J Med* 1997, 337:77–82.

3. Morris FL, Naughton GA, Gibbs JL, *et al.*: Prospective ten-month exercise intervention in premenarcheal girls: positive effects on bone and lean mass. *J Bone Miner Res* 1997, 12:1453–1462.

4. Lloyd T, Rollings NJ, Chinchilli VM: The effect of enhanced bone gain achieved with calcium supplementation during ages 12 to 16 does not persist in late adolescence. In *Nutritional Aspects of Osteoporosis.* Edited by Burkhardt P, Dawson-Hughes B, Heaney R. New York: Springer-Verlag, 1998:11–26.

5. Johnston CC, Miller JZ, Slemenda CW, *et al.*: Calcium supplementation and increases in bone mineral density in children. *N Engl J Med* 1992, 327:82–87.

6. Hopper JL, Seeman E: The bone density of female twins discordant for tobacco use. *N Engl J Med* 1994, 330:387–392.

7. Wasserman RH, Chandler JS, Meyer SA, *et al.*: Intestinal calcium transport and calcium extrusion processes at the basolateral membrane. *J Nutr* 1992, 122:662–671.

8. Heaney RP, Smith KT, Recker RR, Hinders SM: Meal effects on calcium absorption. *Am J Clin Nutr* 1989, 49:372–376.

9. Recker RR: Calcium absorption and achlorhydria. *N Engl J Med* 1985, 313:70–73.

10. Knox TA, Kassarjian Z, Dawson-Hughes B, *et al.*: Calcium absorption in elderly subjects on high- and low-fiber diets: effect of gastric acidity. *Am J Clin Nutr* 1991, 53:1480–1486.

11. Cochet B, Jung A, Griessen M, *et al.*: Effects of lactose on intestinal calcium absorption in normal and lactase-deficient subjects. *Gastroenterology* 1983, 84:935–940.

12. Bouhtiauy I, LaJeunesse D, Brunette MG: The mechanism of parathyroid hormone action on calcium reabsorption by the distal tube. *Endocrinology* 1991, 128:251–258.

13. Borke JL, Minami J, Verma A, *et al.*: Monoclonal antibodies to human erythrocyte membrane $Ca^{2+}$-$Mg^{2+}$ adenosine triphosphate pump recognize an epitope in the basolateral membrane of human kidney distal tubule cells. *J Clin Invest* 1987, 80:1225–1231.

14. Massey LK, Whiting SJ: Dietary salt, urinary calcium, and bone loss. *J Bone Miner Res* 1996, 11:731–736.

15. Lemann J, Gray RW, Pleuss JA: Potassium bicarbonate, but not sodium bicarbonate, reduces urinary calcium excretion and improves calcium balance in healthy men. *Kidney Int* 1989, 35:688–695.

16. Prince RL, Dick I: Oestrogen effects on calcium membrane transport: a new view of the inter-relationship between oestrogen deficiency and age related osteoporosis. *Osteoporosis Int* 1997, 7:S150–S154.

17. Prince RL, Smith M, Dick IM, *et al.:* Prevention of postmenopausal osteoporosis: a comparative study of exercise, calcium supplementation, and hormone-replacement therapy. *N Engl J Med* 1991, 325:1189–1195.

18. Prince R, Devine A, Dick I, *et al.:* The effects of calcium supplementation (milk powder or tablets) and exercise on bone density in postmenopausal women. *J Bone Miner Res* 1995, 10:1068–1075.

19. Reid IR, Ames RW, Evans MC, *et al.:* Long-term effects of calcium supplementation on bone loss and fractures in postmenopausal women: a randomized controlled trial. *Am J Med* 1995, 98:331–335.

20. Devine A, Dick IM, Heal SJ, *et al.:* A 4-year follow up study of calcium supplementation on bone density in elderly postmenopausal women. *Osteoporosis Int* 1997, 7:23–28.

21. Chevalley T, Rizzoli R, Nydegger V, *et al.:* Effects of calcium supplements on femoral bone mineral density and vertebral fracture rate in Vitamin-D-replete elderly patients. *Osteoporosis Int* 1994, 4:245–252.

22. Recker RR, Hinders S, Davies KM, *et al.:* Correcting calcium nutritional deficiency prevents spine fractures in elderly women. *J Bone Miner Res* 1996, 11:1961–1966.

23. Chapuy MC, Arlot ME, Delmas PD, Meunier PJ: Effect of calcium and cholecalciferol treatment for three years on hip fractures in elderly women. *Br Med J* 1994, 308:1081–1082.

24. Dawson-Hughes B, Harris SS, Khall EA, Dallal GE: Effect of calcium and vitamin D supplementation on bone density in men and women 65 years of age or older. *N Engl J Med* 1997, 337:670–676.

25. Prince RL: Diet and the prevention of osteoporotic fracture. *N Engl J Med* 1997, 337:701–702.

26. Goulding A: Effects of varying dietary salt intake on the fasting urinary excretion of sodium, calcium and hydroxyproline in young women. *N Z Med J* 1983, 853–854.

27. Devine A, Criddle RA, Dick IM, *et al.:* A longitudinal study of the effect of sodium and calcium intakes on regional bone density in postmenopausal women. *Am J Clin Nutr* 1995, 62:740–745.

28. Draper CR, Edel MJ, Dick IM, *et al.:* Phytoestrogens reduce bone loss and bone resorption in oophorectomized rats. *J Nutr* 1997, 127:1795–1799.

29. Kerr D, Morton A, Dick I, Prince R: Exercise effects on bone mass in postmenopausal women are site-specific and load-dependent. *J Bone Miner Res* 1996, 11:218–225.

30. Australian Bureau of Statistics: Falls risk factors for persons aged 65 years and over, ABS catalogue No. 4393.1. Australian Government Printing Service, Canberra, New South Wales. 1995.

31. Province MA, Hadley EC, Hornbrook MC, *et al.:* The effects of exercise on falls in elderly patients. *JAMA* 1995, 273:1341–1347.

32. Lauritzen JB, Petersen MM, Lund B: Effect of external hip protectors on hip fractures. *Lancet* 1993, 341:11–13.

# 14

# ANTIRESORPTIVE THERAPIES OF OSTEOPOROSIS

## Nelson B. Watts

Most current therapies for osteoporosis work primarily by reducing bone resorption. To fully appreciate the benefits and limitations of antiresorptive agents, it is important to understand normal bone remodeling and the effects of age, estrogen deficiency, and other factors on bone remodeling. An imbalance between resorption and formation and an increase in bone remodeling both contribute to bone loss.

Several agents act through different molecular and cellular mechanisms to reduce bone resorption–estrogen, selective estrogen-receptor modulators (SERMs), calcitonin, and bisphosphonates. These agents have been shown to prevent or restore the bone loss associated with corticosteroid excess, prevent bone loss in recently menopausal women, increase bone mass in women with established osteoporosis, and reduce fractures in women with established postmenopausal osteoporosis.

## Normal and Abnormal Bone Remodeling

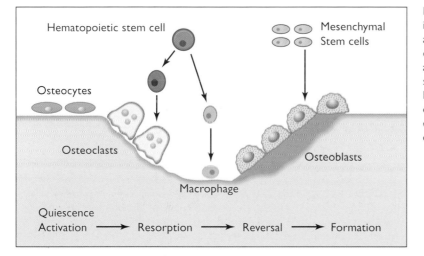

**FIGURE 14-1.** Normal bone remodeling. At any time, most of the skeleton is in the resting phase. Through endocrine, paracrine, and autocrine factors, as well as biomechanical and bioelectrical forces, the remodeling sequence begins with differentiation of hematopoietic stem cells into mature osteoclasts. These cells are responsible for bone resorption. Osteoclasts migrate to bone and attach to surfaces, where they produce acid and enzymes that result in bone resorption. Resorption and formation are coupled, likely through signaling between osteoblasts and osteoclasts. Osteoblastic bone formation follows resorption. In older adults, resorption usually exceeds formation, so that each remodeling cycle results in a net loss of bone.

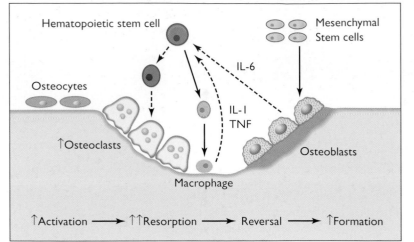

**FIGURE 14-2.** Consequences of estrogen deficiency. The number of osteoclasts and their activity increases with estrogen deficiency, as well as with a number of other conditions and circumstances. This increase in number and activity of osteoclasts is due to increased production of cytokines such as tumor necrosis factor (TNF) and interleukins 1 and 6 (IL-1 and IL-6) by osteoblasts, macrophages, and stromal cells. This increased production of cytokines leads to an increase in remodeling, also called a *high bone turnover state*.

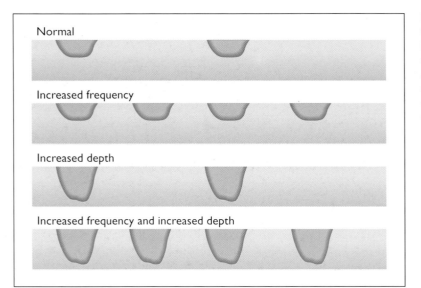

**FIGURE 14-3.** High bone turnover. Because resorption exceeds formation, the higher the rate of bone remodeling (bone turnover), the faster bone is lost. The number of remodeling units (activation frequency) and the activity of osteoclasts (depth of resorption) determine the rate of bone turnover. Antiresorptive drugs improve the balance of bone remodeling through effects on osteoclasts, their precursors, or both. These drugs decrease the numbers osteoclasts (resulting in a lower activation frequency), decrease the activity of individual cells (resulting in reduced remodeling depth), or both.

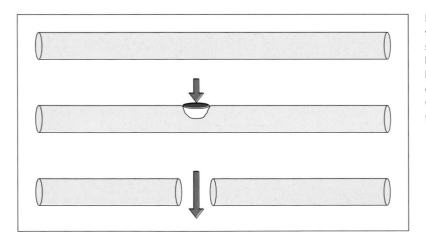

**FIGURE 14-4.** Consequences of high bone turnover. Not only is bone lost with each remodeling cycle but the increased number and depth of remodeling sites lead to bone that is more prone to fracture. An intact broomstick can be broken. Considerable force is required to do so, however, and the site of the break cannot be predicted with certainty. Placing a notch in the broomstick not only makes it easier to break but also marks the site at which it will break. Cutting through the broomstick entirely (similar to increased remodeling leading to interruption of trabecular connections) makes it useless for structural support.

## Antiresoptive Agents

| ANTIRESORPTIVE AGENTS FOR OSTEOPOROSIS |
| --- |

Estrogens
Calcitonin
Selective estrogen-receptor modulators
Bisphosphonates

**FIGURE 14-5.** Antiresorptive medications in current use fall into one of four categories: estrogens, calcitonin, selective estrogen-receptor modulators (SERMs), or bisphosphonates.

| CALCITONIN |
| --- |

Derived from parafollicular thyroid C cells
Inhibits osteoclastic bone resorption by direct action on osteoclasts
Injectable salmon calcitonin available since 1984
Nasal spray introduced in late 1995
Has excellent long-term safety

**FIGURE 14-6.** Calcitonin is a hormone produced by specialized cells in the thyroid. Its role in normal physiology is not clear. In pharmacologic doses, however, calcitonin lowers serum calcium, mainly by inhibition of osteoclastic bone resorption. Salmon calcitonin is used because it is more potent than is human calcitonin. Injectable calcitonin is not widely used because of the cost, discomfort of injections, and side effects (nausea, flushing, or both in about 20% of patients). Nasal spray salmon calcitonin is very well tolerated. The long-term safety of calcitonin is excellent.

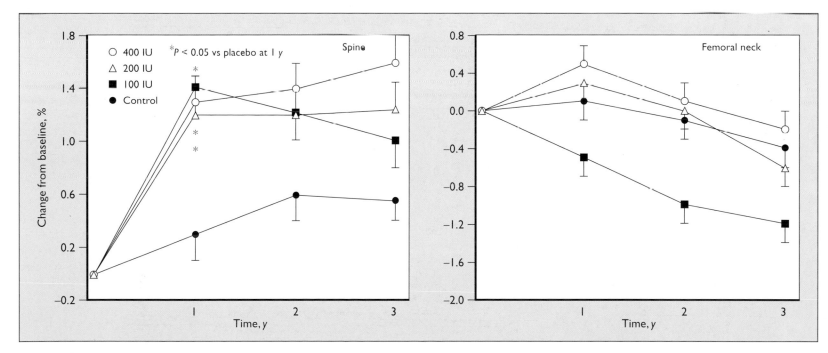

**FIGURE 14-7.** The Prevent Recurrence of Osteoporotic Fractures (PROOF) Study. Nasal calcitonin has been studied in the PROOF Study, a large, double-blind, placebo-controlled, randomized trial. This study consisted of almost 1200 patients, with an average age of 68 years at entry. All were given 1000 mg/d of calcium and either a placebo nasal spray or one of three different dosages of calcitonin nasal spray (100, 200, or 400 IU/d). The trial recently concluded after approximately 5 years. In a preliminary analysis of the 3-year data, changes in bone density at the spine and hip were slight and no different from those seen with placebo. (*From* Stock *et al.* [1]; with permission.)

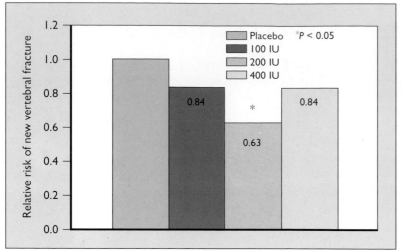

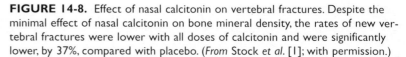

**FIGURE 14-8.** Effect of nasal calcitonin on vertebral fractures. Despite the minimal effect of nasal calcitonin on bone mineral density, the rates of new vertebral fractures were lower with all doses of calcitonin and were significantly lower, by 37%, compared with placebo. (*From* Stock *et al.* [1]; with permission.)

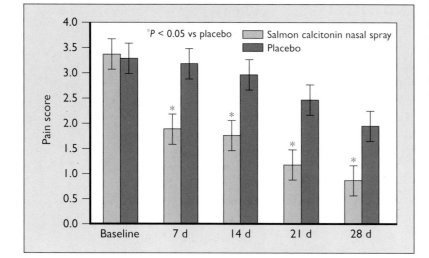

**FIGURE 14-9.** Analgesic effect of calcitonin. Calcitonin appears to have an analgesic effect unrelated to its effect on bone [2]. This effect is thought to be mediated through increased levels of endorphins. It has been shown not only in patients with osteoporosis but also in patients with other painful conditions. Therefore, calcitonin should be considered for patients with acute painful osteoporotic fractures or chronic pain associated with osteoporosis. (*From* Pun and Chan [2]; with permission.)

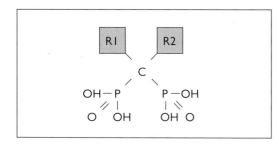

**FIGURE 14-10.** General structure of bisphosphonates. Bisphosphonates consist of two phosphonic acids linked to a carbon, with two side chains, called R1 and R2. The side chains determine the avidity of binding to bone, antiresorptive potency, and side effects.

## CHARACTERISTICS OF BISPHOSPHONATES

Bone-seeking

Effective orally or intravenously

Poor absorption orally

Not metabolized, excreted by the kidney

Long skeletal retention

Side chain determines potency and side effects

**FIGURE 14-11.** Bisphosphonates are poorly absorbed when given orally. Typically, only about 1% of an oral dose is absorbed. Of that, 20% to 50% is adsorbed on bone, and the rest is excreted in urine over the next 12 to 24 hours. Bisphosphonates remain in bone for years; however, after remodeling is complete, they are buried in bone and no longer pharmacologically active. Bisphosphonates have little or no long-term toxicity. The main side effects are gastrointestinal (ie, esophageal irritation), most likely with aminobisphosphonates given orally; and acute phase reactions, hypocalcemia, acute renal failure when given intravenously. Etidronate, given continuously in high doses, may impair bone mineralization. However, this side effect rarely is seen with the doses of other bisphosphonates used to treat osteoporosis.

## MECHANISMS OF ACTION OF BISPHOSPHONATES

Reduce activity of individual osteoclasts:
   Inhibit lactate production
   Inhibit lysosomal enzymes

Reduce activation frequency:
   Inhibit recruitment of osteoclast precursors
   Inhibit differentiation of osteoclast precursors

Accelerate osteoclast apoptosis

**FIGURE 14-12.** After being adsorbed onto hydroxyapatite crystals at sites of active bone formation, bisphosphonates reduce remodeling through several different actions. Bisphosphonates reduce the activity of individual osteoclasts by inhibiting production of lactate and lysosomal enzymes, and reduce activation frequency by inhibiting recruitment and differentiation of osteoclast precursors. Bisphosphonates also accelerate osteoclast apoptosis (programmed cell death).

## GENERATIONS OF BISPHOSPHONATES

| Generation | Side Chain |
|---|---|
| First:<br>Etidronate<br>Clodronate<br>Tiludronate | Short alkyl or halide |
| Second:<br>Alendronate<br>Pamidronate | Amino terminal |
| Third:<br>Risedronate<br>Ibandronate<br>Zoledronate | Cyclic |

**FIGURE 14-13.** Altering the side chains of bisphosphonates changes both their potency and side-effect profile. The antiresorptive potency increases at least 10- to 100-fold between generations. Only alendronate is approved by the Food and Drug Administration for use in osteoporosis; however, etidronate, pamidronate, tiludronate, and risedronate also are available in the United States, and clodronate is available in other countries. Compounds in the late stages of development for osteoporosis include ibandronate and zoledronate.

## POTENTIAL USES FOR BISPHOSPHONATES

Osteoporosis
Hypercalcemia
Paget's disease
Fibrous dysplasia
Osteogenesis imperfecta
Multiple myeloma
Bone metastases
Myositis ossificans
Heterotopic ossification
Periodontal disease
Neuropathic arthropathy (Charcot's joint)

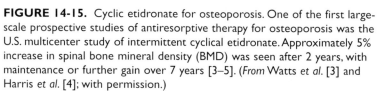

**FIGURE 14-14.** Potential uses for biphosponates. The literature suggests that bisphosphonates may be beneficial in almost any condition characterized by increased bone remodeling.

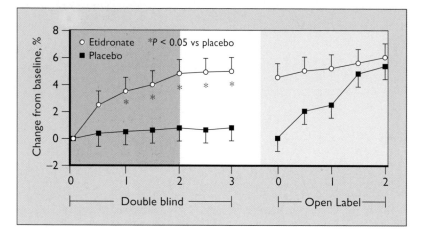

**FIGURE 14-15.** Cyclic etidronate for osteoporosis. One of the first large-scale prospective studies of antiresorptive therapy for osteoporosis was the U.S. multicenter study of intermittent cyclical etidronate. Approximately 5% increase in spinal bone mineral density (BMD) was seen after 2 years, with maintenance or further gain over 7 years [3–5]. (*From* Watts *et al.* [3] and Harris *et al.* [4]; with permission.)

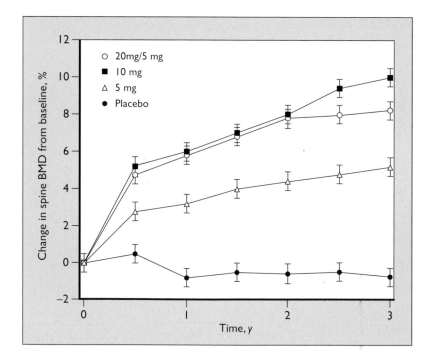

**FIGURE 14-16.** Effect of alendronate (Fosamex; Merck & Co, Inc, West Point, PA) in established osteoporosis. The Phase III trials of alendronate for treatment of postmenopausal osteoporosis consisted of two identical protocols conducted concurrently at 18 centers in the United States and 19 other centers. Almost 1000 postmenopausal women with osteoporosis (spine bone mineral density [BMD] T-score >2.5 standard deviations) were enrolled in a 3-year, double-blind, placebo-controlled study with four treatment groups: placebo; alendronate, 5 mg/d; alendronate, 10 mg/d; and alendronate, 20 mg/d [6]. Even the 5-mg/d dosage of alendronate produced significant gains in BMD; however, the 10-mg/d dosage seemed to provide the optimal effect. The average increase in spine BMD in the U.S. cohort was 6% in the first year and almost 10% by the end of the third year [7]. (*From* Tucci *et al.* [7]; with permission.)

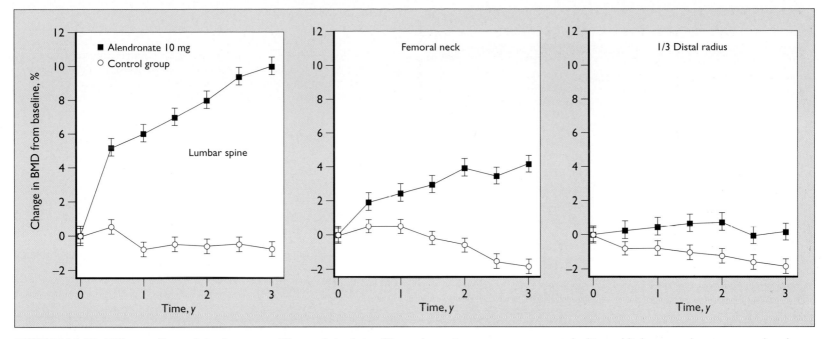

**FIGURE 14-17.** Different effects of alendronate at different skeletal sites. The increase in spinal bone density with alendronate was quite striking; however, lesser increases were seen at the hip, and little or no change occurred at the forearm [7]. (*From* Tucci *et al.*[7]; with permission.)

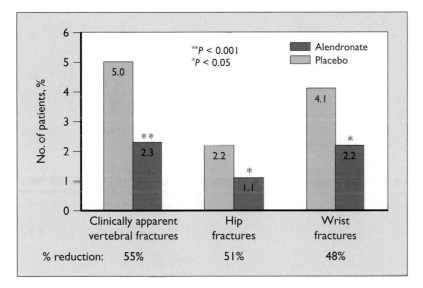

**FIGURE 14-18.** Effect of alendronate treatment on fractures: the Fracture Intervention Trial (FIT). The true proof of effectiveness of any treatment of osteoporosis is reduction in fracture risk. The FIT study enrolled over 2000 women with low bone mineral density (BMD) of the femoral neck and one or more vertebral fractures. The average age of the women was 72 years. They were given either placebo or alendronate and were followed up for 3 years. [8].

The rates of vertebral, hip, and wrist fractures were significantly decreased with alendronate therapy. Of interest, fracture rates were reduced by approximately half at every site, despite changes in BMD that were greatest at the spine, less at the hip, and negligible at the wrist. This result suggests that the reduction in fractures with alendronate is only partially mediated through increases in bone density. (*From* Black *et al.*[8]; with permission.)

## PROPER DOSING OF ALENDRONATE

| Instruction | Reason |
| --- | --- |
| Take on an empty stomach first thing in AM, with water only, and nothing else for 30 minutes. | Avoids binding with divalent cations to ensure adequate absorption. |
| Take with 8 ounces of water. | Minimizes risk of the tablet lodging in the esophagus. |
| | Ensures absorption. |
| Remain upright until food or calcium is consumed to bind the drug. | Minimizes the risk of reflux of the drug into the esophagus. |

**FIGURE 14-19.** Bisphosphonates are poorly absorbed when given by mouth. They must be taken on an empty stomach, with nothing but water for at least 30 minutes. Because alendronate may irritate the esophagus, the tablet should be washed down with water (to avoid sticking). The patient should remain upright (seated or standing) until food or calcium has been taken to bind the drug. Alendronate should not be given to patients with active upper gastrointestinal disease. Alendronate therapy should be discontinued if upper gastrointestinal symptoms develop.

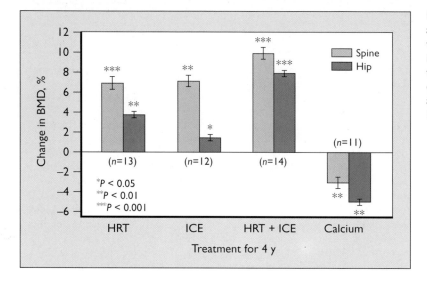

**FIGURE 14-20.** Combination therapy. Although all the agents discussed are antiresorptive drugs, their mechanisms of action differ. Thus, it is possible that they have additive effects. Although several large studies are underway, very little information is available thus far. Results of a small nonrandomized study suggest that the increase in bone mineral density (BMD) seen with the combined use of estrogen and a bisphosphonate (intermittent cyclic etidronate) are better than are the results with either agent alone [9]. HRT—hormone replacement therapy; ICE—intermittent cyclic etidronate. (*From* Wimalawansa [9]; with permission.)

## References

1. Stock JL, Avioli LV, Baylink DJ, *et al.*: Calcitonin-salmon nasal spray reduces the incidence of new vertebral fractures in postmenopausal women: three-year interim results of the PROOF study [abstract]. *J Bone Miner Res* 1997, 12:S149.

2. Pun KK, Chan LW: Analgesic effect of intranasal salmon calcitonin in the treatment of osteoporotic vertebral fractures. *Clin Ther* 1989, 11:205–209.

3. Watts NB, Harris ST, Genant HK, *et al.*: Intermittent cyclical etidronate treatment of postmenopausal osteoporosis. *N Engl J Med* 1990, 323:73–79.

4. Harris ST, Watts NB, Jackson RD, *et al.*: Effects of four years of intermittent cyclical etidronate treatment for postmenopausal osteoporosis. *Am J Med* 1993, 95:557–567.

5. Miller PD, Watts NB, Licata AA, *et al.*: Cyclical etidronate in the treatment of postmenopausal osteoporosis: efficacy and safety after 7 years of treatment. *Am J Med* 1997, 103:468–476.

6. Liberman UA, Weiss SR, Broll J, *et al.*: Effect of oral alendronate on bone mineral density and the incidence of fractures in postmenopausal osteoporosis. *N Engl J Med* 1995, 333:1437–1443.

7. Tucci JR, Tonino RP, Emkey RD, *et al.*: Effect of three years of oral alendronate treatment in postmenopausal women with osteoporosis. *Am J Med* 1996, 101:488–501.

8. Black DM, Cummings SR, Karpf DB, *et al.*: Randomised trial of effect of alendronate on risk of fracture in women with existing vertebral fractures. Fracture Intervention Trial Research Group. *Lancet* 1996, 348:1535–1541.

9. Wimalawansa SJ: Combined therapy with estrogen and etidronate has an additive effect on bone mineral density in the hip and vertebrae: four-year randomized study. *Am J Med* 1995, 99:36–42.

# BONE ANABOLIC AGENTS

## Clifford Rosen

# 15

Pharmacologic agents that suppress bone turnover can produce a secondary increase in bone mineral density (BMD). This occurs because the reduction in activation of new remodeling units, accompanied by the eventual filling in of those resorption spaces that had already been created, results in contraction of the so-called "remodeling space." The increase in BMD achieved by this mechanism leads to a reduction in osteoporotic fractures of the hip and spine. The only drugs currently approved by the United States Food and Drug Administration (FDA) for the treatment of established osteoporosis are agents that work exclusively by inhibiting bone resorption. These include calcitonin, estrogen, raloxifene, and alendronate. Other bisphosphonates, such as etidronate and risedronate, also are available although they are not currently approved by the FDA for this purpose. All of these drugs, as well as calcium supplementation, share the same property, inhibition of bone dissolution, when reaching the bone remodeling unit. Increases in bone mass resulting from antiresorptive therapy are relatively short-lived and generally amount to increments of 2% to 8% before a new steady state is achieved. This plateau effect and concern about the long-term safety of the bisphosphonates in the skeleton have pushed the development of new peptides and growth factors that work on the bone formation component of remodeling.

Anabolic agents in the skeleton are compounds that directly stimulate an increase in bone mass. Sodium fluoride (NaF) was the first skeletally anabolic drug administered to patients, although more than 20 years ago an extract of parathyroid glands was given experimentally to a small group of osteoporotic women. Despite more than two decades of clinical trials, NaF is still considered experimental. This reflects, in part, concerns about the quality of new bone formed in response to fluoride therapy. In at least one large multicenter trial, NaF promoted a substantial BMD increase over 3 years, but more nonvertebral fractures occurred in treated women than in a placebo group [1], indicating that NaF may increase BMD at the expense of bone strength. The use of fluoride for treatment of osteoporosis remains hotly debated.

By the late 1980s, a whole generation of recombinant peptides had been produced for clinical trials of various disorders, including osteoporosis. Currently there are no approved anabolic treatments for osteoporosis. However, several promising agents are currently in phase III trials. For example, parathyroid hormone (PTH) has been shown to increase bone mass and strength in animals [2]. Early phase II trials in humans also were promising. Recombinant human growth hormone (rhGH) and insulin-like growth factor-I (IGF-I) also are experimental agents, although rhGH has been approved for treatment of patients with GH deficiency in whom it can be shown to increase BMD [3]. Short-term use of IGF-I, rhGH, and GH-releasing peptides is currently under investigation for treatment in catabolic states such as burns, hip fracture, and major surgery.

This chapter examines the central pathways that control bone formation and thereby are likely to be operative during anabolic treatment, with particular focus on the IGF regulatory system, because several of these agents, including NaF and PTH, as well as GH, appear to work in part by induction of IGF within bone.

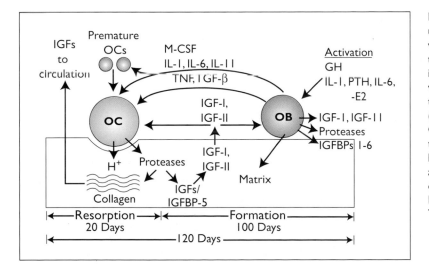

**FIGURE 15-1.** Hormonal regulation of bone remodeling. The bone remodeling unit is a tightly coupled entity. Activation of remodeling occurs with estrogen withdrawal and with administration of growth hormone (GH), thyroxine, parathyroid hormone (PTH), and other cytokines. It is currently thought that the initial regulatory signals exerted by these agents arise from direct interactions with specific receptors in osteoblasts (OB). Release from OB of various cytokines then modulates the maturation, proliferation, and differentiation of osteoclasts (OC), the primary bone resorbing cell. Among the several cytokines that affect OC, interleukins (ILs) 1, 6, and 11 appear to be particularly important. In response to osteoclastic bone resorption, insulin-like growth factor (IGF) I and II, which have been embedded in the bone matrix complexed to matrix binding proteins, are released and likely participate in the recruitment, proliferation, and activation of new osteoblasts, which replace the resorbed bone (see also Ch. 1)[4]. M-CSF—macrophage colony-stimulating factor; TNF—tumor necrosis factor; TGF—transforming growth factor.

# Insulin-like Growth Factor

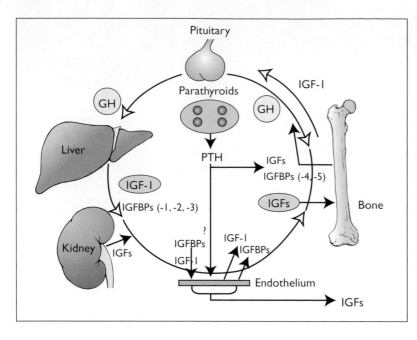

Pituitary

FIGURE 15-2. The circulating insulin-like growth factor (IGF) regulatory system. This system is complex and redundant, being composed of the same elements as is the skeletal IGF system. IGF-I is produced by many cells and constantly shuttles in and out of the circulation. Most circulating IGF exists bound to one of several specific binding proteins (BPs). At least six IGFBPs are known to exist and are produced independently by separate genes. The dominant circulating BP is IGFBP3, which depends on growth hormone (GH) for its production. IGF-I, IGF-II, and BP3 also are bound in the circulation to a 70-kd protein called the acid-labile subunit (ALS), giving rise to a stable ternary complex.

## A. THE IGF REGULATORY SYSTEM IN BONE

Ligands
  IGF-I, IGF-II
High affinity IGF binding proteins (IGFBPs)
  IGFBPs 1-6*
IGF receptors
  IGF-IR
  Type II IGF receptor
IGFBP proteases
  IGFBP-3 proteases (prostate specific antigen and other serine proteases)
  IGFBP-4 proteases (not identified to date)
  IGFBP-5 proteases (matrix metalloproteinases)

*The IGFBPs can shuttle IGF to and from tissue sites; however they can also enhance or antagonize the actions of IGFs at the receptor by competing for binding. IGFBP-4 is a purely inhibitory IGFBP, whereas IGFBP-5 tends to enhance IGF activity while at the same time binding to extracellular matrices including hydroxyapatite. IGFBP-3 is the principle circulating IGFBP; it can enhance or antagonize IGF action.

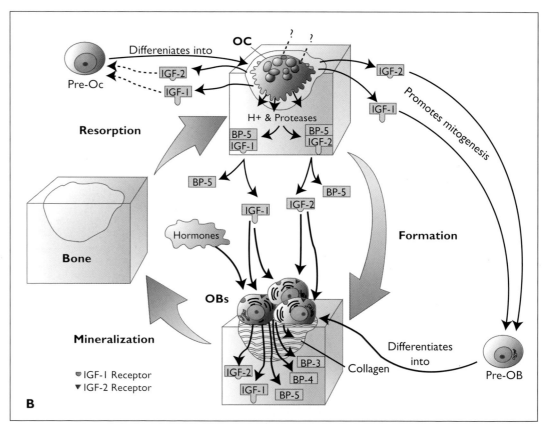

FIGURE 15-3. A, Components of the IGF regulatory system in bone. B, Osteoblasts (OB) synthesize IGFs. IGF-II is more abundant than IGF-I in the skeleton and in the circulation. Circulating IGF-I concentrations decline with age, and skeletal IGF-I content of cortical and trabecular bone is lower in specimens from elderly than from younger individuals. IGFBP-5 anchors IGF to the hydroxyapatite crystal. (Rosen, unpublished data.) BP—binding protein; OC—osteoclasts. (Part B redrawn from Yvonne Walston, CMI, ©1997; with permission.)

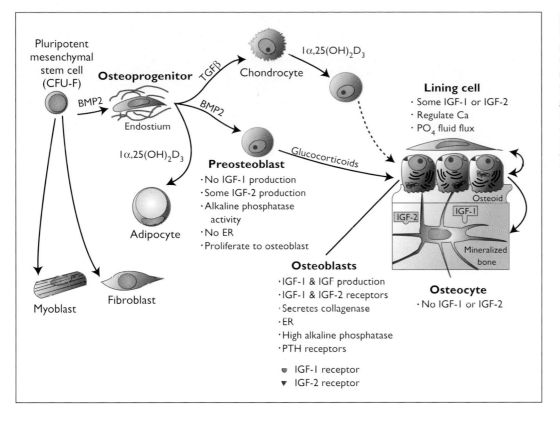

**FIGURE 15-4.** Osteoblast production. The proliferation and differentiation of osteoblasts from pluripotent mesenchymal stem cells (CFU-F) is an elaborate and well orchestrated process under local and systemic regulation. Recently, cbf1, a protein that serves as a transcription factor for numerous genes, has been shown to be a major switch in the initiation of osteoblast differentiation. IGF-1 is also a critical factor later in the differentiation pathway. ER—estrogen receptor; TGF—transforming growth factor. (Rosen, unpublished results). (*Redrawn from* Yvonne Walston, CMI, ©1997; with permission.)

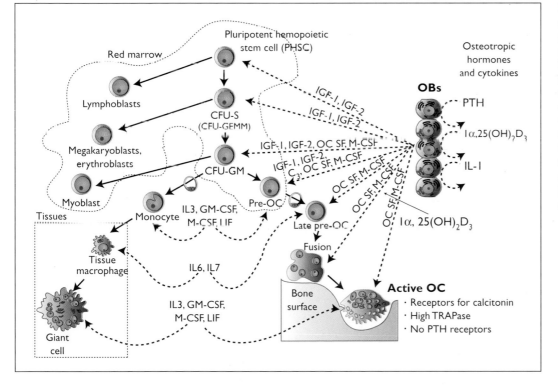

**FIGURE 15-5.** Osteoclast production. Osteoclastogenesis is the process of recruiting hematopoietic stem cells (PHSC) into multinucleated giant cells that can secrete protons and proteases. The formation of osteoclasts (OC) is a complex process involving terminal differentiation and fusion. Several cytokines and growth factors, all originating from osteoblasts (OB), orchestrate the process [4]. CFU—colony forming unit; CFU-S—colony-forming unit stroma; GM—granulocyte monocyte; GM-CSF—granulocyte-monocyte colony-stimulating factor; LIF—leukokinin-inhibiting factor; OC—osteoclast stromal factor; PTH—parathyroid hormone. (*Redrawn from* Yvonne Walston, CMI, ©1997; with permission.)

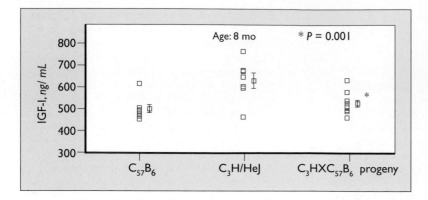

**FIGURE 15-6.** Genetic interaction between IGF-I and bone. Although IGF-I is a key factor in bone remodeling, the relationship between circulating IGF-I and bone mass is not understood. Recent studies in mice have proved very illustrative, however. In two inbred strains of healthy mice there is an approximately 40% difference in BMD, with C34 mice having greater bone mass than C57B6 animals [5]. Circulating IGF-I concentrations differ by the same degree, with C3H mice exhibiting much higher values throughout life [6]. Mating between these two strains results in a first generation of mice in which IGF-I and BMD are closely correlated, and the serum concentrations are intermediate between high and low IGF-I (P = 0.001). IGF-I production also is higher at the osteoblast level in C3H than B6, and there is greater production in vitro of bone-forming colonies from C3H osteoblasts [6].

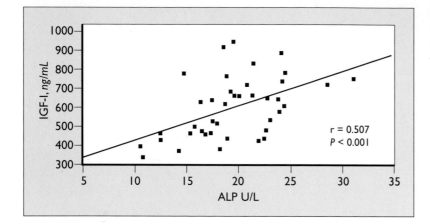

**FIGURE 15-7.** Relationship between circulating IGF-I and osteoblast function in 32-week-old mice. There is a highly significant correlation between serum alkaline phosphatase (ALP) activity and serum IGF-I concentration. Circulating IGF-I reflects skeletal IGF-I content as well as the ability of osteoblasts to synthesize and export alkaline phosphatase [7].

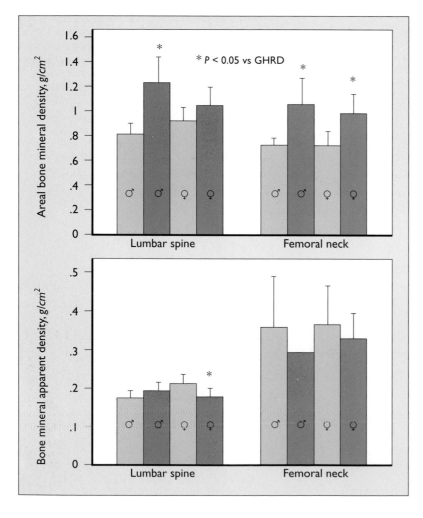

**FIGURE 15-8.** Relationship between IGF status and bone mass. GH-receptor deficiency (GHRD), the syndrome of complete resistance to GH (Laron-type dwarfism), is an autosomal recessive disorder characterized by clinical features of GH deficiency (dwarfism) but normal or elevated GH concentrations. Adults with this condition are extremely short but have normal reproductive, thyroid, and other hormonal status. Circulating IGF-I concentrations in GHRD are extremely low (about 25 ng/mL, compared to normal values of about 250 ng/mL). Bone mineral density (BMD) measured by dual energy x-ray absorptiometry (DXA) is significantly lower in men and women with GHRD than in age-matched controls. However, correction of DXA values for bone size removed this deficit. Thus, differences in bone mass in adults with GHRD are accounted for by differences in the size of bones, not in the mineral content per unit of bone matrix (see also Fig. 1-24 in Chapter 1). Dynamic histomorphometric features of trabecular bone in adults with GHRD are normal. (*Reprinted from* Bachrach et al. [8].)

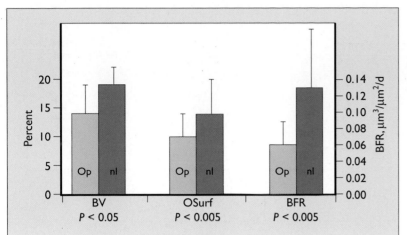

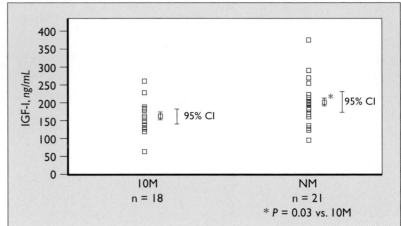

**FIGURE 15-9.** Role of IGF-I in idiopathic osteoporosis in males (IOM). Several reports of postmenopausal women have been unable to show a significant correlation between IGF-I concentrations and bone mineral density (BMD) [9,10]. This contrasts with findings in IOM, a condition associated with normal biochemical evidence of bone turnover but reduced bone formation defined on bone biopsy [11]. This graph shows bone volume (BV), an index of trabecular bone mass; osteoid surfaces (O Surf), the fraction (%) of bone surfaces undergoing bone formation activity; and bone formation rate (BFR) expressed in $\mu m^3$ per $\mu m^2$ of bone area per day. Trabecular bone mass and formation characteristics are lower in osteoporotic men than in normal controls. Op—osteoporotic; nl—normal.

**FIGURE 15-10.** Serum IGF-I concentrations in men with and without osteoporosis. Although there is considerable overlap, average IGF-I concentrations are lower in osteoporotic men. IOM—idiopathic osteoporosis in males; NM—normal men.

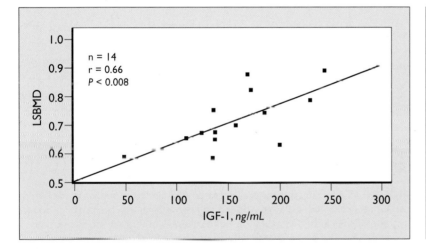

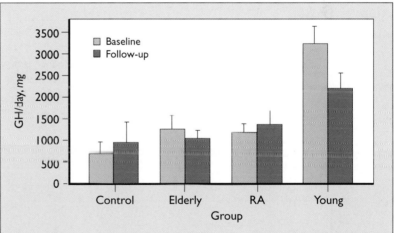

**FIGURE 15-11.** Relationship between circulating IGF-I concentrations and lumbar spine bone mass density (LSBMD) in osteoporotic men. In this series of IOM, a highly significant relationship was found between circulating IGF-I and BMD, as opposed to that in normal men and women. It is likely that the designation IOM applies to a group of heterogeneous disorders. IGF-I may not be an important factor for all of them, accounting for the substantial degree of overlap shown in Figure 15-10. However, it appears that diminished IGF-I status contributes to low bone mass for at least some, or even most, affected men. Whether this effect represents a failure of adequate peak bone mass acquisition or of adult bone maintenance is unknown.

**FIGURE 15-12.** Alterations in the GH–IGF-I axis in health and disease: the effect of age. Normal human aging is associated with a marked decline in growth hormone (GH) secretion, leading to lower circulating levels of IGF-I for each decade after the age of 50 years [12]. This figure shows integrated GH concentrations and an approximation of total daily GH secretion in healthy young and old individuals and in patients with rheumatoid arthritis (RA). GH levels were higher in the young group than the control group ($P = 0.0002$) and the elderly and RA groups ($P = 0.002$). When baseline values was compared to follow-up, there was a significant decrease in the young group compared to the control and RA groups ($P = 0.01$). (*Reprinted from* Roubenoff *et al.* [13].)

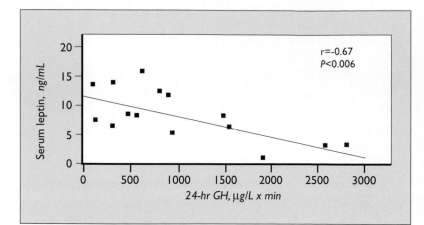

**FIGURE 15-13.** The effect of obesity on growth hormone (GH) status. Obesity has long been known to be associated with diminished GH secretion. Recent evidence suggests this phenomenon may be the result of an inhibitory effect of leptin, a peptide hormone produced by fat cells [14]. This figure shows a strong negative relationship between circulating leptin and 24-hour integrated GH concentrations.

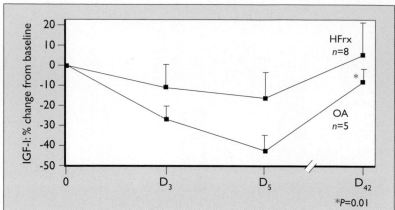

**FIGURE 15-14.** Effect of catabolic illness on IGF-I status. IGF-I production is critically dependent on nutritional state and whole body protein status. In patients with hip fractures, IGF-I concentrations drop within 24 hours of injury and decline further after surgical fixation. This figure shows two groups of patients undergoing surgery for hip fracture or for prosthetic joint replacement for osteoarthritis. $D_3$, $D_5$, $D_{42}$—days 3, 5, and 42 after fracture. Hfrx—hip fracture; OA—osteoarthritis.

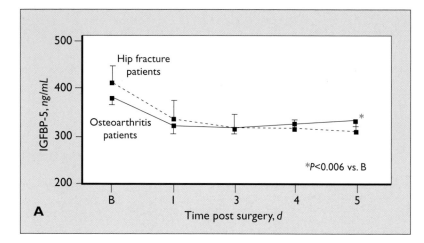

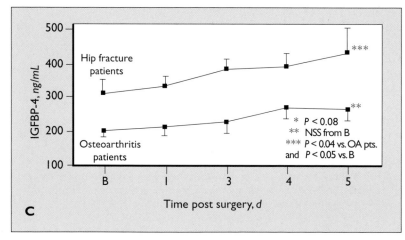

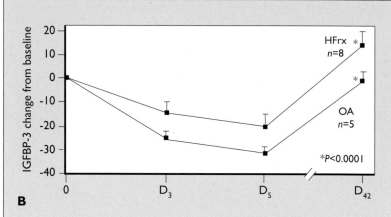

**FIGURE 15-15.** Effect of surgical stress on IGF binding proteins. As explained earlier, circulating IGF-I is largely bound to several binding proteins (BPs). Some of these BPs enhance IGF action on bone, whereas others are inhibitory. Thus, understanding changes in overall IGF-I status is complicated by simultaneous alterations in BP concentrations. This figure shows coordinate changes in IGFBPs 3, 4, and 5 following hip surgery. BPs 3 and 5 drop precipitously, whereas BP4, an inhibitory BP that blocks IGF-I action, actually increases. **A,** Changes in IGFBP-5. **B,** Changes in IGFBP-3. **C,** Changes in IGFBP-4. Hfrx—hip fracture; OA—osteoarthritis. (Rosen, unpublished data).

# Human Growth Hormone

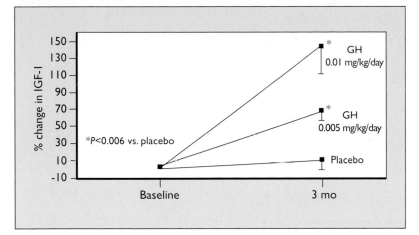

**FIGURE 15-16.** Effect of recombinant human growth hormone (GH) on bone turnover and bone mineral density (BMD) in older individuals. Given the fact of age-related declines in GH and IGF-I status as well as the loss of BMD with age, it seemed possible that replacement of GH might restore BMD in older men and women. This figure shows that treatment of frail older men and women with rhGH for 1 year led to marked increases in IGF-I concentration and, in a dose-dependent manner, also stimulated markers of bone resorption.

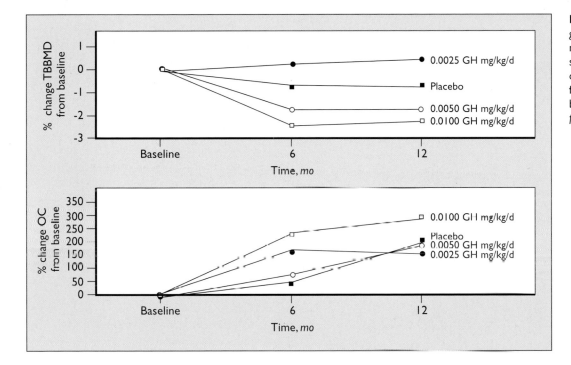

**FIGURE 15-17.** Effect of recombinant human growth hormone (GH) on bone turnover and bone mineral density (BMD) in older individuals. In the same trial described in Figure 15-16, GH stimulated osteocalcin (OC), a biochemical marker of bone formation, but had no beneficial effect on total body bone mineral density (TBBMD). (*Reprinted from* Maclean *et al.* [15]; with permission).

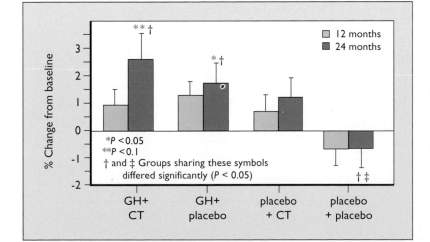

**FIGURE 15-18.** Effect of cyclic growth hormone (GH) with or without calcitonin on bone mineral density (BMD) in osteopenic older women. Because GH administration increases both resorption and formation marker activity, it is likely that GH promotes an increase in new bone remodeling units, with a concomitant increase in the remodeling space. The hypothesis was tested that administration of rhGH together with the antiresorptive hormone, salmon calcitonin, might permit a greater rise in BMD than would rhGH alone. This figure illustrates the effect on lumbar spine BMD of a 2-year program of GH with or without calcitonin (CT) given every two months for 24 months. rhGH stimulated modest increases in BMD, but these were not magnified by CT. The achieved rise in BMD resembles those observed with approved antiresorptive medications. Thus, it appears there is little, if any, therapeutic role for GH in treatment of osteoporosis. (*Reprinted from* Holloway *et al.* [16].]

# Parathyroid Hormone

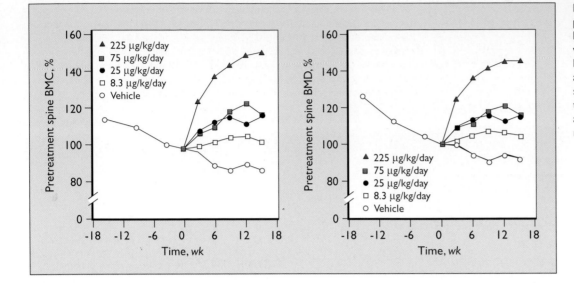

**FIGURE 15-19.** Skeletal effects of exogenous parathyroid hormone (PTH). Although continuously high concentrations of PTH have been associated with bone disease in patients suffering severe primary hyperparathyroidism, intermittent elevation of PTH appears to increase bone mass, particularly in the spine. This figure shows the effects of daily PTH treatment on spine bone mineral content (BMC) and bone mineral density (BMD) in ovariectomized rats. A dose-dependent response is observed [2,17].

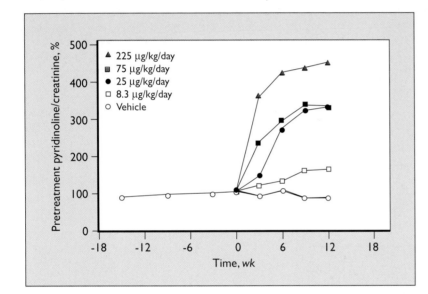

**FIGURE 15-20.** Effect of parathyroid hormone (PTH) on bone turnover in ovariectomized rats. In the same study illustrated in Figure 15-19, PTH led to a dose-related increase in bone turnover indicated by the pyridinoline:creatinine ratio, a resorption marker [2].

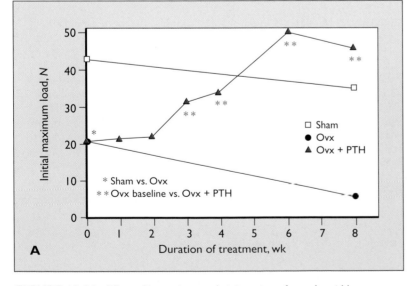

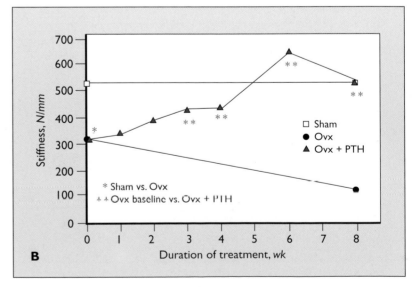

**FIGURE 15-21.** Effect of intermittent administration of parathyroid hormone (PTH) on mechanical competence of bone. In this study rats were sham operated, ovariectomized (OVX) or had OVX plus treatment with a rat PTH analog, PTH(1-34). Sham animals had no significant change in maximum load capacity (**A**) or stiffness

(**B**), two measures of bone strength. OVX animals were significantly lower in both measures by the time PTH(1-34) injections began, and PTH(1-34) restored these to sham values in several weeks. These changes were associated with improvement in cancellous bone volume and trabecular thickness [2,18].

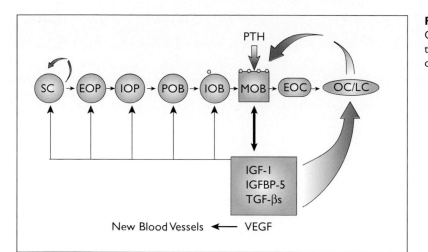

**FIGURE 15-22.** Anabolic actions of parathyroid hormone (PTH) on bone. One mechanism of action by which PTH affects bone is thought to be through the IGF regulatory system with direct induction of IGF-I and several IGFBPs in osteoblasts [19].

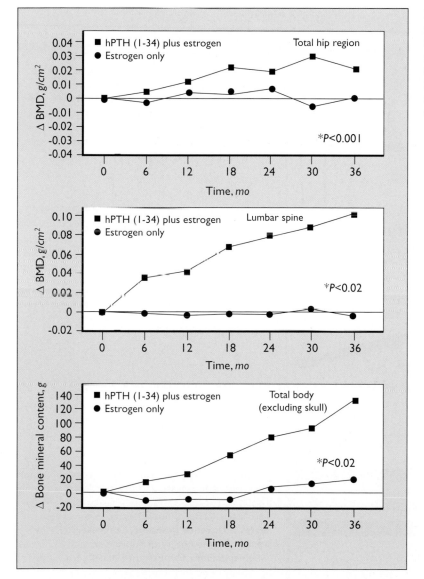

**FIGURE 15-23.** Effects of PTH(1-34) on bone mineral density (BMD) of post-menopausal women. In this randomized trial, human parathyroid hormone (PTH) increased bone mass in postmenopausal women who had been on hormone replacement therapy for at least 1 year [20]. Results were particularly dramatic at the lumbar spine. Although PTH(1-34) alone might predictably decrease cortical bone BMD, the rise in total body BMC in these estrogen-replete women was reassuring. PTH and its analogs are currently in phase II and III clinical trials for treatment of osteoporosis.

# Sodium Fluoride

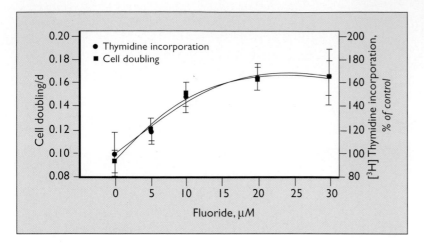

**FIGURE 15-24.** Mitogenic effects of sodium fluoride (NaF) on bone cells. NaF increases 3H-thymidine incorporation and promotes cell doubling in a dose-dependent manner (D. J. Baylink, MD, Loma Linda, CA, personal communication).

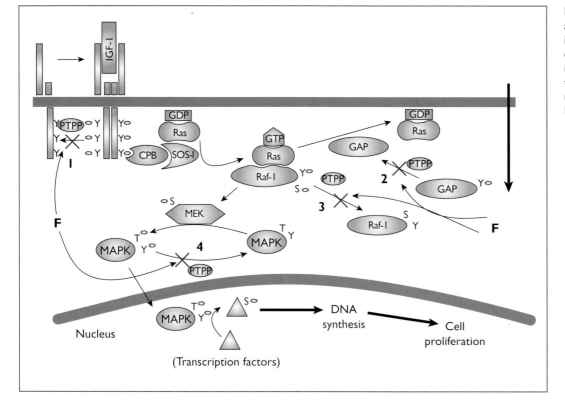

**FIGURE 15-25.** Skeletal actions of NaF. The anabolic effects of NaF are related to alterations in several pathways and second messengers for osteoblasts. In particular, it is thought that fluoride inhibits the action of several tyrosine phosphatases, thereby enhancing the actions of MAP kinases. This may lead to greater signaling amplitude through the IGF-I/IRS-I pathway [21].

## FRACTURE STUDIES USING FLUORIDE:
## RANDOMIZED DOUBLE-BLIND PLACEBO TRIALS

| Study | Reduction in Vertebral Fractures | Fluoride dose |
|---|---|---|
| Riggs, 1990 | No | High dose—NIH |
| Kleerekoper, 1991 | No | High dose—NIH |
| Pak, 1994, 1995 | Yes | With moderate doses—mild low BMD |
| Riggs, 1994 | Yes | Moderate dose |
| Ringe, 1998 | Yes | Males with IOM |
| FAVOS, 1998 | No | High dose |

**FIGURE 15-26.** Summary of the trials of NaF for both sustained release and monosodium fluoride in relation to vertebral fracture efficacy [1,22,23]. The regulatory status of fluoride salts in the United States is currently unsettled. Controversy remains concerning the quality of fluoride-treated bone and whether claims of antifracture benefit are reliable.

# References

1. Riggs BL: Effect of fluoride treatment on the fracture rate in post-menopausal women with osteoporosis. *N Engl J Med* 1990, 322:802–809.

2. Mitlak BH, Burdette-Miller P, Schoenfeld D, Neer RM: Sequential effects of chronic human PTH treatment of estrogen deficiency osteopenia in the rat. *J Bone Miner Res* 1996, 11:430–439.

3. Finkenstedt G, Gasser RW, Hofle G, et al.:: Effects of GH replacement on bone metabolism and bone mineral density in adult onset of GH deficiency: results of a double-blind placebo controlled study with open follow-up. *Eur J Endocrinol* 1997, 136:282–289.

4. Rosen CJ, Donahue LR, Hunter SJ: IGFs and bone: the osteoporosis connection. *Proc Soc Exp Biol Med* 1994, 206:83–101.

5. Beamer WG, Donahue LR, Rosen CJ, Baylink DJ: Genetic variability in adult bone density among inbred strains of mice. *Bone* 1996, 18:397–405.

6. Rosen CJ, Dimai HP, Vereault D, et al.: Circulating and skeletal IGF-I concentrations in two inbred strains of mice with different bone densities. *Bone* 1997, 21:217–223.

7. Dimai HP, Linkhart TA, Linkhart SG, et al.: Alkaline phosphatase levels and osteoprogenitor cell numbers suggest that bone formation may contribute to peak bone density differences between two inbred strains of mice. *Bone* 1998, 22:211–216.

8. Bachrach LK, Marcus R, Ott SM, et al.: Bone mineral, histomorphometry, and body composition in adults with growth hormone receptor deficiency. *J Bone Miner Res* 1998, 13:415–421.

9. Kiel DP, Puhl J, Rosen CJ, et al.: Lack of an association between IGF-I and body composition, muscle strength, physical performance, or self-reported mobility among older persons with functional limitations. *J Am Geriatr Soc* 1998, 46:822–828.

10. Harris TB, Kiel DP, Roubenoff R, et al.: Association of IGF-I with body composition, weight history and past health behaviors in the very old. *J Am Geriatr Soc* 1997, 45:133–139.

11. Kurland E, Rosen CJ, Cosman F, et al.: Osteoporosis in men: abnormalities in the IGF-I axis. *J Clin Endocrinol Metab* 1997, 82:2799–2805.

12. Rall LC, Rosen CJ, Dolnikowski G, Hartman WJ, Roubenoff R: Protein metabolism in rheumatoid arthritis and aging. *Arthritis Rheum* 1996, 39:1115–1124.

13. Rall LC, Rosen CJ, Roubinoff R, et al.: Protein metabolism in RA and aging: effects of strength training. Methotrexate and TNF-X. *Arth Rheum* 1996, 39:1115–1124.

14. Roubinoff R, Rall LC, Veldhuis JD, et al.: The relationship between GH kinetics and sarcopenia in postmenopausal women: the role of fat mass and leptin. *J Clin Endocrinol Metab* 1998, 83:21–24.

15. Maclean DB, Kiel DP, Rosen CJ: Low dose GH for frail elders stimulates bone turnover in a dose dependent manner. *J Bone Miner Res* 1995(Suppl), 10:S48.

16. Holloway L, Kohlmeier L, Kent K, Marcus R: Skeletal effects of cyclic recombinant human growth hormone and salmon calcitonin in osteopenic postmenopausal women. *J Clin Endocrinol Metab* 1997, 82: 1111–1117.

17. Reeve J: PTH: a future role in the management of osteoporosis. *J Bone Miner Res* 1996, 11:440–445.

18. Sogaard CH, Mosekilde L, Thomsen SJ, et al.: A comparison of the effects of two anabolic agents (NaF and PTH) on ash density and bone strength assessed in an osteopenic rat model. *Bone* 1997, 20:439–449.

19. Watson P, Lazowski D, Han V, Hodsman AH: PTH restores bone mass and enhances osteoblast IGF-I gene expression in ovariectomized rats. *Bone* 1995, 16:357–365.

20. Lindsay R, Nieves J, Formica C, et al.: Randomised controlled study of effect of parathyroid hormone on vertebral-bone mass and fracture incidence among postmenopausal women on oestrogen with osteoporosis. *Lancet* 1997, 350:550–555.

21. Ammann P, Rizzoli R, Caverzasio PS, Bonjour JP: Fluoride potentiates the osteogenic effects of IGF-I in aged ovariectomized rats. *Bone* 1998, 22:39–43.

22. Zerwekh JE, Padalino P, Pak CYC: The effect of intermittent slow release NaF and continuous calcium citrate therapy on calciotropic hormones, biochemical markers of bone metabolism, and blood chemistry in post-menopausal osteoporosis. *Calcif Tissue Int* 1997, 61:272–278.

23. Meunier PJ, Sebert JL, Reginster JY, et al.: Fluoride salts are no better at preventing new vertebral fractures than calcium-vitamin D in post-menopausal osteoporosis. The FAVO study. *Osteoporosis Intl* 1998, 8:4–12.

# Index

# G

# Color Plates

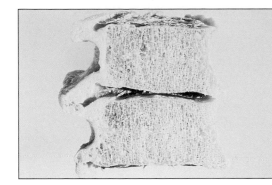

FIGURE 1-3. Page 2

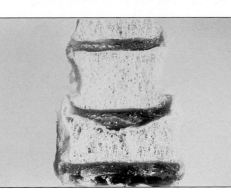

FIGURE 1-4. Page 2

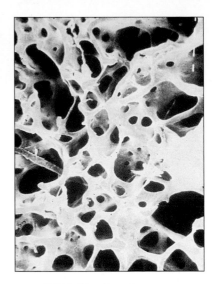

FIGURE 1-5A. Page 2

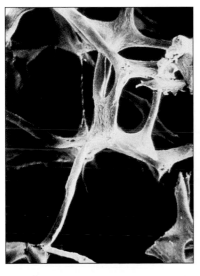

FIGURE 1-5B. Page 2

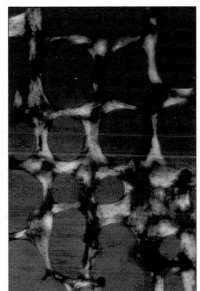

FIGURE 1-15A. Page 6

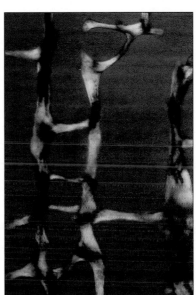

FIGURE 1-15B. Page 6

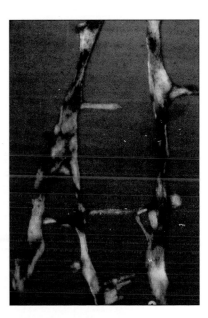

FIGURE 1-15C. Page 7

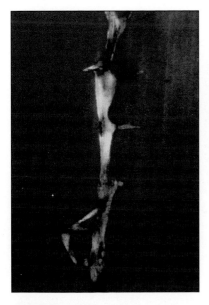

FIGURE 1-15D. Page 7

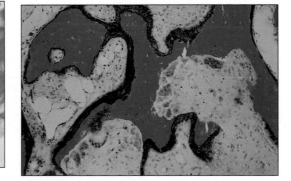

FIGURE 1-21. Page 9

FIGURE 6-9. Page 68

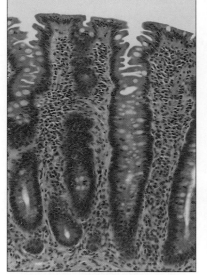

**FIGURE 9-4.** Page 102

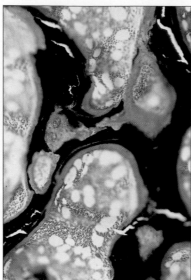

**FIGURE 9-6A.** Page 103

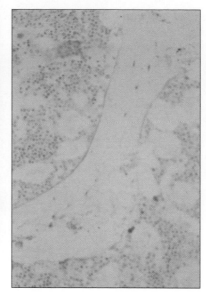

**FIGURE 9-6B.** Page 103

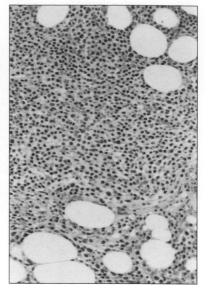

**FIGURE 9-11A.** Page 105

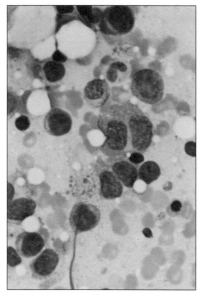

**FIGURE 9-11B.** Page 105

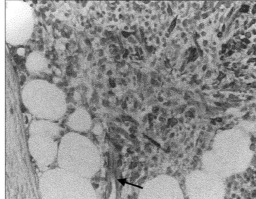

**FIGURE 9-12A.** Page 105

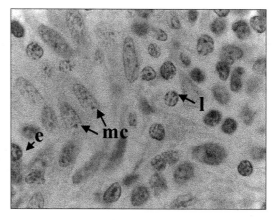

**FIGURE 9-12B.** Page 105

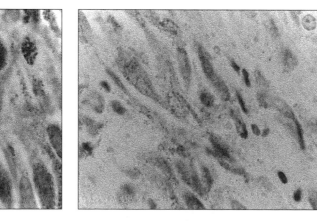

**FIGURE 9-12C.** Page 106

**FIGURE 9-12D.** Page 106

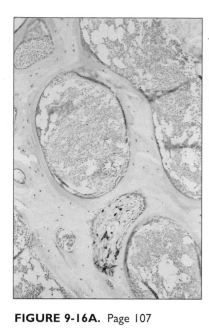

FIGURE 9-16A. Page 107

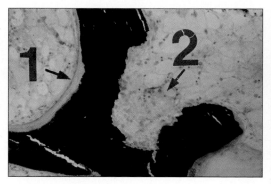

FIGURE 9-16B. Page 107

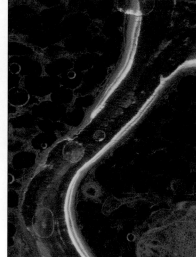

FIGURE 9-16C. Page 108

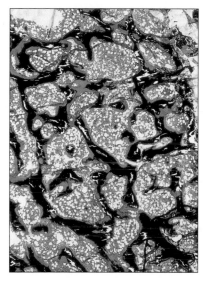

FIGURE 9-24. Page 111

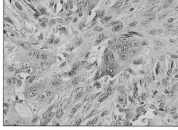

FIGURE 9-27A. Page 113

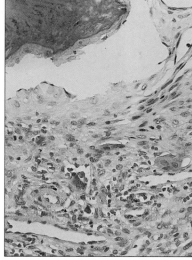

FIGURE 9-27B. Page 113

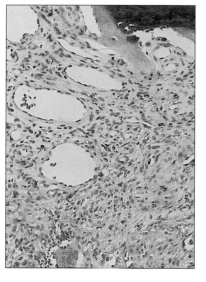

FIGURE 9-27C. Page 113

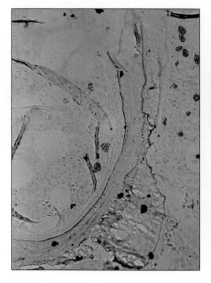

**FIGURE 9-28A.** Page 113

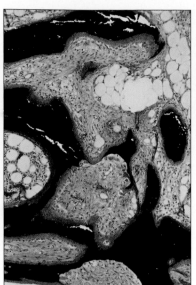

**FIGURE 9-28B.** Page 113

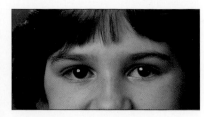

**FIGURE 9-29.** Page 114

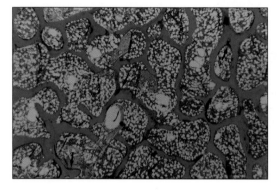

**FIGURE 10-4A.** Page 116

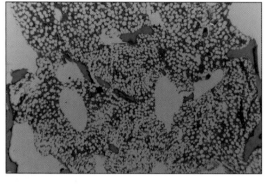

**FIGURE 10-4B.** Page 116